Handbook of HUMAN FACTORS *and the* OLDER ADULT

Handbook of HUMAN FACTORS *and the* OLDER ADULT

Edited by

ARTHUR D. FISK
School of Psychology
Georgia Institute of Technology
Atlanta, Georgia

WENDY A. ROGERS
Department of Psychology
The University of Georgia
Athens, Georgia

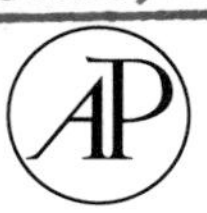

ACADEMIC PRESS
San Diego London Boston
New York Sydney Tokyo Toronto

Find Us on the Web! http://www.apnet.com

This book is printed on acid-free paper. ♾

Academic Press, Inc.
A Division of Harcourt Brace & Company
525 B Street, Suite 1900, San Diego, California 92101-4495

United Kingdom Edition published by
Academic Press Limited
24-28 Oval Road, London NW1 7DX

Library of Congress Cataloging-in-Publication Data

Handbook of human factors and the older adult / edited by Arthur D. Fisk, Wendy A. Rogers.
p. cm.
Includes index.
ISBN 0-12-257680-2 (alk. paper)
1. Human engineering. 2. Aged. I. Fisk, Arthur D. II. Rogers, Wendy A.
TA166.H2753 1996
620.8'2--dc20 96-5501
CIP

PRINTED IN THE UNITED STATES OF AMERICA
96 97 98 99 00 01 EB 9 8 7 6 5 4 3 2 1

Dedicated to

Delos D. Wickens

In the memory of his devotion to science,
his understanding of the need for practically relevant
research, and his unending dedication to the education of
future generations of scientists and practitioners.

Contents

Part 2
APPLICATIONS

Contributors

Numbers in parentheses indicate the pages on which the authors' contributions begin.

Sara J. Czaja (311) Miami Center on Human Factors and Aging Research, University of Miami, Coral Gables, Florida 33136

Katharina V. Echt (335) Department of Psychology, University of Georgia, Athens, Georgia 30602

K. G. Engelhardt (395) NASA—Far West Regional Technology Center, Los Angeles, California 90007

Geoff Fernie (289) Center for Studies in Aging, Sunnybrook Health Science Centre, Toronto, Ontario M4N 3M5 Canada

Daryle Gardner-Bonneau (231) Michigan State University, Kalamazoo Center for Medical Studies, Kalamazoo, Michigan 49008

John Gosbee (231) Michigan State University, Kalamazoo Center for Medical Studies, Kalamazoo, Michigan 49008

Donald H. Goughler (395) Southwestern Pennsylvania Human Services, Inc., Mon Valley Community Health Center, Monessen, Pennsylvania 15062

Darlene V. Howard (7) Department of Psychology, Georgetown University, Washington, District of Columbia 20057

James H. Howard, Jr. (7) Department of Psychology, The Catholic University of America, Washington, District of Columbia 20064

William C. Howell (1) American Psychological Association, Washington, District of Columbia 20002

Timothy R. Jones (257) Department of Psychology, University of Georgia, Athens, Georgia 30602

Donald W. Kline (27) Department of Psychology, University of Calgary, Calgary, Alberta T2N 1N4 Canada

K. H. E. Kroemer (87) Industrial and Ergonomics Lab., Virginia Polytechnic Institute and State University, Blacksburg, Virginia 24061

Von Leirer (199) Decision Systems, Los Altos, California 94022

M. Jackson Marr (171) School of Psychology, Georgia Institute of Technology, Atlanta, Georgia 30332

Roger W. Morrell (335) Institute of Gerontology, University of Michigan, Ann Arbor, Michigan 48109

Daniel Morrow (199) Psychology Department, University of New Hampshire, Durham, New Hampshire 03824

Paul E. Panek (363) Professor of Psychology, The Ohio State University at Newark, Newark, Ohio 43055

Denise C. Park (257) Institute of Gerontology, University of Michigan, Ann Arbor, Michigan 48109

Wendy A. Rogers (151) Department of Psychology, The University of Georgia, Athens, Georgia 30602

Charles T. Scialfa (27) Department of Psychology, University of Calgary, Calgary, Alberta T2N 1N4 Canada

Patricia A. Tun (125) Department of Psychology and The Volen National Center for Complex Systems, Brandeis University, Waltham, Massachusetts 02254

Max Vercruyssen (55) Department of Medicine, University of Hawaii, Honolulu, Hawaii 96822; ITS Institute, University of Minnesota, Minneapolis, Minnesota; and Technische Universiteit, Eindhoven, The Netherlands

Arthur Wingfield (125) Department of Psychology and The Volen National Center for Complex Systems, Brandeis University, Waltham, Massachusetts 02254

Preface

As is well known, the older segments of populations within developed countries are expanding faster than their younger counterparts. Such a change in demographics brings with it unique challenges and opportunities for both the private and public sectors. Human factors and ergonomics can play a major role in meeting these challenges and capitalizing on the opportunities. At the very least, economic factors, it would seem, will increase the need for human factors and ergonomic input oriented toward older adults for the design of work, home environments, and leisure activity aids. Thus, the topical focus of this book is becoming a central concern of many disciplines. With this increased diversity in interest comes the crucial need for increased communication among the contributing disciplines. The book was conceived as a starting point to share important knowledge of human factors and aging across disciplines.

Although no single book can serve as the sole source for the entire profession of human factors design, we hoped to provide a text that would serve a broad audience. To accomplish this goal, we were motivated to create a balanced treatment of facts and "worked examples." On behalf of this balance, the contributors in Part 1, who were dealing with more abstract principles, were constantly reminded of Part 2, which deals with the substantive human factors application of such principles. At the same time, the contributors of Part 2 were asked to remember and acknowledge the principles from whence their applications grew.

This book was planned as a collection of topics and conceptual foundations within the realm of human factors, ergonomics, and aging. Human factors and ergonomics is a broad discipline. Although we would have liked to have covered all areas relevant to human factors and the older adult, it should be immediately obvious why this was not possible. Leaving gaps in many areas was the only way to proceed to ensure publication before our retirement. Some of these gaps will, no doubt, be filled by future books on the topic of human factors and aging, edited by individuals reluctant to leave silent discussion of topics we have chosen to omit. Other gaps will be recognized, and filled, by future research and application. Certainly further volumes will be written and produced. It must be pointed out (or it most assuredly will be by reviewers of this book) that whereas some chapters deal with highly developed and largely settled issues, other chapters may raise more questions than they can answer, and necessarily aim at a more speculative treatment. The latter type of chapters offer fertile ideas for further attack rather than exact solutions and serve a critical role for the future enterprise of human factors and ergonomics.

The book is meant to serve as a reference for practitioners and scientists within the field of human factors and ergonomics. With this in mind, each contributor was given the task of addressing what the *designer* should take away from the chapter as well as what the human factors *scientist* should think about in order to better motivate his or her research. In addition, we envisioned the book as a source for graduate students interested in learning more about the exciting area of human factors and ergonomics, pursuing thoughts on how to contribute practically relevant research, or broadening their perspective in the field of aging. Thus, the contributors were encouraged to consider what a graduate student interested in cognitive aging or gerontology should take away from the chapter and to highlight such points. Finally, the book was written so that it could function effectively not only as a handbook but also as a reference tool. Thus, each contributor was encouraged to ensure that her or his chapter could stand on its own.

We thank numerous people for their contributions to this volume. Each manuscript was peer reviewed and we thank those reviewers who wished to remain anonymous as well as the following individuals: P. Ackerman, D. Boehm-Davis, S. Bogner, J. Brown, S. Casali, D. Chaffin, G. Corso, A. Graesser, J. Harris, T. Maurer, A. Smith, and N. Walker. Each contribution was strengthened by the careful, constructive criticism provided by the reviewers. We also thank Nikki Levy and her colleagues at Academic Press for their help and their patience with us throughout this project. We also offer a heartfelt "thank you" to each of the contributors for their dedication and hard work; to state the obvious, without their efforts this book would never have been given life.

Arthur D. Fisk
Wendy A. Rogers

Chapter 1

Foreword, Perspectives, and Prospectives

William C. Howell

OUR AGING POPULATION

Demographers have been attempting for several decades to alert America to the fact that, collectively speaking, it is growing older (Soldo & Manton, 1988). Longer life expectancies coupled with a general decline in the birth rate led them to predict a dramatic shift in the proportion of "senior citizens" within the general population. As the 1970s and 1980s unfolded, it became clear that the prediction was no exaggeration, but society did little to prepare itself for this unprecedented development.

Now as we approach the 21st century, the change is upon us and society is struggling to deal with the consequences. The median age of 32.1 in 1990, an all-time high, is expected to grow to 36 by the turn of the century and to 42 by 2030. At nearly 13%, the population segment traditionally associated with retirement (i.e., those age 65 and older) is the largest in history and growing. It should hit a startling 22% by 2030, or about 66 million people. What is more, its fastest growing subgroup is the over-85 (so-called oldest old) contingent, the majority of whom are women. Obviously a shift of this magnitude has profound social implications that America is only beginning to appreciate (Berg & Cassells, 1990).

Already quite visible is a change in the demand for products and services associated with older consumers. Marketers, who monitor consumer demographics closely, were quick to grasp the significance of the aging trend and reacted accordingly. Consequently, what advertisers refer to as the "gray market" is receiving a lot of attention today in the commercial domain (Allen, 1981). Consider, for example, how television has changed. What was once the exclusive province of youth now features aging actresses pitching dental adhesives, documentaries on nursing homes, and seniors golf tournaments. Unfortunately, efforts to reach older consumers are often hampered by a lack of understanding of the requirements and preferences of this population. For instance, we have devices designed to provide home medical care that are prone to serious error by elderly users (Bogner, 1994).

A second important impact area is the workplace (Taeuber, 1984). Passage of legislation prohibiting age discrimination, disability discrimination, and mandatory retirement has enabled older workers to remain on the job longer; and many are now doing so. Whatever its benefits, an aging work force poses some tough questions for employers as they attempt to adapt. What changes, for example, should be incorporated into the design of tasks and the work environment to accommodate the older worker? How must personnel practices such as hiring, training, evaluating, compensating, and firing be modified? If there are net costs to the employer, who is to pay?

The matter of costs, or more precisely the economic ramifications of an aging population, constitutes a third area of major concern. It extends well beyond the workplace into national policy realms as diverse as health care, welfare, and federal "entitlement programs" designed to benefit the elderly (e.g., Social Security, Medicare, veterans benefits). Projected costs are staggering. The estimated bill for health care for older patients came to $162 billion in 1987, a 358% increase over the previous decade, and costs have only accelerated since then (Waldo, Sonnefeld, McKusick, & Arnett, 1989). Medicare costs alone may hit $145 billion by 2020 (Schneider & Guralnick, 1990). Policy makers have been forced to recognize the growing seriousness of the problem but cannot seem to agree on the most equitable way to address it.

The Social Security system presents an even more troubling economic picture. Today there are five persons contributing to the system for every one who is drawing on it, and by early next century the ratio will drop to 3/1 (Jorgensen, 1980). Government is under sustained pressure to control federal spending and the associated tax burden on working Americans, yet without cutting entitlements this is a virtual impossibility—even at the current 5/1 ratio. Because older voters have become such a powerful political force, however, elected officials are reluctant to tamper with the entitlements. And the situation can only get worse as their number (and political clout) increases. Some observers go so far as to predict that the system is headed for insolvency and will produce intense generational conflict (i.e., between the younger contributors and the older beneficiaries) as funding shortfalls approach.

It would take little imagination to construct similar scenarios illustrating the impact of an aging population on virtually any facet of society one might care to name. In addition to those already mentioned, highway safety and daily living requirements seem to be receiving the most attention, probably because the link is so obvious and pressures are already building in these areas. In others, the consequences are indirect but promise to be no less profound. Take public education. Retirees are becoming an increasingly large voting block in certain (usually desirable) communities where they tend to locate. With no children of school age and relatively fixed incomes, these senior citizens sometimes vote against the tax increases and bond issues necessary to sustain quality education. I know personally of several school districts that are in a state of decline as a result of just such a shift in the voting pattern.

Clearly, then, our aging population poses a challenge. While I have relied mainly on *problems* in making the point, one can just as easily conceive of this challenge in terms of *opportunities*. There is unquestionable social value in people living longer, more productive, and fulfilling lives. Serious scholars no longer view aging merely as progressive *impairment,* but as a lifelong *development* process that includes sustained adaptation and growth as well as deterioration (Howell, 1993; Smith, 1990). The challenge for society is to provide a context within which older citizens are encouraged to realize their potential and assisted in doing so rather than being perceived as nothing more than a growing burden. A necessary precondition for creating such an environment, naturally, is a valid understanding of how people age.

UNDERSTANDING THE AGING PROCESS

Most of our scientific knowledge of the aging process is of fairly recent vintage and, while impressive given its short history, is still far from complete. Neither the biomedical nor the psychosocial correlates of aging received much attention prior to the 1970s. Then, stimulated by the establishment of the National Institute on Aging (NIA) within the National Institutes of Health (NIH) and programs within the Department of Veterans Affairs, things started to change. Federal support for age-related research grew rapidly over the next two decades, reaching an estimated $601 million by 1990. Despite its impressive growth, however, the total investment remains minuscule relative to the amount spent on health-related requirements of the elderly. The $601 million, for example, represented less than 0.5% of this total for the same year (Lonergan, 1991)!

Finances aside, the past several decades have produced a wealth of information on the topic as evidenced by compilations such as the *Handbook of the Psychology of Aging* (Birren & Shaie, 1996), several Institute of Medicine publications (e.g., Berg & Cassells, 1990; Lonergan, 1991), and three "special issues" of the journal, *Human Factors* (February 1981, October 1990, October 1991). A collaborative effort by a number of scientific and professional organizations designed to provide policy makers with an informed agenda for investment in behavioral and social research—an activity known as the *human capital initiative*—has identified aging as a high-priority area and produced a succinct document summarizing both what we know and still need to know about the aging process (Cavanaugh, Park, Smith, & Smyer, 1993). And, of course, a prominent section of the present volume (Chapters 2–8) provides somewhat more detailed status reports on our knowledge in each of the major function categories to which aging research has been directed.

While there would be little point in trying to address any of this material here, several conclusions seem worth mentioning. First, it is clear that we know much more about aging than is being usefully applied, but equally clear is that there are huge gaps in our knowledge. Second, in keeping with the developmental perspective, it is becoming apparent that age is not the reliable index of functional impairment that society has customarily taken it to be. For one thing, there are marked individual differences in rate of deterioration (see Chapter 7), and for another, older people often find ways to compensate for declining skills in one area by strengthening their capability in (or relying more heavily on) others. Knowledge, which grows rather than declines with age, often compensates for deficits in other cognitive functions (Cavanaugh et al., 1993).

The final conclusion, which concerns the particular focus of this book, is that much can be done in the design of tasks, devices, systems, and environments to better accommodate the aging user. Often, the aging process simply exacerbates suboptimal design features that, to a lesser extent, affect *everyone's* performance. "Childproof" medicine containers is a good case in point: adults, and particularly the elderly, have trouble opening many of these as currently designed.

AGING AND THE HUMAN FACTORS AGENDA

Human factors, the multidisciplinary endeavor that focuses on user-oriented design, can justly claim an interest in aging effects predating that of the federal government by almost 20 years (Smith, 1990). It began, however, as an extremely limited effort and remained so until the zeitgeist dictated otherwise. Now, like the many disciplines that contribute to its knowledge base, human factors is heavily invested in aging issues as they relate both to research and applications. The diversity of this agenda is well represented in the present volume, particularly in Chapters 10–22, which are organized by areas of application.

The basic premise connecting human factors with information on aging is that much of the world designed for people to function in (i.e., to live, work, play, get around) was created with little systematic regard for the older user. Therefore as people age, they are exposed to an increasing array of threats to their health, safety, performance, and quality of life, many of which could be avoided or minimized through improved design. "Improvement" is achieved mainly by translating fundamental knowledge of age-related changes in human capabilities, tendencies, and preferences into design principles or requirements. To use a simple example, vision decrements might call for increased lighting in the workspace and less cluttered displays.

It is not hard to find evidence to support this basic premise—virtually any office, highway, or home is replete with examples. Part of the problem, of course, can be attributed to gaps in knowledge, but a far larger part, particularly in recent years, has been failure to apply what is known. The human factors philosophy is itself only beginning to attract the attention of design professionals, and that only in very limited domains. Design for the aging user is rarely among them. Even if the interest were there, however, the designer would have great difficulty finding the relevant information because archival knowledge of the aging process and its human factors applications are scattered across many disciplines and publication outlets (Czaja, 1990).

The present book goes a long way toward addressing the access problem by providing in one place an overview of the relevant knowledge domains and an entry point into the varied literatures. Further, it should serve an important alerting function by introducing new elements of society to the role human factors can play toward making life more productive, more rewarding, and safer for our aging population. Just as it has enabled us to live *longer*, science can help us live *better*, and the human factors approach offers a very promising route to that end.

References

Allen, C. B. (1981, April). Over 55: Growth market of the 80's. *Nation's Business*, pp. 25–32.

Berg, R. L., & Cassells, J. S. (Eds.). (1990). *The second fifty years: Promoting health and preventing disability.* Washington, DC: National Academy Press.

Birren, J. E., & Schaie, K. W. (Eds.). (1996). *Handbook of the psychology of aging* (4th ed.). San Diego, CA: Academic Press.

Bogner, M. S. (1994). *Human error in medicine.* Hillsdale, NJ: Erlbaum.

Cavanaugh, J. C., Park, D. C., Smith, A. D., & Smyer, M. A. (1993). *Vitality for life: Psychological research for productive aging.* Washington, DC: American Psychological Association, Science Directorate.

Czaja, S. J. (1990). *Human factors research needs for an aging population.* Washington, DC: National Academy Press.

Howell, W. C. (1993). Engineering psychology in a changing world. *Annual Review of Psychology, 44,* 231–263.

Jorgensen, J. (1980). *The graying of America.* New York: Dial.

Lonergan, E. T. (Ed.). (1991). *Extending life, enhancing life: A national research agenda on aging.* Washington, DC: National Academy Press.

Schneider, E. L., & Guralnick, J. M. (1990). The aging of America. Impact on health care costs. *JAMA, Journal of the American Medical Association, 263,* 2335–2340.

Smith, D. B. D. (1990). Human factors and aging: An overview of research needs and application opportunities. *Human Factors, 32*(5), 509–526.

Soldo, B. J., & Manton, K. G. (1988). Demography: Characteristics and implications of an aging population. In J. W. Rowe & R. W. Besdine (Eds.), *Geriatric medicine* (pp. 12–22). Boston: Little, Brown.

Taeuber, C. (1984). Older workers: Force of the future. In P. K. Robinson, J. Livingston, & J. E. Birren (Eds.), *Aging and technological advances* (pp. 75–87). New York: Plenum.

Waldo, D. R., Sonnefeld, S. T., McKusick, D. R., & Arnett, R. H. (1989). Health expenditures by age group, 1977 and 1987. *Health Care Financing Review, 10,* 111–120.

Part 1

FUNDAMENTALS

Chapter 2

Learning and Memory

James H. Howard, Jr.
Darlene V. Howard

INTRODUCTION

The aging population described in the previous chapter by Howell presents challenges and opportunities for human factors design professionals, especially because these demographic changes coincide with an ongoing explosion in the development of electronic devices. These technological devices can serve as tools for simplifying daily routines, as "intelligent agents" to help people cope with the vast amount of information they encounter, and as aids for maintaining independence and contact with the outside world when failing health impairs mobility. But, to be used effectively, this technology requires that people adapt to frequent change. For example, personal banking has involved a shift from interacting with a teller to using a home computer or ATM machine. Similarly, many people have had to learn the jargon, concepts, and range of skills necessary to use the Internet for work or pleasure.

These changes in technology and demography make it clear that the human factors designer must understand how people of all ages adapt to change—how they learn and how they forget. Such understanding provides

Handbook of Human Factors and the Older Adult

the basis for determining if and how a system should be designed to accommodate an aging user community. This chapter focuses on the question of how normal aging influences our ability to learn. In the next section we develop and criticize a traditional view of learning in old age.

Traditional Views of Learning and Aging

While it is obvious that people continue to learn throughout life, it is equally true that advancing age brings some limitations. For example, self-report surveys of cognitive function in older adults typically reveal complaints of memory and word-finding problems as well as a sense of increased difficulty in learning new skills (e.g., Zelinski, Gilewski, & Thompson, 1980). These cognitive differences associated with age have long been recognized by psychologists. In early work, cognitive aging was often characterized as an inevitable decline that begins in young adulthood and continues through senescence to death (e.g., Hall, 1922; James, 1890/1950).

This perspective dominated psychological thinking for some years. In this view, the role of the psychologist was to measure the decline quantitatively and describe it in terms of prevailing theories. For example, figure 1 shows the differences between young adults (18–25 years) and older adults (62–84 years) in their rate of eyeblink conditioning (Braun & Geiselhart, 1959). Here people learn to blink (CR) in response to a light (CS) after it has been paired repeatedly with an air puff delivered to the eye (UCS). The age differences in learning are indeed striking in even this very simple case of classical conditioning. Findings of this sort led to such generalizations as Thorndike's "ability to learn curve," which displayed a monotonically diminishing ability to learn beyond the late teens (Thorndike, Bregman, Tilton, & Woodyard, 1928). In fact, baby-boomers will find it disconcerting that Thorndike's curve ends at the venerable age of 50. From an applied perspective, the prospect of an inevitable and irreversible decline in learning with age is discouraging at best; "youth is an exhilarating, age a depressing theme" to quote Hall (1922, p. viii).

This early approach to cognitive aging reflects two theoretical positions that no longer seem tenable. First, learning was thought to involve the acquisition of S–R associations during conditioning (e.g., Kausler, 1994). This approach implicitly assumes an underlying singular memory system. Hence, an age-related decline in simple conditioning is interpreted in terms of more general, systemwide changes. Second, the traditional approach tacitly reflects a one-mechanism approach to life-span development. In this view, childhood is characterized by growth, middle-age and beyond by decline.

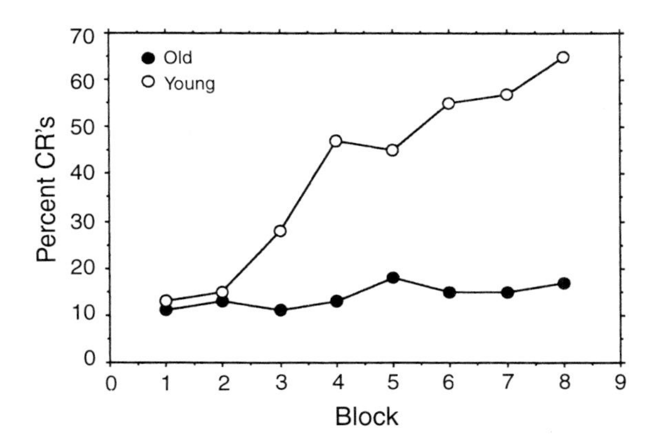

FIGURE 1 Sample data showing age-related deficits in the acquisition of classical eyeblink conditioning. The percent of conditioned responses as a function of practice is shown separately for younger and older adults. Values were estimated from those depicted in Figure 1 of Braun and Geiselhart (1959, p. 386).

Contemporary Views of Learning and Aging

Contemporary approaches are based on two very different assumptions. First, human *memory* is seen as complex and multidimensional (Schacter & Tulving, 1994). As a consequence, age-related change observed in one task will have implications only for the memory processes and systems operative in that context and not for cognitive ability as a whole. Declines in one task may possibly be accompanied by constancy or improvement in others. Second, adult *development* is similarly viewed as the complex interplay of different processes—constancy vs. change, growth vs. decline (e.g., Baltes, 1987). According to this life-span development view, different processes are likely to show different patterns of age-related change and development throughout life is characterized by both gains and losses.

To consider a concrete example, we revisit eyeblink conditioning. Although traditional work consistently demonstrated deficient learning in old age, some more recent work has found comparable conditioning rates for younger and older people when longer interstimulus intervals (CS/UCS interval) are used (Solomon, Blanchard, Levine, Velazquez, & Groccia-Ellison, 1991). This suggests that the young and elderly do not differ in their ability to learn the eyeblink response, but rather in the presentation conditions that are optimal for learning to occur (Solomon et al., 1991). Perhaps older people simply require more time to process the CS than their young counterparts.

This contemporary perspective suggests that it is important to understand why and under what conditions age differences in learning occur. With these general principles in mind, the practitioner is faced with a more encouraging challenge; namely, to design so as to take advantage of the cognitive strengths of the elderly. In the following sections, we highlight some of the theoretical distinctions important for understanding the dynamics of age-related change in learning.

Despite its negative focus, the traditional view of learning in the aged was appealing in its simplicity. One's ability to learn declined as one aged. In contrast, recent work presents a sometimes confusing pattern of results. While, in general, learning efficiency declines with age, this is not always the case. In this section we develop a number of theoretical constructs that have been useful for understanding this pattern of exceptions. While these constructs have been proposed as elements of emerging theories of cognitive aging, they may also be viewed as a set of organizational principles for a complex literature.

MEMORY SYSTEMS AND PATTERNS OF AGING

It is clear that learning, forgetting, and memory are intimately related. Material is accumulated in memory as learning occurs, and forgetting results from either the loss or the inability to recover material from memory. However, contemporary cognitive theory assumes a much more central and varied role of memory than suggested by these seemingly obvious relationships. More than a simple repository of what we know, memory lies at the core of thinking and learning. In a recent review, Schacter and Tulving (1994) identified five major systems of human memory. Four of these proposed systems are particularly important for issues in human factors, and so they will be considered here. These systems are working memory, episodic memory, semantic memory, and procedural memory.

The working memory system underlies our ability to retain and manipulate the limited amount of material that falls within our attentional focus. In this sense it incorporates both William James's notion of a transient store, the primary memory, and Baddeley's idea of an active conceptual workbench (e.g., Baddeley & Hitch, 1994). In contrast, the remaining three systems to be considered here retain information over substantially longer periods. The episodic memory system, for example, is involved in the retention and recollection of our personal experience (Schacter & Tulving, 1994; Tulving, 1993). In other words, the material stored here is linked to a specific time and place, whether an everyday experience or an arbitrary list learned in a laboratory experiment. Semantic memory, on the other hand, is our storehouse of world knowledge. This memory system enables us to use words and language and provides us with an abstract representational system for thought (e.g., Tulving, 1993). Both of these latter memory systems are *declarative* in that they involve knowing *that*. For example, I know *that* I had eggs for breakfast on Sunday morning (episodic) and *that* eggs are high in cholesterol (semantic).

In contrast, procedural memory is concerned with knowing *how,* which Squire (1994) has referred to as *nondeclarative*. For example, I know *how* to scramble an egg or *how* to play chess. Procedural memory is involved with our learning and memory of everything not supported by one of the other memory systems (Schacter & Tulving, 1994). In the following sections, we summarize briefly some of the major age-related findings for each of these four memory systems.

Working Memory

In general, age differences are small or nonexistent for tasks that simply require people to retain small amounts of information for short periods but are larger when people must simultaneously process, or manipulate, the material (Craik, 1994). For example, the digit span task emphasizes the storage aspect of working memory; people are presented with a list of digits that must be recalled in the order presented—much like the everyday experience of retaining a telephone number long enough to dial it. The list is increased over trials to determine the maximum length that yields error-free recall. Many studies have reported no age differences at all in digit span. Even when age differences do emerge, the digit-span deficit is generally less than 10%, implying that the elderly fall well within Miller's "magical number seven" range for working memory capacity (6.0–6.5 digits) (cf. Kausler, 1994).

Conclusions about aging are different when tasks are used that place a greater emphasis on the role of working memory in mental processing and manipulation, as occurs, for example, when we calculate the 15% gratuity on a restaurant check. This chore requires that we hold the results of partial calculations in mind while we perform yet other calculations. For example, the restaurant goer, after calculating that 10% of $36.58 is about $3.60, must hold that value in mind, while dividing it in half to get $1.80, and then add the retained value of $3.60 to $1.80 to produce the total tip amount.

To examine age differences in the processing capacity of working memory, Salthouse and his colleagues have asked people to perform a series of single-digit addition and subtraction problems while simultaneously remembering the second digit from each problem. As in the traditional digit-span task, the computation span reflects the number of digits the person is

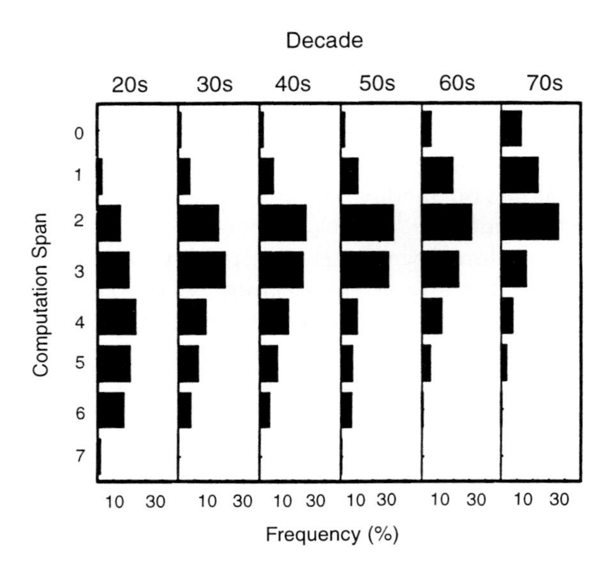

FIGURE 2 The distribution of computation span by age decade from Salthouse's (1994) study of 1132 individuals. [From Figure 3 of Salthouse (1994 p. 538). Copyright 1994 by the American Psychological Association. Reprinted by permission.]

able to recall without error. Figure 2 shows the computation span distribution by age obtained in five experiments involving a total of 1132 volunteers (Salthouse, 1994). As is evident in this figure, a substantial decrease occurred with advancing age. This age deficit in computation span, when contrasted with age similarities in digit span, suggests the processing efficiency of working memory—not its passive storage capacity—declines with advancing age. Salthouse and his colleagues have also reported more direct evidence for this same conclusion using yet other working memory tasks (e.g., Salthouse & Skovronek, 1992). In addition, by calling upon a wide range of evidence and statistical modeling techniques, Salthouse (e.g., 1994) has argued that this age-related decline in working memory efficiency is due to a more general age-related decline in processing speed that is known to accompany aging.

In conclusion, the processing component of working memory appears to be particularly important in understanding age-related change. When the processing demands of a task are light, elderly people perform as well or nearly as well as younger ones. On the other hand, in situations that involve simultaneous processing, a substantial working memory deficit would be expected for the older person. These age-related limitations in working memory can be of practical significance, because of the central role that working memory plays in many activities.

Episodic Memory

The extensive literature on aging shows that, when people are asked to recollect material from episodic memory, performance declines with age. In the following we illustrate this finding for several learning contexts.

Although the designation "episodic memory" was first introduced by Endel Tulving in 1972, age deficits have been reported for verbal learning studies since the 1930s (see Kausler, 1994, for a review). In a representative experiment, young and elderly volunteers would be asked to memorize a list of word pairs (e.g., DOG–CHAIR) such that in a subsequent test they could produce the response member of the pair (CHAIR) when given the stimulus member (DOG). Age related deficits are typical in such tasks, with people in their 70s recalling as few as half the items of college-age participants.

Many of these early studies ignored potential cohort effects and other confoundings in their subject samples. For example, they usually used small convenience samples of elderly volunteers who could have been more poorly educated or of lower verbal ability than their college student volunteers. But age deficits in episodic memory have still appeared in more recent research that overcomes such problems by using large sample sizes (Hultsch, Masson, & Small, 1991), by selecting matched or stratified samples (Herzog & Rodgers, 1989), or by repeated (longitudinal) testing of the same individuals (Colsher & Wallace, 1991). Thus, episodic memory differences still appear even when cohort effects and subject ability are controlled.

Much of the early work on episodic memory involved arbitrary and unfamiliar memorization tasks, raising the possibility that smaller age deficits or age constancy would occur for more meaningful material. However, the results of a number of recent studies indicate that this usually is not the case. For example, Hultsch et al. (1991) administered a battery of several tasks to a large sample of 584 community dwelling adults from three age groups, young (19–36 years), middle (55–69 years), and old (70–86 years). Two episodic memory tasks were used that differ in meaningfulness, story, and word recall. The word task required subjects to memorize and recall a list of nouns in the traditional manner, whereas in the story task, performance was based on the proportion of propositions recalled from the original narrative. In other words, in the latter case, subjects need report only the gist of sentences rather than their verbatim wording. Despite this, the middle-aged and older groups recalled fewer propositions than the young (.428, .329, and .299 for the young, middle, and old groups, respectively). As expected, an age deficit was also found for word recall (.668, .614, and .545

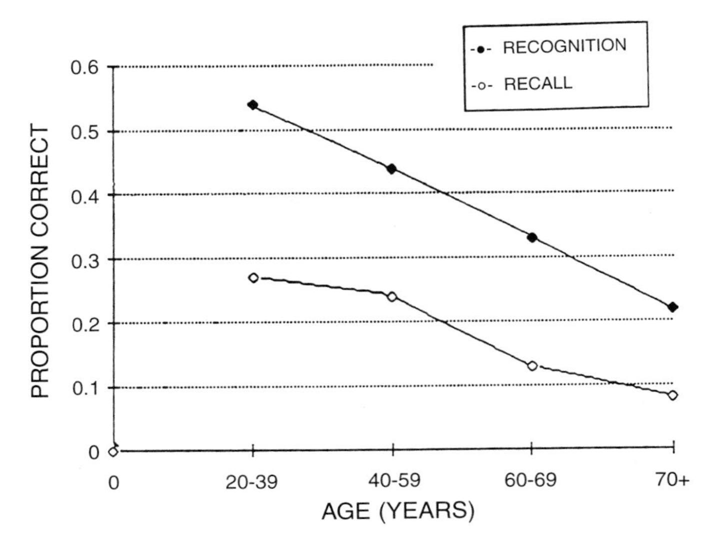

FIGURE 3 Proportion correct on incidental recall and recognition tests regarding the contents of an interview, as a function of age. [Data taken from Table 3 of Herzog and Rodgers (1989, p. 178).]

mean proportion correct for young, middle, and old, respectively). Similar findings have been reported by Stine and Wingfield (1987) for people of high and average verbal ability. Hence, it is clear that there are age deficits in episodic memory even for meaningful material.

The studies reviewed so far in this section have all investigated laboratory learning of words and text. Age deficits in episodic memory, however, are not restricted to either verbal material or the laboratory setting. Older people have difficulty with a range of nonverbal material such as faces (Crook & Larrabee, 1992) and maps (Lipman & Caplan, 1992), and such deficits occur whether measured in the laboratory or in a realistic setting (Uttl & Graf, 1993). For example, Herzog and Rodgers (1989) investigated what people happened to remember of the questions asked in an immediately preceding interview. A stratified sample of 1491 households was selected to complete a personal interview on a variety of health, economic, political, and other topics. Immediately following the interview, the respondents' memory for the interview questions was examined using both a recognition and a recall procedure. The results of these memory tests, plotted as a function of respondent age appear in Figure 3. Clear age deficits occurred for both measures with the magnitude of the deficit increasing nearly linearly with age.

An aspect of episodic memory especially vulnerable to aging is termed *source memory.* Source memory has to do with our ability to remember where or when information was originally acquired. For example, many of us know that former president Jimmy Carter was a peanut farmer, but cannot remember where or when we learned this. Failures of this sort have been called *source amnesia* or *source forgetting* (Schacter, Harbluk, & McLachlan, 1984). Craik and his colleagues have demonstrated greater source forgetting in the old than young that cannot be explained by a general memory impairment (Craik, Morris, Morris, & Loewen, 1990; McIntyre & Craik, 1987). Failures of source memory can be of practical significance in distinguishing imagined from experienced events or in differentiating reliable and unreliable information. For example, did my physician tell me to take two aspirin daily to prevent heart attacks or did I read it in a supermarket tabloid?

In summary, then, episodic memory consistently reveals age-related deficits, which appear to emerge gradually over the adult life span. These declines in episodic memory appear to be due at least in part to the age deficits in working memory discussed in the previous section, because processing by the working memory system is necessary if some event or stimulus is later to be recollected from episodic memory (e.g., Baddeley & Hitch, 1994). Indeed, a number of recent studies have used causal modeling, path analysis, and regression to show that processing-capacity measures of working memory predict episodic memory performance (e.g., Hultsch, Hertzog, & Dixon, 1990; Stine & Wingfield, 1987).

Semantic Memory

The semantic memory system is our repository of relatively stable world knowledge. This system underlies our ability to use language and to understand the relationships among concepts.

While age deficits are commonplace in episodic memory, they are rare in semantic memory (Bowles, 1993; Light, 1992). For example, studies using a variety of methods have consistently demonstrated age constancy in both the organization and content of semantic knowledge (cf. Light, 1992). In some instances, age reversals can be shown to occur; older people are frequently superior to younger in vocabulary tests. This suggests that our lexical and conceptual knowledge remains constant or improves throughout the life span.

On the other hand, the everyday observation that the elderly experience increased word or name finding difficulties (tip-of-the-tongue experiences) suggests that some declines in the functioning of semantic memory may occur with age, even though its organization remains intact. Laboratory investigations of semantic processing are consistent with this observation; older people respond more slowly than younger when naming pictures (Bowles, 1993) and when producing low-frequency words in response to definitions (Burke, MacKay, Worthley, & Wade, 1991). Interestingly, while older subjects reported tip-of-the-tongue states more frequently than young, with time they produced more correct words than their younger counterparts. In other words, age deficits in semantic memory functioning seem to relate more to decreases in processing speed with age than to memory content or organization per se. As a practical matter, this suggests that semantic memory may become a problem for older people only in situations where processing time is limited.

Procedural Memory

In contrast to episodic and semantic memory (which are often termed *explicit memory*) the procedural memory system is nondeclarative (or implicit) in that memories subserved by this system cannot necessarily be declared or described by the rememberer. In this sense, then, the memories considered in this section are not what we usually call *memory* in everyday language, when the term usually refers to conscious recollection. Procedural memory refers instead to a diverse class of abilities in which earlier experience alters subsequent performance in the absence of conscious awareness (Squire, 1994). The set of abilities included in this implicit, nondeclarative category is so diverse that this form of memory likely encompasses more than one system, and so it is not surprising that some aspects of procedural memory decline with aging whereas others do not. For present purposes, we will consider three kinds of nondeclarative, or implicit, learning and memory; these are classical conditioning, skill learning, and priming.

The case of *classical conditioning* has already been discussed. We noted that although age deficits in the rate of such conditioning usually occur, these deficits can be eliminated by increasing the time between the conditioned and unconditioned stimulus (e.g., Solomon et al., 1991). So age seems to be characterized not so much by a decreasing ability to be conditioned, as by a narrower range of temporal conditions under which conditioning occurs.

Skill learning encompasses everything from a motor skill like dancing to a cognitive skill such as computer programming. As a general rule age deficits are observed in skill learning, particularly when unfamiliar tasks are used. Much of the early research on skill learning in the elderly focused on the ability to learn motor tasks. For example, Thorndike and his colleagues (1928) investigated the ability of young to middle-aged adults to learn typing, nondominant-hand writing, line drawing, and other skills. Their findings were consistent with Thorndike's general notion of a decline in "sheer modifiability" with age across even the relatively narrow age range of their subjects.

A popular laboratory task for investigating motor skill learning is rotary pursuit. In a variation of this task, Wright and Payne (1985) required younger (aged 18–22 years) and older (aged 57–86 years) volunteers to track a target manually using mirror vision. Their results revealed a large age deficit both in tracking performance and in the rate of tracking improvement with practice. In other words, although learning occurred for both the young and old, the advantage of youth actually increased during the experiment. These findings are typical of those obtained with laboratory tasks of this sort.

Not all skill learning involves motor tasks. Daily experience suggests that the elderly maintain complex cognitive skills such as chess playing into very old age. But what about acquiring cognitive skills? Recent research has documented age differences for the learning of these skills that are similar to those observed for motor skills. For example, a number of studies have examined age as a factor in learning everyday tasks such as using a computer spreadsheet or word processing program (see Charness & Bosman, 1992). In general, the elderly are able to learn these skills, but often require additional time to do so. Age deficits in these tasks are sometimes difficult to interpret because of cohort differences in prior familiarity with task components such as general computer familiarity and typing experience. However, similar results have been reported for even very simple cognitive tasks, such as searching working memory for the presence of a target item (Salthouse & Somberg, 1982). Overall, there is ample evidence that cognitive skill learning proceeds more slowly for older than for younger people (see Kausler, 1994, for a review).

Charness (1989) has argued that the relative importance of an age deficit in skill learning may be quantified by the amount of additional practice time required to reduce or even reverse the effect. After investigating this index for a number of laboratory studies, he concluded that "3 min of practice per year of age difference is all that it takes to eliminate age effects. . . " (p. 452). While this conclusion is clearly an oversimplification, it does make the point that in some instances age differences in skill acquisition can be reduced and even eliminated with practice.

The various kinds of skill learning all have in common the requirement that some general skill be learned, whether it be how to track a target, how to program a computer, or how to type. In contrast, the final type of nondeclarative memory we will consider, *priming,* refers to the facilitation of performance resulting form an earlier encounter with some *specific* stimulus. In general, and in contrast to skill learning, priming appears to decline little, if at all, with aging (Howard, 1996; Howard & Wiggs, 1993; Mitchell, 1993). Age-related deficits are sometimes observed on priming tasks, but even then the deficits are very small and seem to appear only when either very large numbers of subjects are included (e.g., Hultsch et al., 1991), when priming of newly learned associations between words is tested (e.g., Howard, 1996; Howard & Wiggs, 1993), or when there is reason to suspect that explicit memory is "contaminating" the results. This relative age constancy in priming occurs even though there are usually substantial age deficits in explicit, episodic memory, for the same stimulus. Here we describe two examples of age constancy, priming of category exemplar generation, and priming of serial patterned sequences.

In a study of category exemplar generation, Light and Albertson (1989) asked younger (mean age = 22) and older (mean age = 70) people to rate the pleasantness of each of the words on a study list that included 18 target items—three exemplars from each of six categories. For instance, the target words BADGER, ELEPHANT, and DEER might have been scattered throughout the list, but the category name, ANIMAL, was never presented. People were then given an implicit priming test in which they were asked to generate several exemplars for each of a number of categories (e.g., ANIMAL). The earlier list was not mentioned at this point. Finally, an explicit cued recall test was administered in which people were given the names of the categories again and asked to recall any category members they remembered from the original study list. In both tests, exemplar generation and cued recall, the number of target exemplars produced from the study list (e.g., ELEPHANT) were counted. The results revealed a large and unsurprising age deficit for explicit cued recall, illustrating again the age differences in episodic memory discussed earlier. In contrast, there was only a very small, statistically nonsignificant, deficit for implicit exemplar generation. Thus, the older people were poorer than the younger in consciously recollecting that ELEPHANT had occurred on the earlier list, but that earlier encounter with ELEPHANT influenced which animals came to mind just as much for the older as for the younger people.

We have observed a similar pattern of age differences in conscious recollection, but not in priming, in a very different situation, that of learning a repeating serial spatial pattern (Howard & Howard, 1989, 1992). We used a serial reaction time task (from Nissen & Bullemer, 1987) in which people observed a series of asterisks, each presented at one of four spatial locations on a computer screen. Their task was to respond to each asterisk as quickly as possible by pressing a corresponding key. Unknown to the subjects, the location of the asterisks was determined by a repeating spatial pattern. When we assessed learning of this pattern using an explicit (episodic) test,

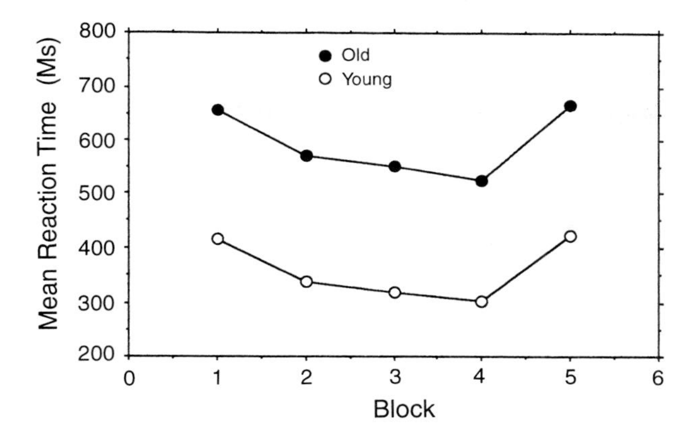

FIGURE 4 Mean reaction times over practice blocks in a serial reaction time task for younger and older groups. The stimulus followed a repeating pattern for blocks 1 through 4, but this pattern was removed on block 5, resulting in a disruption of performance for both age groups, revealing that they had learned the pattern. [Data redrawn from those reported in Howard and Howard (1989).]

we found age-related deficits. That is, when people were asked to predict the location of each asterisk based on their experience on the response trials, we found that older participants (mean age = 71 years) performed at only 76% the accuracy level of the younger ones (mean age = 22 years).

On the other hand, when we used an implicit measure, older people revealed as much pattern learning as younger. The implicit measure is based on how much reaction times in the serial pattern learning task itself are disrupted when the pattern is removed. These data from one of our experiments are shown in Figure 4. Notice that reaction times decreased over the first four testing blocks as people gained experience with the repeating pattern (the earlier responses to the pattern priming subsequent ones), but that reaction times increased dramatically on the fifth block when the pattern was removed and the asterisk locations determined randomly. This increase in response time when the pattern is removed provides an implicit measure of pattern learning since it reflects the influence of pattern knowledge on reaction time, and most important here, this increase is at least as large for the older people as it is for the younger. Therefore, people of both ages revealed equivalent priming due to the pattern's presence, even though the older people were poorer than the younger ones at conscious recollection of the pattern.

In summary, some kinds of procedural memory, such as skill learning, show age-related deficits, but others, such as priming, do not.

MODERATING FACTORS

In the preceding sections we have discussed age-related change in learning in general terms by summarizing the major patterns that emerge. But, despite these generalizations, no two people learn or age in exactly the same way. Further, on almost all learning and memory tasks, the age groups overlap. This can be seen clearly in Figure 2, where the distributions of computation span are shown; although the central tendency of the oldest group is lower than that of the youngest, many of the oldest people tested had higher computation spans than did many of the youngest people.

In this section we review some of the factors that have been shown to moderate age-related differences in learning and memory. We consider expertise, strategy learning, extended practice, and individual differences.

Expertise

It is not unusual to encounter older experts. For example, ship or airline captains, distinguished writers or scientists, and successful business executives are often relatively advanced in age. These people excel in their areas of expertise despite the deficits so often observed in laboratory research. A number of studies have investigated age and expertise for skills such as bridge and chess playing, miniature golf or transcription typing (see Charness, 1989, for a review). A theme that has emerged from this work is that elderly experts maintain high levels of performance in their skill by using compensatory processing to overcome the limitations of age. For example, expert typists maintain their typing speed into old age by looking farther ahead as they grow older (Bosman, 1993; Salthouse, 1984), even though these same individuals display the usual age-related declines that are seen in a simple choice reaction time task.

Charness (1989) has pointed out that experts develop highly efficient encoding or chunking strategies and specialized procedural knowledge, which both increase the efficiency and reduce the attentional demands of expertise-relevant processing. These skills enable the older expert to compensate for some of the working memory limitations summarized previously. The following section examines whether new learning of compensatory strategies can occur in the elderly.

Strategy Learning and Mnemonics

A number of studies have investigated the ability of older adults to learn and use mnemonic techniques to improve learning (see West, 1989, for a review). These studies have shown that although mnemonics training rarely eliminates age differences altogether, such training can lead to substantial improvements in performance of the elderly. In one study, for example, Baltes and Kliegl (1992) taught young (aged 20–30 years) and old (aged 66–80 years) people to use the method of loci for word list learning. This method involves associating each item with a specific location in an imagined place (e.g., one's house or home town). At the time of test, learners retrace their mental steps through the place recalling items as they go. The authors found that the technique enabled both age groups to improve their word learning and that performance continued to improve for both groups with practice. However, the older people performed more poorly than the younger throughout and this difference persisted even after 38 hours of practice with the mnemonic over 16 months (Baltes & Kliegl, 1992). Despite this, for practical purposes it is noteworthy that older people with the technique performed better than younger ones without it. Similar findings have been reported for other mnemonic techniques. Overall, it is clear that adults of all ages can benefit from training in the use of mnemonic techniques.

Extended Practice and Automatization

Another important characteristic of expertise is that certain tasks or task components have become automated through extended practice. Fisk and his colleagues have investigated the development of automatic processes in elderly volunteers. An automatic process is one that, by definition, places relatively few demands on cognitive resources (such as working memory) and occurs without intent (see Fisk, Ackerman, & Schneider, 1987; Hasher & Zacks, 1979). Fisk's research has shown that, while previously learned automatic processes are maintained in the elderly, older people experience more difficulty than younger in either acquiring new automatic processes (Fisk, Rogers, & Giambra, 1990) or inhibiting existing automatic processes (Rogers & Fisk, 1991). In the latter case, Rogers and Fisk (1991) compared young and elderly participants on an arithmetic Stroop task over 45 testing blocks. Here, subjects are required to validate simple single-digit arithmetic problems (e.g., 2 + 5 = 8) as either true or false. People were slower and less accurate on Stroop problems (e.g., 3 + 3 = 9) than on non-Stroop (e.g., 3 + 4 = 9), reflecting interference form their automatic retrieval of simple arithmetic tables (multiplication for the examples given). Most important, however, this interference effect diminished with practice for the young but remained constant for the old. Fisk and Rogers interpreted this to mean that older people experience greater difficulty than younger in inhibiting previously learned automatic processes.

In several other studies, Rogers, Fisk, and their colleagues examined the ability of young and old to acquire automaticity in a newly learned visual search task (Rogers, Bertus, & Gilbert, 1994; Rogers, Fisk, & Hertzog, 1994). In this task, individuals must identify the location of a target in a rectangular display of four words, three of which are distractors and one of which is a target. The target is distinguished from the distractors by its semantic category; for example, an animal term (target) could occur with an item of furniture, a weapon, and a fruit (distractors). As in earlier studies, Rogers, Fisk, and Hertzog (1994) demonstrated that with practice, young individuals develop an automatic attention response in this task when the target and distractor categories remain constant throughout the experiment (the consistent mapping condition). Under identical conditions, elderly individuals reveal a dramatic improvement in performance with practice but do not display automaticity. Rogers and her colleagues have interpreted this to mean that "the mechanism by which new automatic processes develop in visual search is disrupted for old adults" (Rogers, Fisk, & Hertzog, 1994, p. 735). Similar results were obtained by Rogers, Bertus, and Gilbert (1994) using visual search in a dual task procedure. On the whole, the findings from these experiments support the argument that established automatic processes are preserved in old age, but that new ones are difficult to acquire.

Individual Differences

Within group variability in cognitive tasks is typically substantial. In this section, we briefly summarize some of the individual factors that contribute to such variability and cognitive function in the elderly.

While most studies focus on "healthy" volunteers, such people can vary tremendously in their degree of physical and mental health. Some people, for instance, enjoy a greater level of aerobic fitness than others. There is substantial evidence that general health factors such as aerobic fitness can contribute significantly to cognitive function in the elderly (Bashore & Goddard, 1993). For example, lifelong fitness has been shown to correlate with mental processing speed in the elderly. Furthermore, aerobic exercise undertaken as an intervention in old age can also lead to improved performance on a range of neuropsychological tests (Bashore & Goddard, 1993). Similarly, mental health has been shown to play a role in cognitive performance. For example, elderly persons suffering from depression frequently complain of memory problems, and in some cases the symptoms of depression can be difficult to distinguish from those of dementia (see Kaszniak, 1990, for a review). Such physical and mental health factors contribute to the variability observed in learning.

People are also likely to differ in cognitive ability. A number of studies have investigated the role of verbal ability, a factor of particular interest since many laboratory studies use verbal tasks and vocabulary tends to increase with age. This research has shown that verbal ability can moderate age effects with age deficits occurring more frequently for people of lower verbal ability than for those with higher (Meyer & Rice, 1989). More recent work has employed structural statistical methods such as path analysis to estimate the relative contribution of a variety of ability measures to cognitive performance (e.g., Rogers, Fisk, & Hertzog, 1994).

From a practical standpoint, it is important to recognize that the performance of anyone, regardless of age, will reflect a variety of factors and that healthy, high-ability older people may outperform younger but less fit and less able persons, and this is particularly likely to be true when people are operating within their domains of expertise. Our understanding of how such individual differences moderate age-related change is in its infancy, but is improving with the use of new analytical techniques and larger sample sizes.

SUMMARY AND CONCLUSIONS

The traditional view was that one's ability to learn and remember declined with increasing age and that this decline was universal and inevitable. Contemporary research has shown that, while, in general, the elderly do learn less efficiently than the young, this is not always the case. Age-related decline as well as its important exceptions can be understood by considering learning situations in terms of the underlying memory systems involved. From this vantage, we see that, while working memory processing and episodic memory decline with age, semantic memory and some aspects of procedural memory remain quite stable. The ultimate effects of age on any given learning task will depend on the interplay of these systems. Furthermore, not all individuals age in the same way. Improved efficiency can be achieved through specific strategy training, extended practice, or the expertise acquired in a lifetime of experience. In many cases these individual differences in experience can compensate for declines that might otherwise occur with age. Health and abilities factors also play a role in learning, especially for the older learner.

From a practical standpoint, the contemporary approach to cognitive aging reviewed in this chapter suggests that the practitioner's challenge is as much to design for what is retained in aging as for what is lost. In some cases, age-related deficiencies can be addressed by adding a simple memory aid, by allowing increased time to respond or by providing additional practice. Our understanding of cognitive aging and life-span development has improved dramatically in recent years and the basic theory emerging from this understanding will continue to guide the practitioner concerned with age-related change.

Acknowledgment

Preparation of this chapter was supported in part by National Institute on Aging grant R37 AG02751 awarded to Darlene Howard. Correspondence should be addressed to James H. Howard, Jr., Department of Psychology, The Catholic University of America, Washington, DC 20064, or via electronic mail to HOWARD@CUA.EDU.

References

Baddeley, A. D., & Hitch, G. J. (1994). Developments in the concept of working memory. *Neuropsychology, 8,* 485–493.

Baltes, P. B. (1987). Theoretical propositions of life-span developmental psychology: On the dynamics between growth and decline. *Developmental Psychology, 23,* 611–626.

Baltes, P. B., & Kliegl, R. (1992). Further testing of limits of cognitive plasticity: Negative age differences in a mnemonic skill are robust. *Developmental Psychology, 28,* 121–125.

Bashore, T. R., & Goddard, P. H. (1993). Preservative and restorative effects of aerobic fitness on the age-related slowing of mental processing speed. In J. Cerella, J. Rybash, W. Hoyer, & M. L. Commons (Eds.), *Adult information processing: Limits on loss* (pp. 205–228). San Diego, CA: Academic Press.

Bosman, E. A. (1993). Age-related differences in the motoric aspects of transcription typing skill. *Psychology and Aging, 8,* 87–102.

Bowles, N. (1993). Semantic processes that serve picture naming. In J. Cerella, J. Rybash, W. Hoyer, & M. L. Commons (Eds.), *Adult information processing: Limits on loss* (pp. 303–326). San Diego, CA: Academic Press.

Braun, H. W., & Geiselhart, R. (1959). Age differences in the acquisition and extinction of the conditioned eyeblink response. *Journal of Experimental Psychology, 57,* 386–388.

Burke, D., MacKay, D., Worthley, J., & Wade, E. (1991). On the tip of the tongue: What causes word finding failures in young and older adults? *Journal of Memory and Language, 30,* 542–579.

Charness, N. (1989). Age and expertise: Responding to Talland's challenge. In L. Poon, D. C. Rubin, & B. A. Wilson (Eds.), *Everyday cognition in adulthood and late life* (pp. 437–456). New York: Cambridge University Press.

Charness, N., & Bosman, E. A. (1992). Human factors and age. In F. I. M. Craik & T. A. Salthouse (Eds.), *The handbook of aging and cognition* (pp. 495–552). Hillsdale, NJ: Erlbaum.

Colsher, P. L., & Wallace, R. B. (1991). Longitudinal application of cognitive function measures in a defined population of community-dwelling elders. *Annals of Epidemiology, 1,* 215–230.

Craik, F. I. M. (1994). Memory changes in normal aging. *Current Directions in Psychological Science, 3,* 155–158.

Craik, F. I. M., Morris, L. W., Morris, R. G., & Loewen, E. R. (1990). Relations between source amnesia and frontal lobe functioning in older adults. *Psychology and Aging, 5,* 148–151.

Crook, T. H., & Larrabee, G. S. (1992). Changes in facial recognition memory across the adult life span. *Journal of Gerontology, 47,* P138–P141.

Fisk, A. D., Ackerman, P. L., & Schneider, W. (1987). Automatic and controlled processing theory and its applications to human factors problems. In P. A. Hancock (Ed.), *Human factors psychology* (pp. 159–197). Amsterdam: North-Holland.

Fisk, A. D., Rogers, W. A., & Giambra, L. M. (1990). Consistent and varied memory/visual search: Is there an interaction between age and response-set effects? *Journal of Gerontology: Psychological Sciences, 45,* P81–P87.

Hall, G. S. (1922). *Senescence: The last half of life.* New York: Appleton.

Hasher, L., & Zacks, R. T. (1979). Automatic and effortful processes in memory. *Journal of Experimental Psychology: General, 108,* 356–388.

Herzog, A. R., & Rodgers, W. L. (1989). Age differences in memory performance and memory ratings as measured in a sample survey. *Psychology and Aging, 4,* 173–182.

Howard, D. V. (1996). The aging of implicit and explicit memory. In F. Blanchard-Fields & T. M. Hess (Eds.), *Perspectives on cognitive changes in adulthood and aging* (pp. 221–254). New York: McGraw-Hill.

Howard, D. V., & Howard, J. H., Jr. (1989). Age differences in learning serial patterns: Direct versus indirect measures. *Psychology and Aging, 4,* 357–364.

Howard, D. V., & Howard, J. H., Jr. (1992). Adult age differences in the rate of learning serial patterns: Evidence from direct and indirect tests. *Psychology and Aging, 7,* 232–241.

Howard, D. V., & Wiggs, C. L. (1993). Aging and learning: Insights from implicit and explicit tests. In J. Cerella, J. Rybash, W. Hoyer, & M. L. Commons (Eds.), *Adult information processing: Limits on loss* (pp. 512–528). San Diego, CA: Academic Press.

Hultsch, D. F., Hertzog, C., & Dixon, R. A. (1990). Ability correlates of memory performance in adulthood and aging. *Psychology and Aging, 5,* 356–368.

Hultsch, D. F., Masson, M. E. J., & Small, B. J. (1991). Adult age differences in direct and indirect tests of memory. *Journal of Gerontology, 46,* P22–P30.

James, W. (1950). *Principles of psychology.* New York: Dover. (Original edition published 1890)

Kaszniak, A. W. (1990). Psychological assessment of the aging individual. In J. E. Birren & K. W. Schaie (Eds.), *Handbook of the psychology of aging* (3rd ed., pp. 427–445). San Diego, CA: Academic Press.

Kausler, D. H. (1994). *Learning and memory in normal aging.* San Diego, CA: Academic Press.

Light, L. L. (1992). The organization of memory in old age. In F. I. M. Craik & T. A. Salthouse (Eds.), *The handbook of aging and cognition* (pp. 111–166). Hillsdale, NJ: Erlbaum.

Light, L. L., & Albertson, S. A. (1989). Direct and indirect tests of memory for category exemplars in young and older adults. *Psychology and Aging, 4,* 487–492.

Lipman, P. D., & Caplan, L. J. (1992). Adult age differences in memory for routes: Effects of instruction and spatial diagrams. *Psychology and Aging, 7,* 435–442.

McIntyre, J. S., & Craik, F. I. M. (1987). Age differences in memory for item and source information. *Canadian Journal of Psychology, 41,* 175–192.

Meyer, B. J. F., & Rice, G. E. (1989). Prose processing in adulthood: The text, the reader, and the task. In L. W. Poon, D. C. Rubin, & B. A. Wilson (Eds.), *Everyday cognition in adulthood and late life* (pp. 157–194). New York: Cambridge University Press.

Mitchell, D. B. (1993). Implicit and explicit memory for pictures: Multiple views across the lifespan. In P. Graf & M. E. J. Masson (Eds.), *Implicit memory: New directions in cognition, development, and neuropsychology* (pp. 171–190). Hillsdale, NJ: Erlbaum.

Nissen, M. J., & Bullemer, P. (1987). Attentional requirements of learning: Evidence from performance measures. *Cognitive Psychology, 19,* 1–32.

Rogers, W. A., Bertus, E. L., & Gilbert, D. K. (1994). Dual-task assessment of age differences in automatic process development. *Psychology and Aging, 9,* 398–413.

Rogers, W. A., & Fisk, A. D. (1991). Age-related differences in the maintenance and modification of automatic processes: Arithmetic Stroop interference. *Human Factors, 33,* 45–56.

Rogers, W. A., Fisk, A. D., & Hertzog, C. (1994). Do ability-performance relationships differentiate age and practice effects in visual search? *Journal of Experimental Psychology: learning, Memory, and Cognition, 20,* 710–738.

Salthouse, T. A. (1984). Effects of age and skill in typing. *Journal of Experimental Psychology: General, 113,* 345–371.

Salthouse, T. A. (1994). The aging of working memory. *Neuropsychology, 8,* 535–543.

Salthouse, T. A., & Skovronek, E. (1992). Within-context assessment of age differences in working memory. *Journal of Gerontology: Psychological Science, 47,* P110–P120.

Salthouse, T. A., & Somberg, B. L. (1982). Skilled performance: Effects of adult age and experience on elementary processes. *Journal of Experimental Psychology: General, 111,* 176–207.

Schacter, D. L., Harbluk, J. L., & McLachlan, D. R. (1984). Retrieval without recollection: An experimental analysis of source amnesia. *Journal of Verbal Learning and Verbal Behavior, 23,* 593–611.

Schacter, D. L., & Tulving, E. (1994). What are the memory systems of 1994? In D. L. Schacter & E. Tulving (Eds.), *Memory systems 1994* (pp. 1–38). Cambridge, MA: MIT Press.

Solomon, P. R., Blanchard, S., Levine, E., Velazquez, E., & Groccia-Ellison, M. E. (1991). Attenuation of age-related conditioning deficits in humans by extension of the interstimulus interval. *Psychology and Aging, 6,* 36–42.

Squire, L. R. (1994). Declarative and nondeclarative memory: Multiple brain systems supporting learning and memory. In D. L. Schacter & E. Tulving (Eds.), *Memory systems 1994* (pp. 208–231). Cambridge, MA: MIT Press.

Stine, E. L., & Wingfield, A. (1987). Levels upon levels: Predicting age differences in age recall. *Experimental Aging Research, 13,* 179–183.

Thorndike, E. L., Bregman, E. O., Tilton, J. W., & Woodyard, E. (1928). *Adult learning.* New York: Macmillan.

Tulving, E. (1972). Episodic and semantic memory. In E. Tulving & W. Donaldson (Eds.), *Organization of memory* (pp. 381–403). New York: Academic Press.

Tulving, E. (1993). What is episodic memory? *Current Directions in Psychological Science, 2,* 67–70.

Uttl, B., & Graf, P. (1993). Episodic spatial memory in adulthood. *Psychology and Aging, 8,* 257–273.

West, R. L. (1989). Planning practical memory training for the aged. In L. W. Poon, D. C. Rubin, & B. A. Wilson (Eds.), *Everyday cognition in adulthood and late life* (pp. 573–597). New York: Cambridge University Press.

Wright, B. M., & Payne, R. B. (1985). Effects of aging on sex differences in psychomotor reminiscence and tracking proficiency. *Journal of Gerontology, 40,* 179–184.

Zelinski, E. M., Gilewski, M. J., & Thompson, L. W. (1980). Do laboratory tests relate to self-assessment of memory ability in the young and old? In L. W. Poon, J. L. Fozard, L. S. Cermak, D. Arenberg, & L. W. Thompson (Eds.), *New directions in memory and aging: Proceedings of The George A. Talland Memorial Conference* (pp. 95–112). Hillsdale, NJ: Erlbaum.

Chapter 3

Sensory and Perceptual Functioning: Basic Research and Human Factors Implications

Donald W. Kline
Charles T. Scialfa

INTRODUCTION

Age-related changes in the ability to detect, interpret, and respond to visual and auditory information are often sufficient to compromise performance on a wide range of daily tasks (Garstecki, 1987; Hakkinen, 1984; Kline et al., 1992; Slawinski, Hartel, & Kline, 1993). For some, these deficits are profound (e.g., Davis, 1991; Lowman & Kirchner, 1988; Moscicki, Elkins, Baum, & McNamara, 1985). More typically, they develop gradually and are moderate in degree (e.g., Corso, 1987; Schieber, 1992; Spear, 1993; Willott, 1991). The goal of this chapter is to review such visual and auditory changes, as well as their consequences in real-world settings.

Handbook of Human Factors and the Older Adult

VISUAL AGING

In the United States, about 46% of those who are legally blind (corrected acuity below 20/200 and/or visual fields of 20 degrees or smaller) and approximately 68% of those with severe visual impairment (inability to read newspaper reprint with best correction) are 65 or older. Such deficits are more common among women than men (Kirchner & Lowman, 1988) and among institutionalized elderly (Klein, Klein, Linton, & De Mets, 1991). The leading causes of severe age-related losses are cataract, diabetic retinopathy, glaucoma, and macular degeneration (Kahn et al., 1977). Normal changes in the transparent anterior segments of the eye may be noticeable in the 30s and quite evident by the 40s. Nonpathological alterations in the sensorineural processes at and beyond the retina are not generally evident until somewhat later.

The Visual System

Optical Mechanisms

Cornea, Aqueous Humor, and Vitreous Humor Age-related yellowing (Lerman, 1984) and thickening (Weale, 1982) of the cornea normally have negligible effects on its role as the eye's principal refractive surface. The aqueous humor, the clear liquid behind the cornea filling the anterior chamber of the eye (see Figure 1), provides metabolic support for the lens and cornea. Aqueous outflow may decline with age (Linner, 1976) and could contribute to the increase in intraocular pressure associated with glaucoma. Although the vitreous tends to liquefy with age, its clarity is usually maintained (Spear, 1993).

Pupil The iris sets the pupil to its optimum diameter for ambient light levels, thereby maximizing depth of focus, decreasing optical aberration, and to some degree, controlling retinal illuminance. The pupil's resting diameter declines with age (*senile miosis*), reducing retinal illuminance proportionate to the change in area. This decline is greatest and is most likely to disadvantage older observers under low illumination conditions (Winn, Whitaker, Elliott, & Phillips, 1994).

Lens With aging, the lens yellows and becomes thicker, less flexible (i.e., *sclerotic*), and more opaque (Kashima, Trus, Unser, Edwards, & Datiles, 1993), changes that appear to be hastened by exposure to sunlight (Schein et al., 1994). The range over which the lens can adjust its focus (*accommodation*) appears to decline linearly (Sun et al., 1988), and by age 60 or so, little accommodative capacity remains (*presbyopia*). Before it is lost, onset laten-

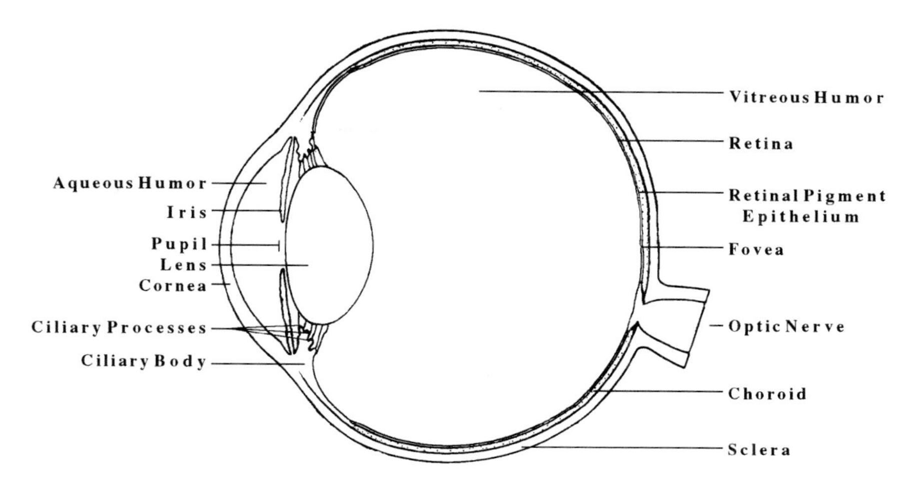

FIGURE 1 Structure of the eye.

cy of accommodation appears to change little with age, although its velocity declines, particularly under degraded viewing conditions (Elworth, Larry, & Malmström, 1986). As a result of its greater opacity, the senescent lens transmits less light to the retina; due to lenticular yellowing, absorption is greatest for short wavelengths (blues).

Refractive Errors The prevalence of refractive errors that necessitate the use of corrective lenses increases with age. For example, Wang, Klein, Klein, and Moss (1994) found that farsightedness (*hyperopia*) in the right-eye in excess of 0.5 diopters rose from 22.1% in those 43–54 years to 68.5% among those 75 and older. Conversely, the prevalence of near-sightedness (*myopia*) greater than −0.5 diopters declined from 43.0 to 14.4% in the same age groups. An association with higher levels of education suggests that extended near work contributes to myopia, at least in younger observers (e.g., Owens, 1991).

Retinal Illumination Due to changes in the ocular media, light reaching the retina is attenuated, scattered, and altered spectrally. There is about a 0.5 log unit (67%) decline in retinal illuminance from age 20 to 60 (Weale, 1961). Elliot, Whitaker, and MacVeigh (1990) estimate that this is accounted for by additive reductions of 0.3 log units (50%) and 0.2 log units (38%) at the pupil and lens, respectively. Increased light scatter in the older eye reduces retinal image contrast (e.g., van den Berg, 1995). These changes in retinal illuminance can affect performance on tasks that are low in contrast or carried out in low illuminance (Kline, 1991).

Sensorineural Mechanisms

Photoreceptors Retinal cones, which are smallest and most densely packed in the visual center of the retina (i.e., fovea) mediate spatial resolution and color perception. Rods, concentrated more peripherally, are responsible for sensitivity in low light. Although the age-related loss of foveal cones appears to be minimal, some decline has been noted in the peripheral retina (Curcio, Millican, Allen, & Kalina, 1993; Gao & Hollyfield, 1992). Curcio et al. (1993) also reported a 30% decline in rod density near the central retina, although the net responsiveness of rods to light appeared to be maintained.

Neural Components A decline in the amplitude of the photopic pattern electroretinogram (ERG) in older observers suggests a deficit in cone-fed retinal ganglion cells (Porciatti, Burr, Morrone, & Fiorentini, 1992). Little is known about age differences in retinal ganglion cells with rod inputs or the effects of aging on the lateral geniculate nucleus, the thalamic relay in the geniculostriate pathway.

As assessed by the latency of visually evoked potentials (VEPs), the speed with which visual information reaches the cortex declines with age (e.g., Morrison & Reilly, 1989). And binocular summation, the extent by which binocular task performance exceeds monocular performance beyond probability summation, may be reduced in elderly observers (Owsley & Sloane, 1990).

Voluntary Eye Movements

Objects in continuous motion are tracked using smooth pursuit eye movements (PEMs). When PEMs cannot maintain fixation, they are interspersed with high-velocity, ballistic saccadic eye movements (SEMs). SEMs also occur during the inspection of different locations in stationary scenes. With rapid motion, the lag in PEMs is greater among older observers and there is a decline of almost 30% in presaccadic acceleration, postsaccadic velocity, and peak pursuit velocity (e.g., Morrow & Sharpe, 1993; Zakon & Sharpe, 1987). Consistent with their difficulties in selective attention (Plude & Doussard-Roosevelt, 1989), the PEMs of older adults are more likely to be interrupted during the performance of a concurrent, cognitive task (Lapidot, 1987).

The deficits in PEMs and reduced ability to use information presented in the periphery (see the section on "Seeing in the Visual Periphery") mean that a larger number of SEMs may be required to acquire a target (Sharpe & Zakon, 1987). Studies report an increase in saccadic latencies and a decline in both peak saccadic velocity and accuracy among the elderly (e.g., Huaman & Sharpe, 1993). It is likely that such changes adversely affect performance on everyday tasks. For example, Scialfa, Thomas, and Joffe (1994) found that age-related deficits in a visual search task were eliminated when age differences in SEMs were removed statistically. The degree to which these deficits affect performance on such visual tasks as dynamic resolution and industrial inspection remains to be determined. Tasks involving stable gaze, however, are unlikely to be a problem since this is little affected by aging (Kosnik, Kline, Fikre, & Sekuler, 1987)

Visual Functioning

Light and Visual Performance

Light Sensitivity To be detected, more light must reach the front of the older eye. Because of older differential absorption by the ocular media, particularly the lens, dark adapted thresholds are most elevated for short-wavelength light (e.g., Pitts, 1982). Even with a long-wavelength test light and observers with good acuity, however, Eisner, Fleming, Klein, and Mauldin (1987) observed a threshold elevation of 0.09 log units (19%) per decade. Although the increase in minimum light threshold is attributable largely to a decline in retinal illuminance, deficits in photopigment regeneration and/or the neural pathways are probably also involved (Sturr, Hannon, Zhang, & Vaidya, 1992). This may explain why increased illuminance does not usually eliminate age differences on visual tasks.

Susceptibility to Glare While older observers usually benefit from increased light levels (e.g., Boyce, 1973), their increased vulnerability to disability glare makes it important to assure that lighting is appropriately directed. Olson and Sivak (1984) found that both steady-state and transient glare from rear-view mirrors affected visibility more adversely among old than young drivers. Schieber and Kline (1994) found that transient glare under nighttime conditions reduced the legibility of highway signs among elderly drivers, although it had no adverse effects on young and middle-aged ones. Steen, Whitaker, Elliott, and Wild (1994) reported that disability glare increased age differences in sensitivity for red–green, but not yellow–blue gratings. This effect may be associated with the spectral properties of the glare source. The only effective solution for disability glare is to prevent it from reaching the eye (Vos, 1995).

Recovery from glare is more protracted among older observers. Elliott and Whitaker (1991) found that photostress recovery time increased from 20 years of age onward, even when age differences in retinal illuminance were controlled. Schieber (1994) found that older observers required three times longer than the young to regain sensitivity for low-contrast letters following exposure to intense glare.

Color Perception Color discrimination seems to decline modestly with age, at least for short wavelengths. For example, Knoblauch et al. (1987) observed that errors increased with age along the tritan (i.e., blue–yellow) axis on the Farnsworth–Munsell 100 Hue Test, particularly under reduced illumination. Cooper, Ward, Gowland, and McIntosh (1991) found a similar decline after 60 years of age with the Lanthony New Color Test. Age deficits of smaller magnitude were seen for reds and yellows. Both optic and sensorineural factors contribute to age-related changes in color discrimination (Werner & Steele, 1988).

Spatial Vision

Static Acuity Whether assessed cross-sectionally (e.g., Yang, Elliott, & Whitaker, 1993) or longitudinally (Gittings & Fozard, 1986) acuity (the smallest detail that can be discriminated in stationary high-contrast targets) declines with age, independent of visual pathology. Gittings and Fozard found that a decline in uncorrected acuity was evident by age 30, but for corrected acuity, not until the 70s. About 12% of those over 75 had acuities worse than 20/50 and a majority of the participants maintained acuity levels of 20/40 or better into their 80s.

Age deficits in acuity are increased by low light levels. Sturr, Kline, and Taub (1990) reported that 77% of drivers under 65 had acuity of 20/40 or better at 2.4 cd/m^2. For those 65–75 and over 75, the corresponding proportions were 28 and 4%. Low-contrast acuity is also reduced among visually screened old observers, even when they are similar to young observers at high contrast (Owsley, Sloane, Skalka, & Jackson, 1990). Although reduced retinal illuminance contributes to the acuity decline, sensorineural factors also appear to be involved (Adrian, 1995).

Static Contrast Sensitivity and Discrimination Spatial contrast sensitivity is a measure of the ability to discern luminance differences, usually in a stationary grating in which luminance varies sinusoidally. Sensitivity for gratings of varied coarseness (i.e., spatial frequency) is represented by the contrast sensitivity function (CSF), a comprehensive summary of an observer's spatial vision. At high spatial frequencies, the CSF contains information about a person's acuity (e.g., resolution of a 30 c/deg grating is equivalent to 20/20 acuity); sensitivity at lower frequencies provides an index of the ability to perceive larger, low-contrast objects (e.g., a truck in fog). Since many real-world tasks depend on sensitivity to large or low-contrast targets, CSF measures are often more suitable than acuity for predicting performance on them. For example, the contrast sensitivity measures have been shown to be more strongly associated with detection and identification of common objects (Owsley & Sloane, 1987), the discriminability of highway signs (Evans & Ginsburg, 1985), and the self-reported visual problems of aging drivers (Schieber, Kline, Kline, & Fozard, 1992).

Aging is associated with a decline in contrast sensitivity, particularly at intermediate and higher spatial frequencies (e.g., Crassini, Brown, & Bowman, 1988; Elliott et al., 1990; Scialfa, Adams, & Giovanetto, 1991). These deficits are reduced but not eliminated when observers are optimally corrected (Owsley, Sekuler, & Siemsen, 1983; Scialfa, Adams, & Giovanetto, 1991). As well, because sensitivity to intermediate and higher spatial frequencies is affected by retinal illuminance (Patel, 1966), age-related losses in this range of the CSF are minimized by using stronger light sources (Owsley et al., 1983; Sloane, Owsley, & Alvarez, 1988).

Although the discrimination of contrast at suprathreshold levels is impaired among older observers, this can be explained by the sensitivity loss at threshold (Tulunay-Keesey, Ver Hoeve, & Terkla-McGrane, 1988). Beard, Yager, and Neufeld (1994) found no age difference in the contrast discrimination threshold once the data of older observers had been normalized to their contrast detection levels. These findings indicate that the performance of older persons on everyday suprathreshold visual tasks can be optimized by high-contrast stimuli and adequate illumination.

Dynamic Acuity and Spatial Contrast Sensitivity As might be expected, age-related deficits in static resolution and the execution of eye movements affect dynamic visual tasks such as dynamic visual acuity (DVA) adversely (Burg, 1966). Scialfa, Garvey, Tyrrell, and Leibowitz (1992) examined age differences in CSFs for sine-wave gratings traveling at varying speeds. Older adults had higher thresholds for stationary gratings of intermediate and higher spatial frequency, a deficit which increased with object motion. While inadequate pursuit gain may be responsible for these losses, Long and Crambert (1990) have suggested that reduced retinal illuminance among the elderly may be involved. If so, increases in ambient illumination may enhance older persons' performance on dynamic tasks.

Since the upper limit on dynamic sensitivity is determined largely by sensitivity for stationary targets, they are related positively to each other and inversely to age (Scialfa et al., 1988). Thus, the dynamic resolution levels of older adults can be enhanced by optimizing their static acuity, although it is unlikely to bring them up to the level of their younger counterparts.

Seeing in the Visual Periphery A great deal of important environmental information comes to us from the peripheral visual field. This is most commonly measured with the visual field test (also known as *visual perimetry*) in which the observer is required to detect a luminance target at varying retinal distances from fixation. Using this measure, binocular visual fields average 180 deg for young adults, but by the age of 70 years decline to 140 deg (Johnson, 1986).

Age-related declines in acuity for peripheral targets have also been shown to be greater than for central targets (Collins, Brown, & Bowman, 1989). Optical lenses, more frequently worn by the elderly, exhibit off-axis image distortion, and lenses do not provide best correction over the entire visual field, leaving the eyeglass wearer uncorrected in the periphery. Both factors may contribute to age-related declines in peripheral visual function, some of which are discussed here.

Depth Perception Research has examined age effects on stereopsis, the depth information available from perspective differences in the two retinal images, but there has been little research on other depth cues. Although failure rates on tests of stereopsis increase among the elderly (e.g., Wright & Wormaid, 1992), thresholds show little (Gittings & Fozard, 1986) or no decline with age (Yekta, Pickwell, & Jenkins, 1989). Green and Madden (1987) observed higher thresholds among old participants on the Randot stereopsis test, but the age difference was eliminated with the exclusion of data from four elderly participants without measurable depth perception.

Perception of Stimulus Change

Flicker Sensitivity Older persons tend to be disadvantaged by visual tasks that depend on the perception of quickly changing stimuli. Many early studies indexed age differences in temporal sensitivity using the critical flicker frequency (CFF) threshold, the lowest rate at which a pulsing light source appears to be continuous. Virtually all studies show an age decline in the CFF threshold (e.g., Coppinger, 1955). Although reduced, an age decrement in CFF occurs in studies that have employed high luminance levels or light/dark ratios (e.g., McFarland, Warren, & Karis, 1958) or which have controlled for pupil size (Falk & Kline, 1978; Weekers & Roussel, 1946). This suggests that not all of the decline in CFF can be attributed to reduced retinal illuminance.

Recent investigations of age differences in flicker sensitivity have frequently employed the *temporal contrast sensitivity function* (TCSF), a measure of the minimum contrast needed to detect sinusoidal modulation of a light source over time. Although the largest age differences occur at intermediate and high temporal frequencies, studies disagree on whether this reflects a loss of sensitivity to the amplitude of the temporal change or an actual slowing of the senescent visual system. Mayer, Kim, Svingos, and Glucs (1988) concluded that observers over 65 were less sensitive to flicker from 10 to 45 Hz, but showed little evidence of visual slowing. Tyler (1989) found both a decline in sensitivity to high temporal frequencies and a shift of the overall function to lower frequencies suggestive of an increase in the time constant of the senescent visual system. A similar finding has been reported by Kuyk and Wesson (1991). Age deficits in temporal modulation sensitivity seem to be most pronounced for peripheral targets (Casson, Johnson, & Nelson-Quigg, 1993), suggesting that flickered peripheral targets will be less salient for them.

The age decline in temporal resolution varies with the spatial characteristics of the stimuli. No age deficit was seen by Tulunay-Keesey et al. (1988) at low spatial frequencies, but there was a prominent loss at high spatial frequencies. Elliott et al. (1990), however, found that significant age differences also occurred at lower spatial frequencies if counterphase flicker rate was increased sufficiently. The sensitivity of young observers was unaffected when they performed the task under conditions of simulated pupillary and lenticular aging, suggesting a neural explanation.

Perception of Moving Stimuli As for many tasks involving stimulus change, older observers have relative difficulty perceiving motion at a threshold. Oscillatory displacement thresholds appear to increase markedly past middle-age (Elliott, Whitaker, & Thompson, 1989). To evaluate oscillation detection free of changes in spatial resolution, Kline, Culham, Bartel, and Lynk (1994) compared the static and oscillatory vernier thresholds of young and old observers. The displacement thresholds of young and old observers were similar for high- and low-contrast static targets, but oscillation produced a marked age deficit. These findings suggest that older persons would perform less effectively on tasks involving the detection of small target excursions (e.g., on dials or indicators).

Motion perception has also been evaluated by determining motion coherence thresholds, the proportion of elements in an array that must move together to produce a global perception of motion. One study found that motion coherence thresholds increased directly with age (Trick & Silverman, 1991). More recently, Wojciechowski, Trick, and Steinman (1995) reported that age differences in motion coherence thresholds were more pronounced in the central than peripheral field.

Despite the evidence of age deficits on threshold motion tasks, the extent to which older adults are disadvantaged in "real-world" conditions is not clear. Scialfa, Guzy, Leibowitz, Garvey, and Tyrrell (1991) compared age differences in verbal estimates of the velocity of a single automobile. The older observers velocity scales suggested a lessened sensitivity to speed, but between 15 and 55 mph, there were no age differences. Schiff, Oldak, and Shah (1992) found that older women gave higher and thus more cautious verbal estimates of the speed of a filmed automobile. Older men and women were more cautious, though less accurate, in their direct estimates of time to arrival. Given the importance of accurate speed and distance judgments in many daily tasks, it is an area worthy of further research.

The flow of stimuli over the retina provides moving observers with critical information regarding direction, velocity, and orientation. Any decline in the quality of this information or its less effective integration with vestibular or somatosensory information could impair the mobility or postural stability of older persons. Warren, Blackwell, and Morris (1989) compared young and old observers on the ability to estimate apparent direction of motion from computer-presented, random-dot optical flow patterns that simulated translational or curvilinear motion. Small but significant increases in error were found among older adults for both motion types. Wade, Lindquist, Taylor, and Treat-Jacobson (1995) utilized a force-measuring platform to evaluate the effects of radial (central retina), lamellar (peripheral retina), and global (central and peripheral retina) optical flow on the postural stability of younger (20–59) and older (60–83) participants. Age differences were seen in the latter two conditions, suggesting that as a result of slower or reduced somatosensory feedback, older persons rely increasingly on the visual system for postural control. The authors noted that a lack of visual anchors in the task environment may make older persons more prone to falls. Consistent with this, Turano, Rubin, Herdman, Chee, and Fried (1994) found that the contribution of vision to postural stability is greater among those with a history of falls than those without. One response to this problem may be to provide conspicuous high-contrast visual anchors in high-risk areas.

Attention and Vigilance

Visual Search Efficient task performance depends on the selection and subsequent processing of task-relevant stimuli, as well as the rejection of irrelevant information. But research has repeatedly shown that older adults have more difficulty with visual search, a difficulty that increases with the number of items to be searched (Plude & Doussard-Roosevelt, 1989; Scialfa & Essau, 1993). Age differences in search are slight when targets are featurally distinct from background objects, but increase with target–background similarity (Plude & Doussard-Roosevelt, 1989).

Typically, observers are given minimal practice on visual search tasks, which increases age differences because display size effects are reduced or eliminated when target identity is constant during training (Schneider & Shiffrin, 1977). Such automaticity develops, in part, because targets gain and distractors lose the ability to attract attention. In fact, middle-aged persons who have become proficient at domain-specific search seem to attend automatically to targets (Clancy & Hoyer, 1994). However, Fisk and his colleagues (Fisk & Rogers, 1991; Rogers, 1992) have consistently found attenuated priority learning in the elderly. This deficit may be due to a failure to inhibit processing of distractors (Kane, Hasher, Stoltzfus, Zacks, & Connelly, 1994).

The costs and benefits associated with advance cueing provide additional indices of attentional selectivity. Generally, only small age differences are observed in the magnitude and time course of attentional allocation (Folk & Hoyer, 1992; Hartley, Kieley, & Slabach, 1990; Madden, 1992). The elderly often benefit more than the young from advance information, perhaps because the cue allows them to more effectively inhibit processing of irrelevant locations. The search performance of older operators can be improved if task-relevant objects are made conspicuous, and if adequate practice and advance information are provided to guide them to target objects or locations.

Vigilance Tasks such as driving and industrial inspection require vigilance over extended durations. This, in turn, requires attentional control and continued arousal (Davies & Parasuraman, 1982). Giambra and Quilter (1988) examined age effects on vigilance using the Mackworth Clock Test (Mackworth, 1948), in which a chronometer's infrequent "double jumps" had to be detected. Neither hit rate nor vigilance decrement were related to age. Monk, Buysse, Reynolds, Jarrett and Kupfer (1992) gave a computerized version of the Mackworth Clock Test to young and old men over 36 hours of wakefulness. Hit rates showed neither a main effect of age, nor an age by time interaction. Age deficits emerge, however, when the stimuli are degraded optically (Parasuraman, Nestor, & Greenwood, 1989) or temporally (Parasuraman & Giambra, 1992).

The Useful Field of View Attention can be selective only to the extent that the observer is capable of perceiving the features making up task-relevant objects, many of which are some distance from fixation. The *useful field of view* (UFOV) is defined as "the total visual field area from which target characteristics can be acquired when eye and head movements are precluded" (e.g., Scialfa, Kline, & Lyman, 1987). Unlike static visual field measures, the size of the UFOV changes as a function of target–distracter similarity, primary task demands (i.e., detection vs. identification vs. localization), and secondary task characteristics. There is considerable evidence that the UFOV is restricted in older observers (e.g., Ball, Beard, Roenker, Miller, & Griggs, 1988; Scialfa et al., 1994; Sekuler & Ball, 1986). Ball et al. (1988, Exp. 1) have shown that practice expands the UFOV in older adults but not more than in the young or middle-aged.

There is evidence that UFOV restrictions contribute to age deficits on other tasks, including nonsearch detection (Cerella, 1985, Exp. 3), visual search (Plude and Doussard-Roosevelt, 1989), and driving (Owsley, Ball, Sloane, Roenker, & Bruni, 1991). Scialfa et al. (1994) demonstrated that older adults were more likely than young ones to make a saccade prior to identifying an eccentric feature search target if it was presented amid distractors. Finally, Anandam (1994) trained young and old observers in CM visual search. After training, older adults still showed reliable display size effects; younger adults did not. However, when restricted to the central 2 deg of the display, analyses of the reaction times of older adult's were also independent of display size, indicating that they too had achieved automaticity, although over a more limited spatial extent.

Age-related reductions in the UFOV have several implications for task and environment design. Target objects should be presented near to anticipated fixation. Additionally, their conspicuity should be maximized by reducing visual clutter and increasing target contrast (e.g., color, brightness, size, orientation). UFOV measures might also be useful in screening operators for particular tasks.

The Self-Reports of Older Observers

Since they are usually gathered in isolation from one another and under circumstances quite different from those of daily life, objective clinical and laboratory measures are often inadequate predictors of the visual problems of older persons. Hakkinen (1984) employed personal interviews and ophthalmological tests to assess the visual difficulties of older persons in the natural environment. Although she found that the relationship between clinical measures and independent functioning was positive, there were also discrepancies. For example, even when their acuity fell as low as 20/120, most elderly persons coped effectively; many did not use their prescribed visual correction.

When Kosnik, Winslow, Kline, Rasinski, and Sekuler (1988) surveyed healthy adults about their everyday visual problems, they found five dimensions that declined with age: visual processing speed, light sensitivity, dynamic vision, near vision, and visual search. Subsequently, Kosnik, Sekuler, and Kline (1990) reported that those who experienced such difficulty on everyday visual tasks were also more likely than their like-age cohorts to have stopped driving. When Kline et al. (1992) surveyed several hundred drivers regarding their visual problems on a wide range of everyday and driving tasks, they found several that were age-related: unexpected vehicles, vehicle speed, dim displays, windshield problems, and sign reading. The authors noted that some of the visual problems reported by older drivers were consistent with their elevated risk for certain types of accidents. Rumsey (1993) found that visual complaints and decrements on acuity, contrast sensitivity, stereopsis, glare sensitivity, and color vision increased with age. Only the global complaint of decreased vision, however, was directly related to objective performance. Rubin, Roche, Prasada-Rao, and Fried (1994), however, found quite specific relationships between spatial vision losses and self-reported disability on everyday tasks. Acuity declines were associated with problems requiring good resolution and adjustment to changing light conditions; declines in contrast sensitivity, with distance judgment, night driving, and mobility. Possible reasons for the inconsistency in vision–disability relationships across studies include high variability in individual and circumstantial factors, differences in the specificity of self-report measures, and variation in self-knowledge of visual loss. In relation to the latter, self-reports appear to underestimate the prevalence of cataract and age-related macular degeneration (Linton, Klein, & Klein, 1991) as well as binocular field loss (Johnson & Keltner, 1983).

Enhancing the Visual Performance of Older Observers

The visual deficits of older observers, which vary markedly with task type and conditions, suggest the following guidelines for optimizing their visual performance:

1. Task design or selection should be guided by the visual abilities of the end-users, including a recognition of the high variability among older persons.
2. Tests of visual ability should be matched carefully to the visual task(s).
3. Self-report and observational measures are valuable supplements to visual tests in assessing the fit of end-users to their visual environment.
4. For older observers, legibility is enhanced by increased illumination and contrast, particularly for finely detailed stimuli presented in poor light or glare.
5. Glare and UV exposure should be avoided.
6. Use larger color contrast steps where short-wavelength discriminations are required.
7. Where possible, the need to discriminate near stimuli should be avoided, and task-specific information presented at a constant depth plane.
8. On tasks where accurate depth perception is important, provide nonphysiological cues (e.g., texture gradient, interposition, relative size, linear perspective).
9. Observers should be optically corrected for the viewing distance.

10. Stimuli demanding careful inspection should be large, simple, uncrowded, and presented in the central visual field.
11. The need to process rapidly changing or moving stimuli should be minimized.
12. Conspicuity of critical stimuli can be enhanced through changes of size, contrast, color, or motion.
13. Conspicuous high-contrast visual anchors should be provided in areas where there is a high risk of falling (e.g., halls, stairways, foyers, etc.)

HEARING

In audition, as in vision, the prevalence of loss is strongly age related. Davis (1991) found that almost 90% of the seriously hearing impaired in England and Wales were over age 60. More typically, however, elderly individuals, experience moderate hearing loss (Gates, Cooper, Kannel, & Miller, 1990).

The Auditory System

The Ear

The pinna and auditory canal of the external ear (see Figure 2) funnel acoustic energy to the middle ear, amplifying frequencies of about 1800–7000 Hz, a range that overlaps much of the speech spectrum (approximately 550–5000 Hz). In old age, excess wax in the auditory canal often diminishes pure tone sensitivity (Corso, 1963). The collapse of the auditory canal can also bring about hearing loss at some frequencies in the speech range (Schow & Goldblum, 1980).

The *eardrum* is displaced as a function of a sound's intensity and at a rate consistent with its frequency. In the older ear, signal strength is attenuated by diminished elasticity in the tympanic ring (Belal, 1975). The three small bones (*ossicles*) of the middle ear act as a lever system, increasing signal strength some 44X. Calcification of the ossicles in the old ear reduces its amplification and, in turn, its psychophysical sensitivity (Etholm & Belal, 1974).

At the *oval window,* movement of the ossicles sets in motion the fluid held within the *cochlea* of the inner ear. This initiates a pressure wave that travels along the *basilar membrane,* reaching a peak near the oval window in response to high-frequency sounds and near the apex of the basilar membrane for low-frequency sounds (see Gulick, Gescheider, & Frisina, 1989).

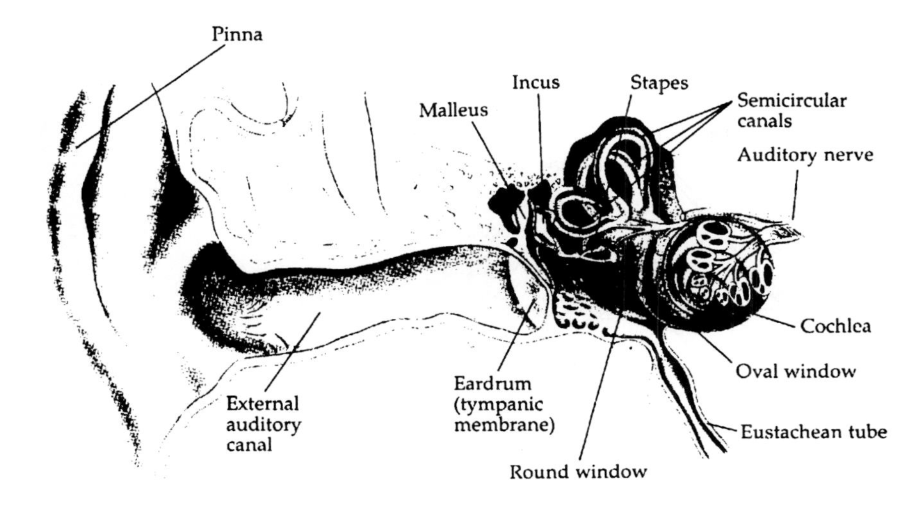

FIGURE 2 Structure of the ear. [From Culic, W. L., Gescheider, G. A., & Frisina, R. D. (1989). *Hearing: Physiological Acoustics, Neural Coding and Psychophysics.* New York: Oxford University Press. Adapted by permission.]

This produces a shearing force on the *inner* and *outer hair cells,* which are the sensory receptors for hearing (see Figure 3). The basilar membrane becomes less compliant with age (Hansen & Reske-Nielsen, 1965), and normal aging is associated with a loss of hair cells, which is more pronounced in the basal region responsible for coding higher frequencies (Johnsson & Hawkins, 1972) and in outer compared to inner hair cells (Bohne, Gruner, & Harding, 1990). Hair cell loss may be responsible for age deficits in high-frequency pitch discrimination (Matschke, 1990), absolute sensitivity and speech recognition. It may also explain older listeners' greater difficulty with women's and children's than with men's voices and more frequent mistakes discriminating some speech sounds (e.g., *s* and *f*).

The Higher Neural Pathways

As the central pathways are ascended, auditory processing increases remarkably in complexity. Like those in the visual cortex, cells in the auditory cortex exhibit considerable stimulus selectivity and appear to code complex features often related to communication (see Gulick et al., 1989). Unfortunately, gerontological studies of higher auditory centers are limited largely to gross anatomical studies (Vaughan & Vincent, 1979) that say little about functional changes.

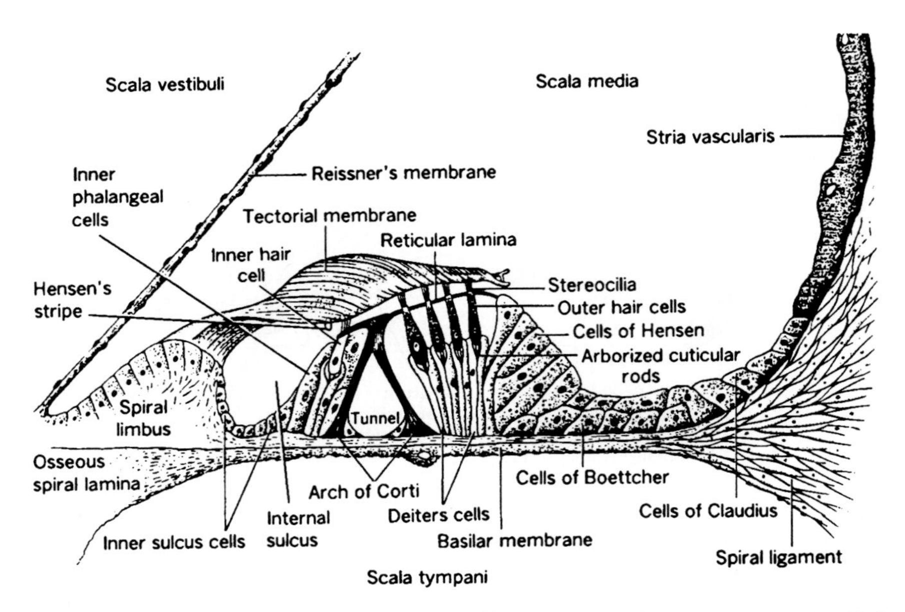

FIGURE 3 Cross-sectional diagram of the cochlea. [From Matlin, M. W., & Foley, H. J. (1995). *Sensation and Perception* (3rd ed.). Needham Heights, MA: Allyn & Bacon. Adapted by permission.]

Auditory Functions

Perception of Loudness

A person's ability to hear low-amplitude sounds is commonly represented by an audiogram, a graphical depiction of hearing level (HL) in decibels (dB) as a function of frequency. Aging is associated with a decline in the audiogram at the higher frequencies, a loss termed *presbycusis*. Although the rate of loss at high frequencies appears to be steady, it increases in the speech frequencies (Brant & Fozard, 1990). Davis, Ostri, and Parving (1991) reported that binaural hearing loss was about 2.5 dB/decade up to age 55, and about 8.5 dB/decade beyond 55.

The loss of sensitivity at higher frequencies is usually greater among men than women, a difference that increases with age (e.g., Pedersen, Rosenhall, & Moller, 1989). This often has been attributed to sex differences in noise exposure (e.g., Moscicki et al., 1985). Pearson et al. (1995), however, found that longitudinal declines in hearing sensitivity proceeded more quickly among men not involved in noisy occupations or showing evidence of noise-induced hearing loss.

Long-term exposure to noise of any type degrades hearing at higher frequencies; at lower frequencies (1 and 2 kHz), the effects appear to be relatively noise specific (Rosler, 1994). The evidence that presbycusis increases susceptibility to noise-induced hearing loss suggests that the avoidance of noise exposure may be particularly important for older listeners (Shone, Altschuler, Miller, & Nuttall, 1991).

Discrimination of Pitch

Frequency discrimination, which is important to many auditory tasks including speech perception, appears to decline with age. Discrimination thresholds for short tones have been reported to increase with age (Cranford & Stream, 1991). Similarly, Lutman, Gatehouse, and Worthington (1991) found that, even after accounting for initial hearing level differences, frequency resolution for a standard 2 kHz tone was related to age. Similar age differences have been seen in the discrimination of complex tones. Matschke (1990) determined that by age 60 there is a decrement in the ability to discriminate speech-range sounds that differ in spectral composition.

Temporal Resolution

Auditory temporal resolution, critical to both speech perception and sound localization, declines with age. For example, time compression impairs speech comprehension more among old than young listeners (Rastatter, Watson, & Strauss-Simmons, 1989). An age-related temporal loss was also observed by Raz, Millman, and Moberg (1990) on the discrimination of two target tones in a backward masking task. Robin and Royer (1989) presented young and elderly listeners with two tones separated by a silent, variable, interstimulus interval (ISI). Fusion occurred at longer first-tone durations among older listeners at all ISIs. Using a temporal gap procedure, however, Moore, Peters, and Glasberg (1992) concluded that an age loss of temporal resolution is not inevitable.

Localization of Sound

Binaural localization of sound sources depends on the ability to make accurate determinations of interaural time and intensity differences, so some loss of localization ability with age might be expected. Studies are generally consistent with this expectation, especially among those with neurally based presbycusis (e.g., Willott, 1991). Nordlund (1964), comparing hearing listeners with and without presbycusis, found that loss of the ability to localize sound in free-field conditions was pronounced in the former group and mild in the latter. Hausler, Colburn, and Marr (1983) observed that participants with good speech discrimination ability showed normal localization abilities, while those with poor speech discrimination were also impaired on localization, even at high intensity levels.

Speech Perception

Given the importance to daily life, it is not surprising that older persons express concern about their communicative disabilities (Jacobs-Condit, 1984). Normal aging, which implies sensorineural hearing loss, is generally associated with deficits in speech perception. The deficits tend to be small when the speech is presented in quiet, but increase when listening takes place in less optimal environments (Helfer, 1992). Until recently, the prevailing view was that age differences in speech perception result largely from damage to the central auditory centers. However, the correlations between measures of pure-tone sensitivity and speech perception, while showing considerable variation, tend to be in the range of 0.5 to 0.9 (e.g., Lutman, 1991). Importantly, once age-related changes in pure-tone sensitivity are taken into account, either by sampling or by statistical means, age deficits in speech recognition are minimal (Helfer, 1992; Lutman, 1991; van Rooij & Plomp, 1992). For example, Lutman (1991) assessed various aspects of hearing in almost 2000 persons aged 17 to 80 years. In addition to providing pure-tone thresholds, participants identified sentences presented in speech-shaped noise at an intensity of 70 dB sound and pressure level (SPL) and a signal-to-noise (S/N) ratio of +5 dB. Measures of frequency resolution and temporal resolution were also obtained. After partialling out the effects of pure-tone sensitivity, age accounted for only 3% of the variance in speech perception.

A finding with considerable human factors relevance is that, compared to the young, older adults make as good or better use of context cues to facilitate speech recognition in both time-gated speech (Craig, Kim, Rhyner, & Chirillo, 1993) and normal carrier sentences (Holtzman, Familant, Deptula, & Hoyer, 1986). Informationally consistent and rich speech, spoken clearly and at a high S/N ratio, optimizes hearing for all listeners, and particularly for the elderly.

Auditory Attention

Since the 1960s numerous studies have examined age differences in auditory attention using dichotic listening tasks (see the review by Tun & Wingfield, 1993). Dichotic listening tasks require a listener to repeat ("shadow") the information presented in one ear, while ignoring the information presented simultaneously to the other ear. Briefly, older adults have difficulty with shadowing if competing information is presented to the other ear (e.g., Barr & Giambra, 1990), perhaps reflective of a divided attention deficit (McDowd & Craik, 1988). They also require more time to switch attention between ears and, consequently, miss information that is heard by younger persons (Wickens, Braune, & Stokes, 1987). This latter finding may be important when considering the perceptual challenges of older listeners in noisy or multitalker environments and also in the design of directionally sensitive hearing aids.

The Self-Reports of Older Listeners

Auditory handicaps among the elderly are explained only partly by audiometric loss, indicating that nonauditory variables are also determinants of perceived handicap (Dancer, Pryor, & Rozema, 1989). These nonauditory factors may include health, other sensory losses, compensatory skills, education level, social support, vocational and avocational activities, and living arrangements. The Hearing Handicap Inventory for the Elderly (HHIE) was developed by Ventry and Weinstein (1982) to assess the emotional and social effects of self-reported impairment among the elderly. When Weinstein and Ventry (1983) administered the HHIE instrument to respondents over 65, they found that audiometric measures accounted for less than 50% of the variance in hearing handicap and suggested that self-report measures are more appropriate for this purpose. Relatedly, Garstecki (1987) found that about 30% of those who passed a pure-tone screening test appeared to be handicapped on the HHIE and, conversely, 20–25% of those who failed the screening test were not. For such reasons, Weinstein (1994) has argued that the most important predictor of hearing-aid candidacy is not degree of hearing loss, but a person's motivation and perception of the extent of handicap. The *Your Hearing* self-report instrument of Slawinski and Kline (1989) was developed to evaluate the impact of age-related auditory changes on task performance in everyday life. When Slawinski et al. (1993) used the instrument to solicit the responses of adults of different ages, seven types of age-related auditory problems emerged: temporal resolution, hearing in background noise, understanding distorted speech, understanding normal speech, and hearing high-pitched sounds. These difficulties were related to self-reported hearing quality. They are also consistent with objective measures, and suggest some promising areas for human factors applications.

Enhancing the Auditory Performance of Older Listeners

The following guidelines for optimizing task effectiveness for older listeners are derived from research on age effects on audition and speech perception:

1. Task design and selection should be based on the auditory and speech-perception abilities of the target listeners, recognizing that variability in both increases with age.

2. Assure congruence between auditory tasks and the tests by which listeners' fitness for them is evaluated.
3. To optimize the auditory environments for older listeners, augment hearing and speech-perception tests with self-report or observational measures.
4. Long-term exposure to noise should be avoided.
5. Where possible, avoid the need for high-frequency detection and discrimination.
6. The discrimination of acoustic cues can be improved by maximizing their pitch, spectral, or location differences.
7. Signal-to-noise ratios can be enhanced through volume adjustment and by minimizing background noise and reverberation.
8. Accurate speech perception is fostered by messages that are clear, reasonably paced, redundant, and rich in context.
9. Sound localization can be improved through maximizing location and frequency differences and by increasing signal on-time.

Acknowledgment

Preparation of this review was supported in part by grants to both the first and second authors from the Natural Sciences and Engineering Research Council of Canada (NSERC).

References

Adrian, W. (1995). Change of visual acuity with age. In W. Adrian (Ed.) *Proceedings of the Third International Symposium, Lighting for Aging Vision and Health* (pp. 65–76). New York: Lighting Research Institute.

Anandam, B. (1994). *Ageing and visual search.* Unpublished Master's thesis, University of Calgary, Department of Psychology, Calgary, Canada.

Ball, K. K., Beard, B. L., Roenker, D. L., Miller, R. L., & Griggs, D. S. (1988). Age and visual search: Expanding the useful field of view. *Journal of the Optical Society of America A, 35,* 2210–2219.

Barr, R. A., & Giambra, L. M. (1990). Age-related decrement in auditory selective attention. *Psychology and Aging, 5,* 597–599.

Beard, B. L., Yager, D., & Neufeld, S. (1994). Contrast detection and discrimination in young and older adults. *Optometry and Vision Science, 71,* 783–791.

Belal, A. (1975). Presbycusis: Physiological or pathological. *Journal of Laryngology, 89,* 1011–1025.

Bohne, B. A., Gruner, M. M., & Harding, G. W. (1990). Morphological correlates of aging in the chinchilla cochlea. *Hearing Research, 48,* 79–92.

Boyce, P. R. (1973). Age, illuminance, visual performance and preference. *Lighting Research and Technology, 5,* 125–144.

Brant, L. J., & Fozard, J. L. (1990). Age changes in pure-tone hearing thresholds in a longitudinal study of normal human aging. *Journal of the Acoustical Society of America, 88,* 813–820.

Burg, A. (1966). Visual acuity as measured by static and dynamic tests: A comparative evaluation. *Journal of Applied Psychology, 50,* 460–466.

Casson, E. J., Johnson, C. A., & Nelson-Quigg, J. M. (1993). Temporal modulation perimetry: The effects of aging and eccentricity on sensitivity in normals. *Investigative Ophthalmology & Visual Science, 34,* 3096–3102.

Cerella, J. (1985). Age-related decline in extra-foveal letter perception. *Journal of Gerontology, 40,* 727–736.

Clancy, S. M., & Hoyer, W. J. (1994). Age and skill in visual search. *Developmental Psychology, 30,* 545–552.

Collins, M. J., Brown, B., & Bowman, K. J. (1989). Peripheral visual acuity and age. *Ophthalmic and Physiological Optics, 9,* 314–316.

Cooper, B. A., Ward, M., Gowland, C. A., & McIntosh, J. M. (1991). The use of the Lanthony New Color Test in determining the effects of aging on color vision. *Journal of Gerontology: Psychological Sciences, 46,* 320–324.

Coppinger, N. W. (1955). The relationship between critical flicker frequency and chronological age for varying levels of stimulus brightness. *Journal of Gerontology, 10,* 48–52.

Corso, J. F. (1963). Age and sex differences in pure tone thresholds. *Archives of Otolaryngology, 77,* 385–105.

Corso, J. F. (1987). Sensory-perceptual processes and aging. *Annual Review of Gerontology and Geriatrics, 7,* 29–55.

Craig, C. H., Kim, B. W., Rhyner, P. M. P., & Chirillo, T. K. B. (1993). Effects of word predictability, child development, and aging on time-gated speech recognition performance. *Journal of Speech and Hearing Research, 36,* 832–841.

Cranford, J. L., & Stream, R. W. (1991). Discrimination of short duration tones by elderly subjects. *Journal of Gerontology, 46,* 37–41.

Crassini, B., Brown, B., & Bowman, K. (1988). Age-related changes in contrast sensitivity in central and peripheral retina. *Perception, 17,* 315–332.

Curcio, C. A., Millican, C. L., Allen, K. A., & Kalina, R. E. (1993). Aging of the human photoreceptor mosaic: Evidence for selective vulnerability of rods in central retina. *Investigative Ophthalmology & Visual Science, 34,* 3278–3296.

Dancer, J., Pryor, B., & Rozema, H. (1989). Hearing screening in a well elderly population: Implications for gerontologists. *Educational Gerontology, 15,* 41–47.

Davies, D. R., & Parasuraman, R. (1982). *The psychology of vigilance.* London: Academic Press.

Davis, A. C. (1991). Epidemiological profile of hearing impairments: The scale and nature of the problem with special reference to the elderly. *Acta Oto-Laryngologica Supplement, 476,* 23–31.

Davis, A. C., Ostri, B., & Parving, A. (1991). Longitudinal study of hearing. *Acta Oto-Laryngologica Supplement, 476,* 12–22.

Eisner, A., Fleming, S. A., Klein, M. L., & Mauldin, W. M. (1987). Sensitivities in older eyes with good acuity: Cross-sectional norms. *Investigative Ophthalmology & Visual Science, 28,* 1824–1831.

Elliott, D. B., & Whitaker, D. (1991). Changes in macular function throughout adulthood. *Documenta Ophthalmologica, 76,* 251–259.

Elliott, D. B., Whitaker, D., & MacVeigh, D. (1990). Neural contribution to spatiotemporal contrast sensitivity decline in healthy ageing eyes. *Vision Research, 30,* 541–547.

Elliott, D. B., Whitaker, D., & Thompson, P. (1989). Use of displacement threshold hyperacuity to isolate the neural component of senile vision loss. *Applied Optics, 28,* 1914–1918.

Elworth, C. L., Larry, C., & Malmström, F. V. (1986). Age, degraded viewing environments, and the speed of accommodation. *Aviation, Space and Environmental Medicine, 57,* 54–58.

Etholm, B., & Belal, A. (1974). Senile changes in the middle ear joints. *Annals of Otology, Rhinology, & Laryngology, 83,* 49–64.

Evans, D. W., & Ginsburg, A. P. (1985). Contrast sensitivity predicts age differences in highway-sign discriminability. *Human Factors, 27,* 637–642.

Falk, J. L., & Kline, D. W. (1978). Stimulus persistence in CFF: Overarousal or underactivation? *Experimental Aging Research, 4,* 109–123.

Fisk, A. D., & Rogers, W. A. (1991). Toward an understanding of age-related memory and visual search effects. *Journal of Experimental Psychology: General, 120,* 131–149.

Folk, C. L., & Hoyer, W. J. (1992). Aging and shifts of spatial attention. *Psychology and Aging, 7,* 453–465.

Gao, H., & Hollyfield, J. G. (1992). Aging of the human retina—differential loss of neurons and retinal pigment epithelial cells. *Investigative Ophthalmology & Visual Science, 33,* 1–17.

Garstecki, D. C. (1987). Self-perceived hearing difficulty in aging adults with acquired hearing loss. *Journal of the Academy of Rehabilitative Audiology, 20,* 49–60.

Gates, G. A., Cooper, J. C., Kannel, W. B., & Miller, N. J. (1990). Hearing in the elderly: The Framingham cohort, 1983–1985. *Ear and Hearing, 11,* 247–256.

Giambra, L. M., & Quilter, R. E. (1988). Sustained attention in adulthood: A unique, large-sample, longitudinal and multicohort analysis using the Mackworth Clock Test. *Psychology and Aging, 3,* 75–83.

Gittings, N. S., & Fozard, J. L. (1986). Age changes in visual acuity. *Experimental Gerontology, 21,* 423–434.

Greene, H. A., & Madden, D. J. (1987). Adult age differences in visual acuity, stereopsis, and contrast sensitivity. *American Journal of Optometry and Physiological Optics, 64,* 749–753.

Gulick, W. L., Gescheider, G. A., & Frisina, R. D. (1989). *Hearing: Physiological acoustics, neural coding, and psychoacoustics.* New York: Oxford University Press.

Hakkinen, L. (1984). Vision in the elderly and its use in the social environment. *Scandinavian Journal of Social Medicine, 35,* 5–60.

Hansen, C. C., & Reske-Nielsen, E. (1965). Pathological studies in presbycusis. *Archives of Oto-Laryngology, 82,* 115–132.

Hartley, A. A., Kieley, J. M., & Slabach, E. H. (1990). Age differences and similarities in the effects of cues and prompts. *Journal of Experimental Psychology: Human Perception and Performance, 16,* 523–537.

Hausler, R., Colburn, S., & Marr, E. (1983). Sound localization in subjects with impaired hearing. Spatial discrimination and discrimination tests. *Acta Oto-Laryngologica, Supplement, 40C,* 6–62.

Helfer, K. S. (1992). Aging and the binaural advantage in reverberation and noise. *Journal of Speech and Hearing Research, 35,* 1394–1401.

Holtzman, R. E., Familant, M. E., Deptula, P., & Hoyer, W. J. (1986). Aging and the use of sentential structure to facilitate word recognition. *Experimental Aging Research, 12,* 85–88.

Huaman, A. G., & Sharpe, J. A. (1993). Vertical saccades in senescence. *Investigative Ophthalmology & Visual Science, 34,* 2588–2595.

Jacobs-Condit, L. (Ed.). (1984). *Gerontology and communication disorders.* Rockville, MD: American Speech-Language-Hearing Association.

Johnson, C. A. (1986, February 25–26). *Peripheral visual fields and driving in an aging population. Invitational Conference on Work, Aging, and Vision.* Washington, DC: National Research Council, National Academy of Science, Committee on Vision.

Johnson, C. A., & Keltner, J. L. (1983). Incidence of visual field loss and its relationship to driving performance. *Archives of Ophthalmology (Chicago), 101,* 371–375.

Johnsson, L. G., & Hawkins, J. E., Jr. (1972). Sensory and neural degeneration with aging, as seen in microdissections of the human inner ear. *Annals of Otology, Rhinology, and Laryngology, 81,* 179–193.

Kahn, H. A., Leibowitz, H. M., Ganley, J. P., Kini, M. M., Colton, T., Nickerson, R. S., & Dauber, T. R. (1977). Original Contributions, The Framingham Eye Study, I. Outline and major prevalence findings. *American Journal of Epidemiology, 106,* 17–32.

Kane, M. J., Hasher, L. Stoltzfus, E. R., Zacks, R. T., & Connelly, S. L. (1994). Inhibitory attentional mechanisms and aging. *Psychology and Aging, 9,* 103–112.

Kashima, K., Trus, B. L., Unser, M., Edwards, P. A., & Datiles, M. B. (1993). Aging studies on normal lens using the Scheimpflug slit-lamp camera. *Investigative Ophthalmology & Visual Science, 34,* 293–269.

Kirchner, C., & Lowman, C. (1988). Sources of variation in the estimated prevalence of visual loss. In C. Kirchner (Ed.), *Data on blindness and visual impairment in the U.S.* (pp. 3–79). New York: American Foundation for the Blind.

Klein, R., Klein, B. E. K., Linton, K. L. P., & De Mets, D. L. (1991). The Beaver Dam Eye Study: Visual acuity. *Ophthalmology, 98,* 1310–1315.

Kline, D. W. (1991). Light, ageing and visual performance. In J. Marshall, & J. R. Cronly-Dillon (Eds.), *Vision and visual dysfunction: Vol. 16. The susceptible visual apparatus* (pp. 150–161). London: Macmillan.

Kline, D. W., Culham, J., Bartel, P., & Lynk, L. (1994). Aging and hyperacuity thresholds as a function of contrast and oscillation rate. *Canadian Psychology, 35*(2a), 14.

Kline, D. W., Kline, T. J. B., Fozard, J. L., Kosnik, W., Schieber, F., & Sekuler, R. (1992). Vision, aging and driving: The problems of older drivers. *Journal of Gerontology: Psychological Sciences, 47,* 27–34.

Knoblauch, K., Saunders, F., Kusuda, M., Hynes, R., Podgor, M., Higgins, K. E., & de Monasterio, F. M. (1987). Age and illuminance effects in the Farnsworth-Munsell 100-hue test. *Applied Optics, 26,* 1441–1448.

Kosnik, W., Kline, D. W., Fikre, J., & Sekuler, R. (1987). Ocular fixation control as a function of age and exposure duration. *Psychology and Aging, 2,* 302–305.

Kosnik, W. D., Sekuler, R., & Kline, D. W. (1990). Self-reported problems of older drivers. *Human Factors, 32,* 597–608.

Kosnik, W. D., Winslow, L., Kline, D. W., Rasinski, K., & Sekuler, R. (1988). Visual changes throughout adulthood. *Journal of Gerontology: Psychology of Aging, 2,* 302–305.

Kuyk, T. K., & Wesson, M. D. (1991). Aging-related foveal flicker sensitivity losses in normal observers. *Optometry and visual science, 68,* 786–789.

Lapidot, M. B. (1987). Does the brain age uniformly? Evidence from effects of smooth pursuit eye movements on verbal and visual tasks. *Journal of Gerontology, 42,* 329–331.

Lerman, S. (1984). Biophysical aspects of corneal and lenticular transparency. *Current Eye Research, 3,* 3–14.

Linner, E. (1976). Ocular hypertension: 1. The clinical course during ten years without therapy. Aqueous humor dynamics. *Acta Ophthalmologica, 54,* 707–720.

Linton, K. L. P., Klein, B. E. K., & Klein, R. (1991). The validity of self-reported and surrogate-reported cataract and age-related macular degeneration in the Beaver Dam eye study. *American Journal of Epidemiology, 143,* 1438–1446.

Long, G. M., & Crambert, R. F. (1990). The nature and basis of age-related changes in dynamic visual acuity. *Psychology and Aging, 5,* 138–143.

Lowman, C., & Kirchner, C. (1988). Sources of variation in the estimated prevalence of visual loss. In C. Kirchner (Ed.), *Data on blindness and visual impairment in the U.S.* (2nd ed., pp. 3–10). New York: American Foundation for the Blind.

Lutman, M. E. (1991). Degradations in frequency and temporal resolution with age and their impact on speech identification. *Acta Oto-Laryngologica, Supplement, 476,* 120–126.

Lutman, M. E., Gatehouse, S., & Worthington, A. G. (1991). Frequency resolution as a function of hearing threshold level and age. *Journal of the Acoustical Society of America, 89,* 320–328.

Mackworth, N. H. (1948). The breakdown of vigilance during prolonged or visual search. *Quarterly Journal of Experimental Psychology, 1,* 6–21.

Madden, D. J. (1992). Selective attention and visual search: Revision of an allocation model and application to age differences. *Journal of Experimental Psychology: Human Perception and Performance, 18,* 821–836.

Matschke, R. G. (1990). Frequency selectivity and psychoacoustic tuning curves in old age. *Acta Oto-Laryngologica, Supplement, 476,* 114–119.

Mayer, M. J., Kim, C. B. Y., Svingos, A., & Glucs, A. (1988). Foveal flicker sensitivity in healthy aging eyes: I. Compensating for pupil variation. *Journal of the Optical Society of America A, 5,* 2201–2209.

McDowd, J. M., & Craik, F. M. (1988). Effects of aging and task difficulty on divided attention performance. *Journal of Experimental Psychology: Human Perception and Performance, 14,* 267–280.

McFarland, R. A., Warren, B. & Karis, C. (1958). Alterations in critical flicker frequency as a function of age and light:dark ratio. *Journal of Experimental Psychology, 56,* 529–538.

Monk, T. H., Buysse, D. J., Reynolds, C. F., Jarrett, D. B., & Kupfer, D. J. (1992). Rhythmic and homeostatic influences on mood, activation, and performance in young and old men. *Journal of Gerontology: Psychological Sciences, 47,* 221–227.

Moore, B. C. J., Peters, R. W., & Glasberg, B. R. (1992). Detection of temporal gaps in sinusoids by elderly subjects with and without hearing loss. *Journal of the Acoustical Society of America, 92,* 1923–1932.

Morrison, J. D., & Reilly, J. (1989). The pattern visual evoked cortical response in human ageing. *Quarterly Journal of Experimental Physiology, 74,* 311–328.

Morrow, M. J., & Sharpe, J. A. (1993). Smooth pursuit initiation in young and elderly observers. *Vision Research, 33,* 203–210.

Moscicki, E. K., Elkins, E. F., Baum, H. M., & McNamara, P. M. (1985). Hearing loss in the elderly: An epidemiologic study of the Framingham Heart Study cohort. *Ear and Hearing, 6,* 184–190.

Nordlund, B. (1964). Directional audiometry. *Acta Oto-Laryngologica, 57,* 1–18.

Olson, P. L., & Sivak, M. (1984). Glare from automobile rear-vision mirrors, *Human Factors, 26,* 269–282.

Owens, D. A. (1991). Near work, accommodative tonus, and myopia. In T. Geosvenor & M. C. Flom (Eds.), *Refractive Anomalies* (pp. 318–344). Stoneham, MA: Butterworth-Heinemann.

Owsley, C., Ball, K. K., Sloane, M. E., Roenker, D. L., & Bruni, J. R. (1991). Visual/cognitive correlates of vehicle accidents in older drivers. *Psychology and Aging, 6,* 403–415.

Owsley, C., Sekuler, R., & Siemsen, D. (1983). Contrast sensitivity throughout adulthood. *Vision Research, 23,* 689–699.

Owsley, C., & Sloane, M. E. (1987). Contrast sensitivity, acuity and the perception of 'real-world' targets. *British Journal of Ophthalmology, 71,* 791–796.

Owsley, C., & Sloane, M. E. (1990). Vision and aging. In F. Boller & J. Grafman (Eds.), *Handbook of the neuropsychology* (Vol. 4, pp. 229–249). Amsterdam: Elsevier.

Owsley, C., Sloane, M. E., & Skalka, H. W., & Jackson, C. A. (1990). A comparison of the Regan Low-Contrast Letter Charts and contrast sensitivity testing in older patients. *Clinical Vision Science, 5,* 325–334.

Parasuraman, R., & Giambra, L. (1992). Skill development in vigilance: Effects of event rate and age. *Psychology and Aging, 6,* 155–169.

Parasuraman, R., Nestor, P., & Greenwood, P. (1989). Sustained-attention capacity in young and older adults. *Psychology and Aging, 4,* 339–345.

Patel, A. S. (1966). Spatial resolution by the human visual system: The effect of mean retinal illuminance. *Journal of the Optical Society of America, 56,* 689–694.

Pearson, J. D., Morell, C. H., Gordon-Salant, S., Brant, L. J., Metter, E. J., Klein, L. L., & Fozard, J. L. (1997). Gender differences in a longitudinal study of age-associated hearing loss. *Journal of the Acoustical Society of America, 97,* 1196–1205.

Pedersen, K. E., Rosenhall, U., & Moller, M. B. (1989). Changes in pure-tone thresholds in individuals aged 70–81: Results from a longitudinal study. *Audiology, 28,* 194–204.

Pitts, D. G. (1982). The effect of aging on selected visual functions: Dark adaptation, visual acuity, stereopsis, and brightness contrast. In R. Sekuler, D. W. Kline, & K. Dismukes (Eds.), *Aging and the human visual function* (pp. 131–159). New York: Alan R. Liss.

Plude, D. J., & Doussard-Roosevelt, J. A. (1989). Aging, selective attention and feature integration. *Psychology and Aging, 4,* 1–7.

Porciatti, V., Burr, D. C., Morrone, C., & Fiorentini, A. (1992). The effects of ageing on the pattern electroretinogram and visual evoked potential in humans. *Vision Research, 32,* 1199–1209.

Rastatter, M., Watson, M., & Strauss-Simmons, D. (1989). Effects of time-compression on feature and frequency discrimination in aged listeners. *Perceptual and Motor Skills, 678,* 367–372.

Raz, N., Millman, D., & Moberg, P. J. (1990). Mechanism of age-related differences in frequency discrimination with backward masking: Speed of processing or stimulus persistence? *Psychology and Aging, 5,* 475–481.

Robin, D. A., & Royer, F. L. (1989). Age-related changes in auditory temporal processing. *Psychology and Aging, 4,* 144–149.

Rogers, W. A. (1992). Age differences in visual search: target and distractor learning. *Psychology and Aging, 7,* 526–535.

Rosler, G. (1994). Progression of hearing loss caused by occupational noise. *Scandinavian Audiology, 23,* 13–37.

Rubin, G. S., Roche, K. B., Prasada-Rao, P., & Fried, L. P. (1994). Visual impairment and disability in older adults. *Optometry and Visual Science, 71,* 750–760.

Rumsey, K. E. (1993). Redefining the optometric examination: Addressing the vision needs of older adults. *Optometry and Visual Science, 70,* 587–691.

Schein, O. D., West, S., Muñoz, B., Vitale, S., Maguire, M., Taylor, H., & Bressler, N. M. (1994). Cortical lenticular opacification: Distribution and location in a longitudinal study. *Investigative Ophthalmology & Visual Science, 35,* 363–366.

Schieber, F. (1992). Aging and the senses. In J. E. Birren, R. B. Sloane, & G. D. Cohen (Eds.), *Handbook of mental health and aging* (2nd ed., pp. 251–306). San Diego, CA: Academic Press.

Schieber, F. (1994). Age and glare recovery time for low-contrast stimuli. *Proceedings of the Human Factors and Ergonomics Society, 1,* 133–136.

Schieber, F., & Kline, D. W. (1994). Age differences in the legibility of symbol highway signs as a function of luminance and glare level: A preliminary report. *Proceedings of the Human Factors and Ergonomics Society, 1,* 133–136.

Schieber, F., Kline, D. W., Kline, T. J. B., & Fozard, J. L. (1992). The relationship between contrast sensitivity and the visual problems of older drivers. *SAE Technical Paper Series, 920613.*

Schiff, W., Oldak, R., & Shah, V. (1992). Aging persons' estimates of vehicular motion. *Psychology and Aging, 7,* 518–525.

Schneider, W., & Shiffrin, R. M. (1977). Controlled and automatic human information processing: I. Detection Search and attention. *Psychological Review, 84,* 1–66.

Schow, R. L., & Goldblum, D. E. (1980). Collapsed ear canals in the elderly nursing home population. *Journal of Speech and Hearing Disease, 45,* 259–267.

Scialfa, C. T., Adams, E. M., & Giovanetto, M. (1991). Reliability of the Vistech Contrast Test System in a life-span adult sample. *Optometry and Vision Science, 66,* 270–274.

Scialfa, C. T., & Esau, S. (1993). *Age differences in feature and conjunction search as a function of display size and target-distractor similarity.* Annual meeting of the Gerontological Society of America, New Orleans, LA.

Scialfa, C. T., Garvey, P. M., Tyrrell, R. A., Goebel, C. C., Deering, L., & Leibowitz, H. W. (1988). Relationships among measures of static and dynamic visual sensitivity. *Human Factors, 30,* 677–687.

Scialfa, C. T., Garvey, P. M., Tyrrell, R. A., & Leibowitz, H. W. (1992). Age differences in dynamic contrast thresholds. *Journal of Gerontology: Psychological Sciences, 47,* 172–175.

Scialfa, C. T., Guzy, L. T., Leibowitz, H. W., Garvey, P. M., & Tyrrell, R. A. (1991). Age differences in judgements of vehicle velocity and distance. *Psychology and Aging, 6,* 60–66.

Scialfa, C. T., Kline, D. W., & Lyman, B. J. (1987). Age differences in target identification as a function of retinal location and noise level: An examination of the useful field of view. *Psychology and Aging, 2,* 14–19.

Scialfa, C. T., Thomas, D. M., & Joffe, K. M. (1994). Age-related changes in the eye movements subserving feature search. *Optometry and Vision Science, 71,* 1–7.

Sekuler, R., & Ball, K. (1986). Visual localization: Age and practice. *Journal of the Optical Society of America A, 3,* 864–867.

Sharpe, J. A., & Zakon, D. H. (1987). Senescent saccades. *Acta Oto-Laryngologica, 104,* 422–428.

Shone, G., Altschuler, R. A., Miller, J. M., & Nuttall, A. L. (1991). The effect of noise exposure on the aging ear. *Hearing Research, 56,* 173–178.

Slawinski, E. B., Hartel, D. M., & Kline, D. W. (1993). Self-reported hearing problems in daily life throughout adulthood. *Psychology and Aging, 8,* 552–561.

Slawinski, E., & Kline, D. W. (1989). *Your hearing: A survey by the audition/speech and vision/aging laboratories of the University of Calgary.* Calgary, Canada: University of Calgary, Department of Psychology.

Sloane, M. E., Owsley, C., & Alvarez, S. L. (1988). Aging, senile miosis and spatial contrast sensitivity at low luminance. *Vision Research, 28,* 1235–1246.

Spear, P. D. (1993). Neural bases of visual deficits during aging. *Vision Research, 33,* 2589–2609.

Steen, R., Whitaker, D., Elliott, D. B., & Wild, J. M. (1994). Age-related effects of glare on luminance and color contrast sensitivity. *Optometry and Visual Science, 71,* 792–796.

Sturr, J. F., Hannon, D. J., Zhang, L., & Vaidya, C. (1992). Psychophysical evidence for neural losses in the rod systems of older observers in good ocular health. *Investigative Ophthalmology & Visual Science, 33,* 1414.

Sturr, J. F., Kline, G. E., & Taub, H. A. (1990). Performance of young and older drivers on a static acuity test under photopic and mesopic luminance conditions. *Human Factors, 32,* 1–8.

Sun, F., Stark, L., Nguyen, A., Wong, J., Lakshminarayanan, S., & Mueller, E. (1988). Changes in accommodation with age: static and dynamic. *American Journal of Opthalmology and Physiological Optics, 65,* 492–498.

Trick, G. L., & Silverman, S. E. (1991). Visual sensitivity to motion: Age-related changes and deficits in senile dementia of the Alzheimer type. *Neurology, 41,* 1437–1440.

Tulunay-Keesey, U., Ver Hoeve, J. N., & Terkla-McGrane, C. (1988). Threshold and suprathreshold spatiotemporal response throughout adulthood. *Journal of the Optical Society of America A, 5,* 2191–2200.

Tun, P. A., & Wingfield, A. (1993). Is speech special? Perception and recall of spoken language in complex environments. In J. Cerella, J. Rybash, W. Hover & M. L. Commons, *Adult information processing: Limits on loss* (pp. 425–457). San Diego, CA: Academic Press.

Turano, K., Rubin, G. S., Herdman, S. J., Chee, E. & Fried, L. P. (1994). Visual stabilization of posture in the elderly: Fallers vs. nonfallers. *Optometry and Vision Science, 71,* 761–769.

Tyler, C. W. (1989). Two processes control variations in flicker sensitivity over the life span. *Journal of the Optical Society of America A, 6,* 481–490.

van den Berg, T. J. T. P. (1995). Analysis of intraocular straylight, especially in relation to age. *Optometry and Visual Science, 72,* 52–59.

van Rooij, J. C. G. M., & Plomp, R. (1992). Auditive and cognitive factors in speech perception by elderly listeners. III: Additional data and final discussion. *Journal of the Acoustical Society of America, 91,* 1028–1033.

Vaughan, P. W., & Vincent, J. M. (1979). Ultra structure of neurons in the auditory cortex of aging rats: Morphometric study. *Journal of Neurocytology, 8,* 215–228.

Ventry, I. M., & Weinstein, B. E. (1982). The Hearing Handicap Inventory for the Elderly: A new tool. *Ear and Hearing, 3,* 128–134.

Vos, J. J. (1995). Age dependence of glare effects and their significance in terms of visual ergonomics. In W. Adrian (Ed.), *Proceedings of the Third International Symposium, Lighting for Aging Vision and Health* (pp. 11–25). New York: Lighting Research Institute.

Wade, M. G., Lindquist, R., Taylor, J. R., & Treat-Jacobson, D. (1995). Optical flow, spatial orientation, and the control of posture in the elderly. *Journal of Gerontology: Psychological Sciences, 50B,* P51–P58.

Wang, Q., Klein, B. E. K., Klein, R., & Moss, S. E. (1994). Refractive status in the Beaver Dam eye study. *Investigative Ophthalmology & Visual Science, 35,* 4344–4347.

Warren, W. H., Blackwell, A. W., & Morris, M. W. (1989). Age differences in perceiving the direction of self-motion from optical flow. *Journal of Gerontology: Psychological Sciences, 44,* 147–153.

Weale, R. A. (1961). Retinal illumination and age. *Transactions of the Illuminating Engineering Society, 26,* 95–100.

Weale, R. A. (1982). Senile ocular changes, cell death, and vision. In R. Sekuler, D. W. Kline, & K. Dismukes (Eds.) *Aging and human visual function* (pp. 161–171). New York: Alan R. Liss.

Weekers, R., & Roussel, F. (1946). Introduction à l'étude de la fréquencée de fusion en clinique. *Ophthalmologica, 112,* 305–319.

Weinstein, B. E. (1994). Age-related hearing loss: How to screen for it, and when to intervene. *Geriatrics, 49,* 40–47.

Weinstein, B. E., & Ventry, I. M. (1983). Audiometric correlates of the hearing handicap inventory for the elderly. *Journal of Speech and Hearing Disorders, 48,* 379–384.

Werner, J. S., & Steele, V. G. (1988). Sensitivity of human foveal color mechanisms throughout the life span. *Journal of the Optical Society of America A, 5,* 2122–2130.

Wickens, C. D., Braune, R., & Stokes, A. (1987). Age differences in the speed and capacity of information processing: 1. A dual-task approach. *Psychology and Aging, 2,* 70–78.

Willott, J. (1991). *Aging and the auditory system.* San Diego, CA: Singular Publishing Group.

Winn, B., Whitaker, D., Elliott, D. B., & Phillips, N. J. (1994). Factors affecting light-adapted pupil size in normal human subjects. *Investigative Ophthalmology & Visual Science, 35,* 1132–1137.

Wojciechowski, R., Trick, G. L., & Steinman, S. B. (1995). Topography of the age-related decline in motion sensitivity. *Optometry and Vision Science, 72,* 67–74.

Wright, C. E., & Wormald, R. P. (1992). Stereopsis and ageing. *Eye, 6,* 473–476.

Yang, K. C. H., Elliott, D. B., & Whitaker, D. (1993). Does logMAR VA change linearly with age? *Investigative Ophthalmology & Visual Science, 34,* 1422.

Yekta, A. A., Pickwell, L. D., & Jenkins, T. C. A. (1989). Binocular vision, age and symptoms. *Ophthalmic and Physiological Optics, 9,* 115–120.

Zakon, D. H., & Sharpe, J. A. (1987). Smooth pursuit in senescence. Effects of target acceleration and velocity. *Acta Oto-Laryngologica, 104,* 290–297.

Chapter 4

Movement Control and Speed of Behavior

Max Vercruyssen

INTRODUCTION

As one gets older the neuromuscular system changes in ways that influence cognitive and motor behavior as well as general well-being. Most noticeable is an increasing delay in reacting to environmental stimuli and making voluntary movements. Such slowing of most behaviors in later life is inevitable. Usually, rapid movements are more slowly initiated, controlled, and concluded. The ability to maintain continuous movements or to execute complex behaviors also declines and coordination is disrupted. Control of posture and balance degrades, putting older adults at greater risk of falling and other movement control errors. Eventually, for a large portion of older adults, many complex motor skills, such as driving, and even simple daily tasks, such as dressing, eating, toileting, and bathing, are no longer possible without assistance. Loss of neuromuscular control may impair personal and interpersonal functions to the point of threatening one's self-image, self-esteem, quality of life, and the ability to manage daily activities independently. Often older individuals judge the quality of their life by their ability to independently and effectively conduct daily tasks, social activities, and

Handbook of Human Factors and the Older Adult

recreational pursuits with vigor. Age-related declines in functioning diminish such abilities and often lead to such negative outcomes as physical deterioration and disease, poor mental health (e.g., depression), an increased risk of accidents and injury, social isolation, and dependence on others (e.g., Cummings & Nevitt, 1989; Rowe & Kahn, 1987). Hence, it is understandable why so many older adults fear the consequences of an aging motor system, particularly the loss of movement control, motor skills, and the ability to live unassisted (see Spirduso, 1995b).

The purpose of this chapter is to (1) briefly describe some of the changes with age in movement control, specifically speed of behavior as measured by laboratory and daily tasks; and (2) identify attempts at diminishing the negative aspects of expected changes, emphasizing the benefits of practice, a physically and mentally active lifestyle, and effective human factors design. Age-related changes in motor behavior may be expressed at least in terms of capacity characteristics and their changes within the organism, demand characteristics of tasks to be performed within a specified environment, and how science (and technology) might influence the interaction of the organism and environment. Space constraints limit the scope and preclude mention of theoretical development.

CAPACITIES AND SKILLS OF THE PERFORMER

Generally, human behavior is manifest in the observable responses made to environmental stimuli, and they are greatly influenced by previous experience and skills acquired during earlier encounters with similar stimuli. Underlying physiological and psychological processes and mechanisms combine to produce the movements and actions taken, including sensation, attention, perception, cognition, memory, motor preparation, and response execution. Laboratory tasks may be constructed to load individual processes such that performance levels obtained serve as an index of capacity for that process. The research literature is filled with debates over age differences in performance on such tasks and capacity limits. However, compensatory mechanisms within the individual can offset declines with age in many of these processes, resulting in performance on real-world tasks being nominally affected. Therefore, it becomes especially important to view research findings in terms of their contribution to understanding the way in which capacities contribute to skilled performance and how they interact with the demands of different tasks to reveal in predictable ways what exactly limits performance. This point becomes particularly pertinent if performance on some tasks serves as criteria for determining whether an individual can live independently.

Trait and State Differences (Variability)

Traits

Humans are characterized in a variety of ways, but most relevant here is the distinction between interindividual traits that are relatively permanent and intraindividual states that are frequently changing. Individual differences in trait characteristics include cohort age, sex, ethnicity, education, culture, physical and mental fitness, health status, and personality. Some individuals perform many tasks at outstanding levels because of inherent traits. Numerous issues surround each trait with respect to its contributions to research outcomes, but this chapter will only address one—age. The interaction of age with life experiences increases inter- and intraindividual variability in many capacities and performance measures across the life span (e.g., Sprott, 1988; Welford, 1958). Within group (inter-individual/cohort) variability increases with age such that, while average performance of the elderly, at say 80 years of age, may be very different from the average of young adults, at say 20 years of age, some older individuals will show performances at least equal to that of younger adults. Within group variability in motor performance ranges from an 80-year-old frail adult living in a care facility, who experiences extreme difficulty walking, bathing, and dressing, to an 80-year-old active adult living independently, who occasionally runs a marathon race and competes in masters' track meets. Thus, descriptions of "average" behavior for specific age groups (cohorts) becomes less and less accurate as cohort age increases (Spirduso & MacRae, 1990).

States

An individual's performance also changes as a function of day-to-day, even moment-to-moment, variations in physical, psychological, and emotional states. For instance, medications are likely to interact with symptoms of the disorders for which they were prescribed in complex ways, causing dose–response effects on many behaviors. Irregular and wrong dosages during self-administration plus problems of taking other medications that in combination may have serious contraindications (polypharmacy), cause only further intraindividual variations and confound the age index. Motivation and attitude varies as a state characteristic (e.g., Welford, 1958/1973, 1976). Finally, skill and experience (e.g., Salthouse, 1990; Welford, 1958/1973, 1985b, 1993) may regulate an individual's reaction to stress, resources needed to perform, and the very way in which tasks are approached.

Variability

The study of aging and the aged has been hampered by difficulties in differentiating the effects of aging from disuse (declining physical activity), disease, decreased motivation, and reduced societal expectations. Of the over 31 million Americans over age 65, 86% have one or more chronic disease conditions, many of which influence central nervous system (CNS) function and motor performance; 34% are restricted in their activities by long-term physical conditions or health problems; and among those in this group not institutionalized, 74% experience limitations in their home activities because of these conditions (Fernie, 1994). Of those over 65, 70% have limitations in general mobility from mild arthritis to paralysis from stroke (Fernie, 1994; Hobson, 1994). Three million need assistance performing basic daily activities, four million have difficulty traveling outside the home, two million have mobility problems inside the home, nine million have hearing loss, and nine million have sharply impaired vision (Bowe, 1988). The number of factors influencing performance increases with age, producing disproportionate variability in most performance measures between and within older compared with young adults.

Trait and state differences in performance among individuals of a given age may be larger than performance differences between young and old performers, thereby confounding interpretation of the results of empirical studies. Although untrue, for convenience, it is assumed such factors are controlled. The list seems endless of factors that intervene with aging to make comparisons within and between individuals of the same and different ages difficult to interpret. Chronological age is a very ambiguous, confusing, and potentially misleading descriptor, possibly only reinforcing the need for understanding the covariates with age before embarking on summarizing age-related changes in any behavioral measure (see Birren & Fisher, 1995, p. 347, where they call chronological age a "fickle mistress").

Changes in the Neuromuscular System with Age

Muscle Strength, Endurance, and Tone

Loss of muscular strength, endurance, and tone, especially in the lower extremities, are the most obvious age-related motor limitations (e.g., Khalil, Abdel-Moty, Diaz, Steele-Rosomoff, & Rosomoff, 1994; Mortimer, Pirozzolo, & Maletta, 1982; Spirduso & MacRae, 1990). Muscles become less elastic and more tense, have difficulty relaxing, and are more prone to cramping. Flexibility in connective tissues and joints decreases. Bones weaken, become more porous, less dense, less capable of supporting the body, and easily broken. Maximum force exerted, in a single and across multiple repetitions, by a wide range of muscle groups declines from 15 to 50% from the 20s to the 60s, mostly due to the loss of motor units, especially after age 60, changes in metabolism of the motor units that remain, and higher thresholds for neural excitation of muscles. By age 60, maximum speed of movement may decline by as much as 90% and often continues to slow at an increasing rate as one gets older. Especially after age 50, the amount of maximal muscular work performed over an extended period declines; however, submaximal work does not change substantially with increasing age. Stiffness in joints and pain from arthritis may also influence performance. (See Spirduso, 1995, for age-related changes in basic mechanisms of motor control.)

Changes in the Nervous System

Accompanying aging of the motor system are (1) morphological degradation of neural tissues in motor centers like the cerebellum; (2) decreased number of Type II (fast twitch) muscle fibers and their associated motor neurons, causing reduced peak muscular strength and speed of muscular contractions; (3) decline in dopaminergic function in the basal ganglia; (4) decline in sensory function, such as decreased visual acuity and stereopsis, which limits the performance of more complex tasks; (5) disturbances in temporal organization of motor synergies and postural reflexes; (6) decrease in the maximum rate of sequential repetitive movements; and (7) impaired performance on tasks requiring complex programming and transformations (see Hamerman, 1990; Mortimer et al., 1982; Spirduso & MacRae, 1990).

Slowing of Behavior

Probably the most pronounced and ubiquitous age-related declines in physical and mental functioning are those observed in movement control, especially the slowing of most behaviors. While there are marked declines in peripheral (sensory and motor) mechanisms and processes, such input–output deficits account for relatively little of the overall slowing of performance with age (Welford, 1977a, 1977b). There is consensus among researchers that the effects of aging are greater on cognitive components of performance than on perceptual–motor components, and age differences in response speed are mediated predominantly by central rather than peripheral factors (Salthouse, 1985). Clearly, the locus of diminished reactive capacity and movement control with age lies in the central nervous system and these differences increase with the degree to which higher order neurocognitive functions are invoked.

Among the many explanations for the slowing of decisions and movements in older adults two general types of overlapping categories emerge: the neurobiological ("hardware") and psychological ("software") perspectives (Vercruyssen, 1994). One example from each category will be briefly mentioned with supporting references.

Neurobiological ("Hardware") Perspective

This category includes such explanations as slowing is (1) throughout the nervous system but greater in the central than peripheral portions (e.g., Birren & Fisher, 1995); (2) due to interference from distracting neural noise, like background sounds from neuronal irregularities and task-unrelated subvocal thoughts (e.g., Welford, 1977a, 1981, 1982, 1984); (3) correlated with speed of the internal clock and alpha waves (e.g., Surwillo, 1968); (4) generalized across nearly all neuropsychological processes (e.g., Birren & Fisher, 1995); (5) due to structural and system decomposition from cell loss and disease (e.g., Salthouse, 1985); (6) due to genetic and other factors; and (7) due to disuse.

Deciding within which category a particular explanation falls is somewhat arbitrary since some explanations merit membership in several categories. An example is the *neural noise hypothesis*. Neural impulses in the central nervous system occur in an environment of random neural noise such that the effectiveness of a neural signal depends on the ratio between strength of the signal and background noise. With age, the signal level decreases and the noise level increases. Older individuals can compensate for the lower signal-to-noise ratio given extra time to complete the task, but if the task requires a series of rapid decisions or movements the elderly will encounter difficulties. Thus, age-related slowing and several other cognitive and motor tendencies may be attributed somewhat to a reduction of signal-to-noise ratios in the sense organs and brain. Some slowing occurs because signal strengths have to accumulate over longer times to reach levels sufficient to initiate action while some errors may be caused by the relative increase in random brain activity (noise). Further, signal-to-noise problems may be in the early (sensory, perceptual), middle (cognitive), or later (motor) stages of processing or any combination. For instance, because of their having more difficulty in distinguishing signals from noise in sensory and perceptual incoming information, older adults can be expected to be slower on tasks that require feedback for appropriate deceleration (homing in) during final approach to a target due to increased errors from imprecise monitoring and adjustment of impulse components of the movement. Presumably there is competition as well between signals and noise in decision making, response selection, and other such cognitive activities. Assuming that motor noise increases with the amplitude of force generated, and that this effect is exaggerated in the elderly, slower movements are a means of compensation to reduce noise and thereby maintain accuracy (see Seidler & Stelmach, 1996; see also Welford, 1977a, 1981, 1984, for discussion of signal-to-noise ratios). Whether neurobiological or psychological in origin, neural noise is likely to account for some of the behavioral slowing characteristic of older adults.

Psychological ("Software") Perspective

This category includes such explanations as slowing is due to (1) information overload and task complexity (e.g., Cerella, 1990; Salthouse, 1985); (2) memory changes (e.g., Salthouse, 1985; Welford, 1984a, 1984b); (3) the elderly preferring accuracy to speed (e.g., Salthouse, 1985; Salthouse & Somberg, 1982c); (4) older adults' rigidity and lack of flexibility in using alternative strategies; (5) reduced arousal/activation and inability to maintain preparedness (e.g., Birren, Vercruyssen, & Fisher, 1990); (6) society and individual expectations—older adults are expected to slow with age; (7) declining attentional capacities (e.g., McDowd & Birren, 1990; McDowd, Vercruyssen, & Birren, 1991); and (8) depression or reduced motivation.

An example of this perspective is *cautiousness (speed–accuracy tradeoff)*. Part, but not all, of the observed age-related behavioral slowing is due to the tendency for older people to employ more cautious response strategies that make them more accurate than younger cohorts. Despite instructions to the contrary, older adults tend to favor accuracy over speed. Older performers require additional time for verification of accuracy, presumably because they lack confidence but maintain well the skills learned early in life. Across a series of choice reactions, people respond faster and faster until they make an error, whereupon they slow for a while and then again respond ever faster until they make another error, and so on. Errors thereby provide feedback information about whether performance is at the right balance of speed and accuracy. Older people slow more than do the young following an error, suggesting that they are less sensitive to error feedback and therefore make more powerful, and sometimes inappropriate, compensatory adjustments to errors. Consequently, older adults often make fewer errors overall and their reaction times are longer and more variable than the young. Thus, age-related deficits in attentional capacity, specifically the ability to monitor speed and accuracy to perform according to a specified response criteria, may be responsible for some response slowing with increasing age. Unfortunately, age differences in response speed persist even when subjects of different ages are compared at exactly the same level of accuracy thereby suggesting that differences in speed–accuracy strategy cannot explain all of the age-related slowing (Salthouse & Somberg, 1982c).

The nature and extent of the limits imposed on task performance by age-related declines in fundamental processes depend on task demands in relation to capacities available. Achievement is independent of potential capacity until it declines to a point at which it becomes limiting. Beyond this point, achievement is functionally dependent on the capacity considered. For many reasons, measuring physical deficiencies and declines will not predict achievement on complex tasks; that is, the degree of deterioration will be a poor indicator of inefficiency or impaired performance. Physical deficiencies associated with age are associated with a decrease in the range of activities for a single individual as well as an increased variation between individuals.

DEMANDS OF THE TASK

Older adults do not show performance declines in all types of tasks. They change little in their ability to perform single, discrete actions that are planned in advance of the stimulus (e.g., Welford, 1977b) and even some repetitive and reciprocal movements (e.g., Welford, Norris, & Shock, 1969), but age may limit actions requiring a series of different movements (e.g., Welford, 1977c) and produce large age differences when the task is complex, unfamiliar, and uninteresting. Correlations of the speed in performing everyday tasks and age of the performer range from 0.23 for clerical perceptual speed to 0.64 for dialing a telephone and zipping a garment (see the review by Salthouse, 1985). A clear dissociation exists between traditional laboratory tasks and real-world activities (e.g., typing; Salthouse, 1984, 1988; Wickens, Braune, & Stokes, 1987) often due to the presence of age-related declines in neuropsychological processes and mechanisms that are offset by compensatory mechanisms (skill and strategies), making age and age-related declines in measured capacities only indirectly related to performance on real-world tasks. Also, correlations between measures of speed across different tasks increase with age and factor analyses indicate that the performance of older adults is characterized by a general speed factor, whereas that of younger adults is not (e.g., Birren, Riegel, & Morrison, 1962). Performance of laboratory tasks assessing psychomotor skill by the elderly compared with that of the young is usually slower, less accurate (unless they are extremely cautious, in which case responses will be much slower yet), and more variable, especially for complex and difficult tasks, with the rate and style of learning the same regardless of age (e.g., Salthouse & Somberg, 1982b; Welford, 1977b, 1985a). While changes in performance with age are predictable for simple laboratory tasks and sometimes for complex everyday tasks, the ability of laboratory tasks to predict real-world performance is limited.

Rapid Discrete and Repetitive Movements

Rapid movements are executed quickly (ballistically) with no feedback of results until the movement is complete and can be done in a single burst (discrete) or a repeating series (repetitive). Such actions can be further divided into reaction and movement capacities.

The time required to respond (react and move) to a stimulus, called *response time,* is subdivided into *reaction time* (the time required to recognize and interpret the stimulus, select and program a response, and initiate execution of the response) and *movement time* (the time required to initiate, control, and end the response). Declines in reactive and movement capacity are among the most ubiquitous and reliable markers of the aging process (e.g., Birren & Fisher, 1995; Salthouse, 1985; Vercruyssen, 1994). In fact, slow performance of manual tasks better predicts loss of functional autonomy in daily living skills than abnormalities on medical examinations, number of chronic diseases, and social network strength (Williams, Gaylord, & McGahie, 1990).

Older adults plan, execute, and revise discrete and continuous movements in the same way as the young, except slower, often trading off speed for accuracy of execution. However, the elderly may have difficulties with sensory discrimination, perceptual encoding, response selection, movement preparation, and movement execution, resulting in slowing of reaction and movement time. Movements of older adults have different acceleration and deceleration patterns than younger adults and are more dependent on feedback control. Also, their inability to precisely control and modulate force limits many activities (Seidler & Stelmach, 1996).

Reactive Capacity (Reaction Time)

The rise and fall of information processing rates and movement speed over the life span (e.g., Cerella & Hale, 1994; Fozard, Vercruyssen, Reynolds, Hancock, & Quilter, 1994; Kail & Salthouse, 1994) is viewed as a fundamental characteristic of the cognitive and motor systems that is limited by a general mechanism and is clinically useful because of its diagnostic and functional sensitivity to cognitive decline (e.g., Birren, Woods, & Williams, 1980; Borkan & Norris, 1980; Goggin & Stelmach, 1990; Mahurin & Pirozzolo, 1986). Slowing of reaction time (RT) with age in adulthood has been associated with age-related declines in such common movement skills as restoration of posture following an unexpected perturbation of balance (Stelmach & Worringham, 1985) to complex activities such as driving automobiles (e.g., Barrett, Mihal, Panek, Sterns, & Alexander, 1977; Stelmach & Nahom, 1992; see also the driving chapter in this book by Barr and

Morrow). The following are some factors that influence slowing of behaviors with age.

Task Complexity Simple RT, which involves programming only a single movement in response to a single stimulus, can be maintained well through most of life, especially if novelty, practice, stimulus features, and performance expectations are controlled (e.g., Gottsdanker, 1982). However, for complex (choice) RT, which involves presentation of two or more stimuli to which two or more response possibilities exist, age differences are robust through adult life except when compensatory mechanisms intervene (Salthouse, 1985). The more complex, difficult, or complicated the stimulus and response, the longer it takes one to react (e.g., Henry & Rogers, 1960) and the greater will be the age differences (e.g., Cerella, Poon, & Williams, 1980; Spirduso, 1995).

For a wide range of tasks, levels of task difficulty, and response durations, decision times for the old can be computed by simply multiplying the decision times required for the young by a constant. Brinley (1965) showed that response speed for older adults is a simple linear function of speed in the young. Across a wide variety of tasks, RT of older individuals increases by a constant of 1.4 to 2.0 depending on complexity of the task (e.g., Cerella et al., 1980; Salthouse, 1985). Despite the diversity of tasks employed, the proportion of variance accounted for by the equation describing the linear relationship between RTs of old and young subjects is usually greater than 0.9, which some feel supports the theories of generalized slowing. However, the use of Brinley analyses of reaction time studies is controversial (see Bashore, 1994). Many have argued that behavioral slowing with age is general and task independent, which may be expressed through Brinley plots (e.g., Cerella, 1991, 1994; Cerella & Hale, 1994; Kail & Salthouse, 1994; Myerson, Hale, Wagstaff, Poon, & Smith, 1990; Myerson, Wagstaff, & Hale, 1994), while others argue that slowing is likely to be task specific, involving multiple slowing factors that, coincidentally, may be monotonically represented in Brinley plots (e.g., Fisk & Fisher, 1994; Fisk, Fisher, & Rogers, 1992; Perfect, 1994). It is very appealing to represent changes in performance with age by a simple function based on the performance of young participants. While the theoretical significance of this simplification may be challenged, Brinley plots may have great value for designers, who can use them to predict not only average decision times but also the *range* of decision times within individuals, across groups of individuals, and over a many different tasks. Interested readers should consult current literature to monitor this heated debate.

Stimulus Choice Reaction time increases with increases in the absolute and potential number of stimulus choices (or response alternatives) according to the equation RT = $a + b$ log$N$ (Hick, 1952), where N is the number of choices and a and b are constants (see also Crossman, 1953; Luce, 1986; Welford, 1980a). Older adults compared to young cohorts have a higher y-axis intercept (a) with proportional increases in RT (i.e., near equal slopes or b values) as a function of the number of choices or disproportionate increases in RT (i.e., a steeper slope), depending on exposure time of the stimulus (Welford, 1984a). Proportional increases in RT suggest the old process information in the same way as the young just slower; disproportionate increases point to the elderly having difficulties with response selection.

Stimulus Predictability (Uncertainty) Choice RT (CRT) is slower than simple RT (SRT) partly because of the added element of uncertainty. Age differences present with increasing movement complexity in uncertain situations may disappear when conditions are predictable (e.g., Plude, Hoyer, & Lazar, 1982). Reducing the degree of uncertainty by precuing a highly probably stimulus and response improves RT by making CRTs more like SRTs (i.e., by removing the choice component), but older adults do not necessarily take advantage of the precue to the same extent in preprogramming the response.

Stimulus Timing and Attention Everyone is limited by his or her ability to process multiple signals and responses simultaneously or in rapid succession, but the elderly are especially restricted in multiple-task performance (see McDowd & Birren, 1990; McDowd et al., 1991) and critical event timing. Once the process of connecting a perceived input signal to its corresponding output response has begun, decisions regarding any further signal and response must wait until after response to the previous signal has begun. Especially for the elderly, responses to new signals are often delayed (e.g., Welford, 1980a). The elderly also have difficulty ignoring irrelevant information (e.g., Rabbitt, 1965, card sorting) and may be easily distracted (Cunningham & Brookbank, 1988). Once action begins, there may be additional delay in responding due to response monitoring, and subsequent signals arising during the monitoring period must wait until monitoring has concluded before another response can begin. Monitoring frequency and duration increases with age causing an increased risk of accident due to preoccupation of attention. Performance on machine-paced tasks, those with signals requiring action delivered at a fixed rate and not under control of the operator, declines from age 50 onward, especially if the signals are presented at high rates (Welford, 1977a, 1977b).

With age also comes an increased difficulty in maintaining attention (and performance) over long periods of time. Characteristic of serial, self-paced choice reaction time performance studies, in which subjects respond to consecutive trials without rest for 10–30 minutes or longer, is the increased frequency of exceptionally slow responses, longer than usual latencies (LULs, also called *blocks, lags,* and *gaps*). These are isolated instances of very slow information processing but may also be a time during which the individual has temporarily stopped taking in any new information, thereby producing a gap in serial performance, while recovering from demands of the task. Older adults have longer and more frequent LULs, which first occur earlier in the course of the task, compared with young adults. Tasks requiring rapid and continuous scanning or serial sequencing of events are exceptionally fatiguing for older individuals, as reflected by slower performance, increased moment to moment variability, and the presence of LULs.

Stimulus–Response Relationship Stimulus–response (S–R) compatibility refers to the mapping or natural (logical) relationship between the stimulus and the response (e.g., Kornblum, Hasbroucq, & Osman, 1990). For instance, a task requiring a left index finger key depression to a light immediately in front of that finger characterizes high S–R compatibility. Incompatible would be a response with the right index finger each time the light in front of the left index finger illuminates. Everyone is slower in performing tasks with incompatible S–R mappings because of the extra time required for spatial–motor translations. Age differences increase with the degree of S–R incompatibility.

Response–response (R–R) compatibility refers to the ease with which two responses can be executed simultaneously or as two alternatives in a two-choice task (e.g., Kornblum, 1965). For instance, RT is faster when using the index finger for each hand simultaneously than one index finger and any other finger simultaneously. Age differences increase disproportionately with the degree of R–R incompatibility.

Response Modality Age differences in RT may disappear if vocal responses are used instead of manual ones (e.g., Nebes, 1978; Salthouse & Somberg, 1982a, 1982b; Thomas, Waugh, & Fozard, 1978); for example, older subjects who say "left" to a left stimulus rather than pressing a microswitch under the index finger of the left hand should have simple and choice RTs similar to young subjects. Similar RTs for young and old may be due to the short duration of responses—RTs from 150 to, say, 400 ms, especially following extensive practice and careful subject selection, regardless of task characteristics (e.g., manual or vocal); (e.g., Gottsdanker, 1982). Vocal responses are possibly the most highly practiced of all motor responses. Also, using foot tapping (familiar) and hand tapping (unfamiliar) tasks, conventional age effects appeared for hand tapping but not for foot tapping (e.g., Stones & Kozma, 1989).

Movement Capacity (Movement Time)

Whenever movement speed is measured independent of reaction time, like in single rapid limb movements to a target, repetitive tapping, even back and forth (reciprocal) tapping limb movements between targets of varied distance and width, advancing age is associated with predictable slowing (e.g., Vercruyssen, Brogmus, Welford, & Fozard, in review; Welford et al., 1969). Age reduces movement speed and increases variance in the timing of discrete movements and the maintenance of repetitive or reciprocal movements. Compared to young cohorts, the elderly (1) take longer to initiate movements, (2) require more time in the mid-flight phase of movements, (3) are less able to efficiently terminate movements, and (4) are less able to calibrate appropriate levels of force (e.g., Haaland, Harrington, & Grice, 1993; Seidler & Stelmach, 1996; Welford, 1980b). However, reduced movement capacities can be somewhat mitigated with practice (e.g., Pratt, Chasteen, & Abrams, 1994).

Rapid Aiming Movements While still controversial, kinematic analyses of rapid aiming movements (usually elbow flexion and extension) in some studies has shown changes with age in two components of the velocity trajectory: the initiation and acceleration phase, from movement initiation to peak velocity of the movement, and the deceleration and termination phase, from peak velocity to the end of the movement. While young adults show symmetrical, bell-shaped velocity curves for the two components, in some studies older adults spent a greater proportion of time in the deceleration phase with this age difference increasing as a function of accuracy requirements of the movement. The acceleration phase is presumed to be executed ballistically, without feedback (in an open loop), to launch the limb in the direction of the target while the deceleration phase involves error detection and correction by way of monitoring sensory and motor information in a closed loop to determine the remaining distance to the target and make motor adjustment to "home in" on it (e.g., Schmidt, 1988). Thus, discrete movements consist of a sequence of force impulses that move the limb toward a target. Variability in amplitude and duration of these pulses result in variability in the movement end points. The elderly make far more modifications in the deceleration phase of movements. The elderly do not project their limbs as forcefully or as far with the primary component, thereby requiring longer and often multiple movements to arrive at the target. Lengthening of the secondary component with age may be due to difficulties in producing force pulses (see Crossman & Goodeve, 1983) or because older adults require more time to process sensorimotor feedback of limb position relative to the target or both (e.g., Seidler & Stelmach, 1996).

Task Complexity and Difficulty Using a standard protocol (e.g., Fitts, 1954; Fitts & Peterson, 1964) that manipulates the distance of limb movement (2–16 inches) and size of the target end points, movement time (MT) has been shown to reliably vary as a function of an index of difficulty (a logarithm of relative accuracy based on target width and intertarget separation); such as $MT = a + b \log_2 (2A/W)$, where a is the intercept, b is the slope, A is the movement amplitude (distance), and W is the target width. Furthermore, analyses of data from 22 years of testing at the Baltimore Longitudinal Study of Aging has revealed changes occurring with age (Brogmus, 1991a, 1991b; Vercruyssen et al., in review; Welford et al., 1969).

Aging adults have increasing difficulty in performing complex movements, those with multiple sequences of movements, presumably because of impaired ability in initiating and terminating bilateral actions simultaneously and difficulties in modifying motor commands while a response is being executed (Stelmach, Amrhein, & Goggin, 1988).

Continuous and Complex Movements

Movements that use error monitoring to sustain an uninterrupted series of actions may be called *continuous*. *Complex* movements may involve combinations of simple movements, discrete or continuous, movements requiring intricate motor preparation, or even simple movement that follow relatively elaborate cognitive action. Most motor behavior does not consist of a single ballistic movement involving a single run-through from sensory input to motor output but is actually a series of movements programmed and coordinated to achieve a desired outcome, with the result of each segment of the series influencing execution of subsequent segments. Usually skills are executed with little environmental uncertainty (in an "open loop" manner); however, some tasks are based almost entirely on reactions to and interactions with environmental uncertainty (in a "closed loop" manner; Schmidt, 1988; Wickens, 1991). For instance, most forms of vehicle control involve continuous tracking. As one gets older, the time for programming and monitoring increases and the maximum length of the motor program shortens, but these age effects often diminish with practice. In fact, it is common in the workplace to find older workers who perform at high levels on familiar tasks involving a complex series of actions.

Simple Tracking (Error Nulling)

Simple tracking (e.g., Schmidt, 1988; Wickens, 1991) is another type of task sensitive to aging. Such paced tasks typically involve the pursuit of a target with frequent adjustments in tracking responses intended to match or compensate movements to minimize distance between target and cursor locations. Typically, older adults lag behind the target and compensatory adjustments are usually smaller than those made by young adults (Jagacinski, Liao, & Fayyad, 1995).

Balance, Falls, and Coordination

Balance Balance (postural stability) may be arbitrarily divided into two types: static balance, the maintenance of stability in stationary positions, usually vertical, and dynamic balance, the maintenance of stability during locomotion or other movements. Generally, older adults have poorer static postural control than young adults (e.g., Spirduso, 1995a; Woollacott & Shumway-Cook, 1989). Static tests of balance can be significant predictors of falling (e.g., Maki, Holliday, & Topper, 1994) and can be improved with balance training in healthy older adults (Hu & Woollacott, 1994a, 1994b). Dynamic balance is usually measured by changes in characteristics of locomotion like patterns of gait. Over age 60 self-selected walking speed slows 10–20% per decade as a compensation for reduced information processing capabilities, increased risk of falling, earlier onset of fatigue, decreased joint range of motion, decreased lower leg strength, increased musculoskeletal pathologies and discomfort, and increased health problems. Most of the reduction in speed results from decreasing stride length as part of a strategy for being more economical with movement while increasing stability and increasing the time to monitor the immediate environment so that defensive actions can be anticipated, a compensation for slowing of reactive capacity (Khalil et al., 1994; Spirduso, 1995b).

Falls Falls are the second leading cause of accidental deaths in the United States behind automobile accidents (Coombs, 1994). In 1988, falls resulted in over 12,000 deaths, 67% of which involved individuals over age 65 (Coombs, 1994). Each year there are 172,000 hip fractures among individuals over 65 years of age at an economic cost of over $7 billion (Shoyer, 1994). Falls resulting in fractures is the major cause of admissions to hospitals and convalescent care programs. Even without suffering physical injury, the fear of falling can be psychologically injurious—36% of those over 75 years of age have a fear of falling so strong that it affects their mobility and independence.

Risk of falling increases with age, possibly more so for women than men

(Downton, 1993; Wolfson, Whipple, Derby, Amerman, & Nashner, 1994), because of compromises in locomotor control, including impaired balance, muscular weakness, inflexibility, slow and inadequate adjustments to environmental perturbations, cardiovascular disease, reduced leg strength, mental confusion, hearing and vision impairments, arthritis, coordination impairments, contraindications of medications, dependency, and obesity (e.g., Downton, 1993; Shoyer, 1994; Spirduso, 1995b). The consequences of falling, especially for those over 70 years, are often catastrophic. Falls cause 87% of all fractures and 65% of accidental deaths in the elderly (Azar & Lawton, 1964). Of those 70 years of age and older who fracture their hip from a fall, 50–70% die within one year of the fall, usually due to secondary complications.

Coordination Older adults have a reduced ability to precisely time the update of information, according to critical windows of availability, and execute movements in coordination. Older individuals require more time to prepare for receiving new information and may have difficulty timing their preparedness with the time information becomes available. This difficulty in synchronizing the timing of optimal receptivity with the availability of information is in addition to the general slowing of behavior that influences neuromotor integration. Inaccurate time keeping and time scheduling, both in momentary and long-term management of attention, causes difficulty in the production of long-duration, precisely timed, sequences of movements for the elderly.

Job Performance and Essential Tasks

Real-world, or everyday, tasks frequently involve complex skills that are combinations of the types of movements presented thus far. Driving an automobile is a good example of a complex skill involving continuous, coordinated movements (see application chapters by Barr and Morrow). Only two broad categories of skill are now mentioned: job performance and essential tasks of independent living.

Job Performance Older workers are not usually found in jobs that make heavy demands on abilities known to decline with age, have higher accident rates than young workers in such jobs, and tend to move to jobs in which these demands are minimized (for work capacity throughout adulthood, see Ilmarinen & Louhevaara, 1994; Kaneko, 1990; Spirduso, 1995b; Welford, 1993). However, progress has been very slow in assessing performance of older workers for work assignments, mostly due to the legal implications of various personnel assessment strategies (e.g., Avolio, Barrett, & Sterns, 1984). The age at which performance will be optimal depends on the demands of the task and the balance of biological declines and experiential improvements within the individual—younger if demands are mainly biological and older if performance requires experiential and knowledge factors (Welford, 1993).

Studies of the relationship of age and work performance report that they are essentially unrelated (e.g., Davies, Matthews, & Wong, 1991; Waldman & Avolio, 1986), yet employers and younger employees often think of older workers to be "less productive, more resistant to change, and less well suited to particular kinds of jobs such as those involving rapid decision-making or the use of complex skills, especially information technology skills" (Davies, Taylor, & Dorn, 1992). They are also thought to be poorer learners and therefore are less likely to be selected for retraining.

Accidents Slowness causes many, possibly most, accidents of older adults (e.g., Welford, 1958, 1973; Whitfield, 1954). Accidents, that is failure to make an adequate or appropriate response in a hazardous situation, may be due to (1) a failure to appreciate demands of the situation (i.e., to perceive the hazard or to decide what response, if any, ought to be made), or (2) a failure to produce the appropriate response, even if the hazard has been perceived and the appropriate action initiated (Whitfield, 1954). Whitfield found that among accident-prone individuals, the young tended to make the first type of failure while older adults tended to error in direction of the second type.

Changes in the motor system help explain why few people over the age of 50 engage in very strenuous muscular work and why athletic performance declines with age (see Charness, 1985; Spirduso, 1995b; Stones & Kozma, 1985). However, such changes seldom limit everyday activities before one's middle 60s. On the job, workers in later middle age seem capable of performing moderately heavy work (muscular demands). Physical activity also sustains cerebral blood flow and cognitive function, particularly after retirement (Rogers, Meyer, & Mortel, 1990).

Regardless of the cause, slowing with age in the choice and control of movements affects a wide range of daily task performance and fosters tendencies for older workers to avoid fast machine-paced work, which presents signals requiring actions at a fixed rate independent of the operator's control, in favor of slower operator-paced tasks (e.g., Welford, 1977b). The increased liability to error is usually compensated for by increased caution which often leads to more deliberate performances, which are characteristically slow.

Essential Tasks of Independent Living One of the criteria for entrance into convalescent care facilities is the inability of older adults to perform activities of daily living (ADL), including bathing, walking, dressing, transferring, toileting, grooming, shopping, light housework, money management, self-medicating, and eating (e.g., M. C. Clark, Czaja, & Weber, 1990; Lawton, 1990; see also Chapter 13 in this book by Czaja). Incidental activities of daily living (IADL) reflect independence in daily self-care, but are not critical to living alone, such as preparing meals, shopping, money management, telephoning, and housework. Any condition that interferes with one's ability to perform on ADL or IADL threatens independent living. Motor skills such as turning knobs to open doors, dialing (keying) a telephone, manipulating small objects, dressing, opening medication bottles, using hobby tools, food preparation, and operating controls on electronic equipment require hand movements and are essential for independent living (see also Spirduso, 1995a). Therefore, loss of hand functions is most predictive of the need for assistance in living either by family support or by an institution (e.g., Jette, Branch, & Berlin, 1990). Further, there appears to be greater disability and somewhat greater use of personal assistive devices among women compared to men, and there are alternating sex differences in relationships between both personal and technical resources and subjective feelings of well-being across levels of functional disability (see also Charness & Bosman, 1990, 1992, 1994).

INTERVENTION: ATTEMPTS TO REDUCE AGE DIFFERENCES

Again, one's ability to meet the requirements of work situations and the challenges of everyday life depend on how well the capacities of psychophysiological mechanisms (sensory, perceptual, cognitive, and neuromuscular) and knowledge (experience) meet the specific demands of the task at hand. Therefore, performance can be optimized by improving capacity, enhancing experience thereby improving skill, or reducing the demands of the task. Numerous attempts have been made to mitigate age-related declines in psychomotor functions and cope with their consequences including (1) practice, training, and skill; (2) health, exercise, and fitness; and (3) task and system design. The first two modify capacity of the performer while the last is an adaptation of the task or environment to reduce demands.

Adapting the Person

Practice, Training, and Skill

Practice improves and stabilizes psychomotor performance but in different ways depending on age; older adults generally take longer to adapt to novel tasks and new situations (e.g., Grant, Storandt, & Botwinick, 1978; Salthouse, 1985, 1988). Laboratory tasks consistently find interactions between age and task complexity, which are reduced by extended practice (e.g., Falduto & Baron, 1986), presumably due to the way they load capacities to their limits (Welford, 1977b, 1978, 1982). However, this is not necessarily present in job performance (e.g., Sparrow & Davies, 1988). Practice and training help individuals to become faster and less variable at reactions and movements, especially the elderly when successful task performance involves remembering and employing strategies and complex rules. Extended practice can diminish age differences in speed, particularly in cases where experience, knowledge, and wisdom are factors determining response rate (e.g., Welford, 1958, 1973, 1968, 1985b), and even eliminate age differences entirely (e.g., Falduto & Baron, 1986; Nebes, 1978). Cerella and Lowe (1984) reanalyzed 27 studies showing cognitive deficits with age and concluded that declines with age came from a practice component (33%) that was reversible and a nonreversible component (66%) that was assumed to be biological. Given sufficient practice, older adults usually attain levels of performance comparable to the young or adequate in practical situations. Furthermore, once learned, skills and expertise are usually retained and behavioral training can enhance the possibility for retraining older individuals for maintaining effective motor skills (Welford, 1982).

During practice, motor performance often becomes more accurate, less variable, smoother, and faster. In a complex tasks, individual actions or movement components tend to consolidate to become a coherent (coordinated) whole motor program. Extensive practice results in a reduction in time taken to process information and thereby reduces task demands. Increased accuracy tends to reduce monitoring frequency and duration so that performance becomes smoother, more efficient, and more automatic. Improved performance reflects better discrimination of relevant from irrelevant sensory information (cues), identification of efficient responses that effectively reduce the number of alternatives to be considered, encoding of associations between stimuli and appropriate responses, and programming responses over extended periods.

Skill and experience interact (see Salthouse, 1984, 1990; Welford, 1985a, 1985b) such that much of the deterioration of motor capacities that accompanies aging can be counteracted by development of new strategies (see Mortimer et al., 1982). Practice and training enhance skill and the efficient deployment of capacities to meet the demands of tasks, and they modify strategies that direct performance over time (Welford, 1982). These strategies are flexible and are concerned more with a goal-directed series of actions than particular aspects of individual actions, thereby enabling performers to do known tasks more efficiently and new tasks better than otherwise expected. Strategies developed through practice and experience cause compensatory changes in the way tasks are performed, which enable older individuals to maintain effective performance despite diminishing capacities. This demonstrates that assessment of merely sensory and muscular functions may lead to inaccurate predictions of performance and underestimate the overall achievement potential of older individuals (Mortimer et al., 1982; Welford, 1984, 1985a, 1985b).

With advancing age, extensive practice permits development of numerous compensatory mechanisms that maintain skilled performance across the life span (Welford, 1985b). On some skills, older workers can outperform younger workers. Further, overpracticed movements, compared with less familiar ones, are more resistant to deleterious effects of aging. Repeating an example, using foot tapping (familiar) and hand tapping (unfamiliar) tasks, conventional age effects appear in hand tapping but no age differences appear in foot tapping (e.g., Stones & Kozma, 1989). Also, improvements in performance gained from practice on one task may transfer to another. For instance, practicing to improve video game performance has been shown to improve two-choice reaction time in the elderly (e.g., J. E.Clark, Lanphear, & Riddick, 1987; Dustman, Emmerson, Steinhaus, Shearer, & Dustman, 1992).

Despite declining sensory, perceptual, cognitive, and motor processes (and performance on many laboratory tasks), the elderly are often able to maintain real world skills through experience or extensive practice and may even perform some tasks better than young adults. In one study, when length of service was controlled, age effects disappeared and when age was controlled, experience effects remained (Giniger, Dispenzieri, & Eisenberg, 1983), making experience a stronger predictor of job performance than age. No differences were reported between old and young experienced workers but the inexperienced young performed better than the inexperienced old in simultaneous language translators (Murrell & Humphries, 1978) and drill-press operators (Murrell, Powesland, & Forsaith, 1962). There are reports to the contrary (e.g., Salthouse, Babcock, Skovronek, Mitchell, & Palmon, 1989), but most evidence supports the beneficial effects of experience and expertise on reducing or even reversing age effects in job performance (Giniger et al., 1983; Salthouse, 1990; Sparrow & Davies, 1988). Salthouse (1984, 1988) eloquently illustrated this practice effect in a study of typing ability that showed older typists (from a group age 19–69 years) were able to type as well as, and often better than, young name even though they showed typical slowing on a choice reaction time task. The proposed advantage for the older typists has been attributed to extensive practice causing a compensation to loss of speed by the development of more effective strategies—in this case the anticipation of responses to be performed by reading further ahead in the text to be typed; that is, better use of available precuing information.

Health, Exercise, and Fitness

Generally, behavior slows with advancing age, but age differences disappear if one compares average young adults to healthy, active, and physically fit older adults over 50 years of age or compares longitudinally a group of healthy fit subjects early and later in life. Physically fit older individuals not only react faster on simple and choice RT tasks than their sedentary peers but may also perform at levels comparable with sedentary 20-year-olds and in some cases are faster than many individuals in the young population (e.g., Spirduso, 1995; Spirduso & Clifford, 1978). Spirduso (1975, 1987) found no difference in simple and choice reaction time in habitual male joggers over age 60 compared with college sophomores. Also, RT variability from trial to trial between and within individuals, which usually increases considerably with age, may remain unchanged across age groups of physically active individuals.

Declines in psychological functioning with age are much due to deteriorating physical fitness, which is partly reversible through appropriate exercise program (e.g., Bashore, 1989; Kaneko, 1990; Spirduso, 1980, 1995). Lifestyle changes with age—usually the levels of physical and mental activity go from high to low, causing atrophy of muscle structure, slowing of neuromuscular control and information processing, and general declines in cognitive and motor abilities. However, increasing one's level of physical and mental activity may slow, or even reverse, the rate of change associated with aging. Older adults who exercise regularly react more quickly than their nonexercising cohorts, although it has not been determined whether the relationship between fitness and speed of behavior is correlational or causal. This relationship may be due to exercise-induced increases in (a) cerebral blood flow, oxygen utilization, and the control of hypertension, (b) morphological plasticity, and (c) neurotransmitter function (Spirduso, 1995a), among other explanations. Since nearly all human movement requires some minimal level of muscular strength, endurance, speed, and joint flexibility, it seems reasonable that exercise and strength training can help maintain motor system integrity and thereby slow age-related declines in psychomotor functions and skill.

General benefits of exercise in old age are becoming well documented (e.g., Kaneko, 1990; Spirduso, 1980, 1995b) and the quality and safety of physical training programs are rapidly improving (e.g., Shephard, 1990). Spirduso (1995b) reviews fitness and exercise effects on age differences in speed of reactions and movements and reports that the physically fit are reliably faster and less variable than the unfit, but exercise programs designed to improve aerobic fitness have not reliably produced improvements in behavioral speed (see also Birren & Fisher, 1995; Spirduso, 1980).

Neuromuscular mechanisms that are not frequently used are the ones most impaired by aging. Since even a minimal level of physical activity activates spinal reflexes, these movements should be the last mechanisms affected by aging (Clarkson, 1978a, 1978b). Through a lifestyle of regular exercise, motor unit function, specifically nerve conduction velocity, can be maintained with advancing age; disuse of muscles—inactivity—causes inconsistency in motor unit firing making more difficult the control of slow, graded muscular contractions and fine motor control (Spirduso, 1995b).

There are at least three possible explanations of beneficial effects of exercise (adapted from Spirduso & MacRae, 1990): (1) the tonic and overpractice effect model—exercise has an age-invariant, invigorating, tonic effect, coupled with the overpractice effect that occurs with daily physical activity that is generalized across physical and psychological domains (Stones & Kozma, 1989); (2) the moderator effects model—exercise moderates the rate of aging (Stones & Kozma, 1989); and (3) the selection factor—exercisers throughout their lives are inherently healthier and/or physically superior to those who do not exercise.

Maintenance of physical fitness through a lifestyle of daily physical and mental activity may prevent age-related deterioration of motor and mental performance and maintain an optimal level of physical work capacity, delaying the age at which environmental demands exceed physical capabilities and reducing the rate of cognitive slowing. The maintenance of physical and mental capacities, specifically those that are *movement-related,* is associated with a longer period of functional autonomy; that is, independence in daily living, an active social calendar, physical and mental fitness, and other indices of functional health and general wellness (e.g., Clarkson-Smith & Hartley, 1989; Greene & Williams, in press; Hultsch, Hammer, & Small, 1993; Spirduso, 1995). Improved physical fitness has beneficial effects on many CNS functions including memory, attention, and information processing speed by acting directly or indirectly on neurotransmitters that influence the reticular activating system (e.g., Spirduso, 1983), among other locations. Maintaining regular physical fitness training through one's retirement years may extend the age at which environmental and task demands exceed one's physical capabilities by as much as eight years (Shephard, 1978).

Adapting the Environment

Task and System Design

Another way to mitigate declines in psychomotor performance with age is to design tasks, products, and other elements of one's environment to make performance independent of age. Since age-related changes occur at different rates within and between individuals, knowledge of physiological and other changes with age cannot be applied universally to all aging workers. The design of job tasks and work environments must be individualized and flexible after the age of 45 years (e.g., Welford, 1993). Generally, designers should not design for the "average" user but for a diverse range of users. Designers must be sensitive to the range of user characteristics, within and between individuals. Designs for the elderly should account for richness of human diversity found within this population, such as the experience and expertise of older workers.

Task, product, and systems design for the elderly are often made by human factors specialists and gerontechnologists. *Human factors* (aka ergonomics, engineering psychology, human engineering, human ergology)is an applied science concerned with the design of jobs, operations, workplaces, equipment, projects, machines, and environments to match the capabilities, limitations, and desires of people, thereby enhancing opportunities for optimizing system performance, productivity, or profit while reducing the risk of accident, injury, illness, and discomfort. In short, human factors is concerned with commonsense engineering and individual differences in a human–machine–environment systems design (Vercruyssen, Graafmans, Fozard, Bouma, & Rietsema, 1996). *Gerontechnology,* the study of technology and aging for the benefit of a preferred living and working environment and adapted medical care for the elderly (e.g., Bouma & Graafmans, 1992; Vercruyssen et al., 1996), conducts applied and basic research on the interaction of the elderly with products and their technical or built environments to explain the challenges and opportunities of normal and pathological aging. *Challenges* refer to age-related changes in physical, physiological, perceptual, cognitive, and motor processes. *Opportunities* refer to increased time to pursue new activities in self-discovery, work, and relationships with grandchildren and others outside the family. Essentially, gerontechnology uses available technology to compress morbidity and extend functional autonomy (independent living). The need for gerontechnology increases with the degree to which society is caught unprepared for "world age growth," the dramatic increase in the elder segment (e.g., 65 years and older) of the world population.

Gerontechnology addresses aging in at least five ways. It provides technology to (1) improve the way in which aging processes themselves are studied; (2) prevent declines in strength, flexibility, and endurance commonly associated with aging; (3) enhance the performance of new roles provided by aging; (4) compensate for declining capabilities with aging; and (5) assist caregivers. (For a list of resources see Vercruyssen et al., 1996.) Gerontechnologists are responsible for many changes in everyday living that improve functional utility, career duration, and performance on the job while decreasing the risk of accidents and health problems.

Because many capabilities of older adults decline with age, designs for many products and environments need to be altered for elderly users. Sensory, perceptual, cognitive, and motor demands of some jobs can be problematic for older workers but can be somewhat alleviated by task and job redesign (e.g., Bouma & Graafmans, 1992; Charness & Bosman, 1990, 1992, 1994; Smith, 1990; Welford, 1993). For instance, decreased visual acuity, speed, and other functions may lead to a state in which performance is limited. When this happens one must look to see if tasks can be redesigned, that is, made less demanding, or the capacity to perform can be enhanced. The greater experience and job satisfaction of the older worker (Davies et al., 1991) are major variables in optimal matching of jobs and tasks to the worker's perceived abilities. Speed of behavior will become increasingly more important for coping with a society that is becoming increasingly complex, automated, and fast paced with high-technology devices. Since older adults take longer to recognize a signal, initiate a response, and benefit less from forewarnings than young adults, when fast responses are required, warnings should be given of upcoming events considerably in advance of the event, bearing in mind that the elderly require more time to process the information. In real-world tasks, older individuals may compensate for biological slowing and perform as well as young adults by taking advantage of experience and previously learned skills.

Declines in psychomotor processes with age do not necessarily translate into impaired performance. Correct anticipation can eliminate reaction time entirely, for young and old alike, and make movements appear natural and reflexive. Experience and practice may lead to expertise and automatic responses that can make performance of older adults better than that of the young, regardless of impairments observed in fundamental processes. Nearly everyone benefits from the design of tasks and environments based on abilities that are enhanced by experience. Aging does *not* have to limit motor behavior. "Growing old is inevitable for all of us. The clever thing is to accept it and always plan your next move well in advance" (Maurice Chevalier, Concluding Remarks chapter quote, Welford, 1958/1973).

CONCLUSION

Movement control and speed of behavior decline with advancing age, especially in sedentary adults, and may become the primary limiting factor in one's quality of life and ability to live independently. Changes in performance with age are different for different individuals, and for different tasks. Much of the deterioration of motor capacities that accompanies aging can be off-set (compensated for) through the development of new strategies for skilled performance. Behavioral training techniques may enhance possibilities for retraining older individuals and maintaining effective motor skills. And, maintenance of fitness through a life-style of daily physical and mental activity may prevent age-related deterioration of biological processes as well as psychomotor and cognitive performance and thereby maintaining high levels of emotional well-being.

Loss of performance may be reduced or possibly eliminated through effective design of tasks, products, and environments. Tasks should be designed so that demands are within the capacity of those who are asked to perform them thereby bringing the task within the capacities of a much wider age range of performers. Such designs are likely to enhance performance of all individuals, especially older adults. To obtain optimal human–machine–environment system performance requires practical designs that accommodate subtle individual differences, whether such differences are called gender/sex, culture/race/ethnicity, intelligence, . . . or age. Thus, a test of effective and efficient design is to measure the degree to which system performance is maintained regardless of the inter- and intra-individual variations in the human. In other words, the challenge for gerontechnologists, ergonomists, and human factors specialists is to design adaptations for the individual and environment such that age-related changes in movement control and speed of behavior have little or no effect on overall performance.

Acknowledgments

The author is especially grateful to the late A. T. Welford for his assistance in interpreting research literature, especially his own work, and for many of the ideas described herein. R. Seidler, G. Stelmach, and W. W. Spirduso provided valuable manuscripts prior to their publication. The editors, copy editor, anonymous reviewers, J. E. Birren, and W. deWeerd provided useful suggestions for improving this chapter.

References

Avolio, B. J., Barrett, G. V., & Sterns, H. L. (1984). Alternatives to age for assessing occupational performance capacity. *Experimental Aging Research, 10,* 101–105.

Azar, G., & Lawton, A. (1964). Gait and stepping as factors in the frequent falls of elderly women. *Gerontologist, 4,* 83–84.

Barrett, G. V., Mihal, W. L., Panek, P. E., Sterns, H. L., & Alexander, R. A. (1977). Information processing skills predictive of accident involvement for younger and older commercial drivers. *Industrial Gerontology, 4,* 173–182.

Bashore, T. R. (1989). Age, physical fitness, and mental processing speed. *Annual Review of Gerontology and Geriatrics, 9,* 120–144.

Bashore, T. R. (1994). Some thoughts on neurocognitive slowing. *Acta Psychologica, 86,* 295–325.

Birren, J. E., & Fisher, L. M. (1995). Aging and speed of behavior: Possible consequences for psychological functioning. *Annual Review of Psychology, 46,* 329–353.

Birren, J. E., Riegel, K. F., & Morrison, D. F. (1962). Age differences in response speed as a function of controlled variations of stimulus conditions: Evidence for a general speed factor. *Gerontologia, 6,* 1–18.

Birren, J. E., Vercruyssen, M., & Fisher, L. M. (1990). Aging and speed of behavior: Its scientific and practical significance. In M. Bergener, M. Ermini, & H. B. Stahelin (Eds.), *Challenges in aging: The 1990 Sandoz lectures in gerontology* (pp. 3–23). San Diego, CA: Academic Press.

Birren, J. E., Woods, A. M., & Williams, M. V. (1980). Behavioral slowing with age: Causes, organizations, and consequences. In L. W. Poon (Ed.), *Aging in the 1980's: Psychological issues* (pp. 293–308). Washington, DC: American Psychological Association.

Borkan, G. A., & Norris, A. H. (1980). Assessment of biological age using a profile of physical parameters. *Journal of Experimental Psychology, 35,* 177–184.

Bouma, H. H., & Graafmans, J. A. M. (1992). *Gerontechnology.* Amsterdam: IOS Press.

Bowe, F. (1988, August/September). Why seniors don't use technology. *Technology Review,* pp. 35–40.

Brinley, J. F. (1965). Cognitive sets, speed and accuracy of performance in the elderly. In A. T. Welford & J. E. Birren (Eds.), *Behavior, aging and the nervous system* (pp. 191–216). Springfield, IL: Thomas.

Brogmus, G. E. (1991a). Effects of age and sex on speed and accuracy of hand movements and the refinements they suggest for Fitts' law. In *Proceedings of the Human Factor Society 35th annual meeting* (pp. 208–212). Santa Monica, CA: Human Factors and Ergonomics Society.

Brogmus, G. E. (1991b). *Effects of age and sex on speed and accuracy of hand movements and the refinements they suggest for Fitts' law.* Master's thesis in Human Factors, University of Southern California, Los Angeles/Ann Arbor, MI: University Microfilms International.

Cerella, J. (1990). Aging and information processing rate. In J. E. Birren & K. W. Schaie (Eds.), *Handbook of the psychology of aging* (3rd ed., pp. 201–221). San Diego, CA: Academic Press.

Cerella, J. (1991). Age effects may be global, not local: Comments on Fisk and Rogers (1991). *Journal of Experimental Psychology: General, 120,* 215–223.

Cerella, J. (1994). Generalized slowing in Brinley plots. *Journal of Gerontology: Psychological Sciences, 49,* P65–P71.

Cerella, J., & Hale, S. (1994). The rise and fall in information-processing rates over the life span. *Acta Psychologica, 86,* 109–197.

Cerella, J., & Lowe, D. (1984). Age deficits and practice: 27 studies reconsidered. *Gerontologist, 24,* 76.

Cerella, J., Poon, L. W., & Williams, D. M. (1980). Age and the complexity hypothesis. In L. W. Poon & K. W. Schaie (Eds.), *Aging in the 1980s: Psychological issues* (pp. 532–540). Washington, DC: American Psychological Association.

Charness, N. (Ed.). (1985). *Aging and human performance.* New York: Wiley.

Charness, N., & Bosman, E. A. (1990). Human factors and design for older adults. In J. E. Birren & K. W. Schaie (Eds.), *Handbook of the psychology of aging* (3rd ed., pp. 446–463). San Diego, CA: Academic Press.

Charness, N., & Bosman, E. A. (1992). Human factors and age. In F. I. M. Craik & T. A. Salthouse (Eds.), *Handbook of aging and cognition* (pp. 495–551). Hillsdale, NJ: Erlbaum.

Charness, N., & Bosman, E. A. (1994). Age-related changes in perceptual and psychomotor performance: Implications for engineering design. *Experimental Aging Research, 20,* 45–49.

Clark, J. E., Lanphear, A. K., & Riddick, C. C. (1987). The effects of videogame playing on the response selection processing of elderly adults. *Journal of Gerontology, 42,* 82–85.

Clark, M. C., Czaja, S. J., & Weber, R. A. (1990). Older adults and daily living task profiles. *Human Factors, 32,* 537–549.

Clarkson, P. M. (1978a). Practice effects on fractionated response time related to age and activity level. *Journal of Motor Behavior, 10,* 275–286.

Clarkson, P. M. (1978b). The relationship of age and level of physical activity with the fractionated components of patellar reflex time. *Journal of Gerontology, 33,* 650–656.

Clarkson-Smith, L., & Hartley, A. A. (1989). Relationship between physical exercise and cognitive abilities in older adults. *Psychology and Aging, 4,* 183–189.

Coombs, F. (1994). Engineering technology in rehabilitation of older adults. *Experimental Aging Research, 20,* 201–209.

Crossman, E. R. F. W. (1953). Entropy and choice time: The effect of frequency unbalance on choice-response. *Quarterly Journal of Experimental Psychology, 5,* 41–51.

Crossman, E. R. F. W., & Goodeve, P. J. (1983). Feedback control of hand movements and Fitts' Law. *Quarterly Journal of Experimental Psychology, 35A,* 251–278.

Cummings, S. R., & Nevitt, M. C. (1989). A hypothesis: The cause of hip fractures. *Journal of Gerontology, 44,* M107–M111.

Cunningham, W. R., & Brookbank, J. W. (1988). *Gerontology: The psychology, biology, and sociology of aging* (pp. 127–143). San Francisco: Harper & Row.

Davies, D. R., Matthews, G., & Wong, C. S. K. (1991). Ageing and work. In C. L. Cooper & I. T. Robinson (Eds.), *International review of industrial and organizational psychology: Vol. 6.* Chichester, UK: Wiley.

Davies, D. R., Taylor, A., & Dorn, L. (1992). Aging and human performance. In A. Smith (Ed.), *Handbook of human performance* (Vol. 3) (pp. 25–61). San Diego, CA: Academic Press.

Downton, J. H. (1993). *Falls in the elderly.* London: Edward Arnold.

Dustman, R. E., Emmerson, R. Y., Steinhaus, L. A., Shearer, D. E., & Dustman, T. J. (1992). The effects of videogame playing on neurophysiological performance of elderly individuals. *Journal of Gerontology: Psychological Sciences, 47,* P168–P171.

Falduto, L., & Baron, A. (1986). Age related effects of practice and task complexity on card sorting. *Journal of Gerontology, 41,* 659–661.

Fernie, G. (1994). Technology to assist elderly people's safe mobility. *Experimental Aging Research, 20,* 219–228.

Fisk, A. D., Fisher, D. L. (1994). Brinley plots and theories of aging: The explicit, muddled, and implicit debates. *Journal of Gerontology: Psychological Sciences, 49,* P81–P89.

Fisk, A. D., Fisher, D. L., & Rogers, W. A. (1992). General slowing alone cannot explain age-related search effects: Reply to Cerella (1991). *Journal of Experimental Psychology: General, 121,* 73–78.

Fitts, P. M. (1954). The information capacity of the human motor system in controlling the amplitude of movement. *Journal of Experimental Psychology, 47,* 381–391.

Fitts, P. M., & Peterson, J. R. (1964). Information capacity of discrete motor responses. *Journal of Experimental Psychology, 67,* 103–112.

Fozard, J. L., Vercruyssen, M., Reynolds, S. L., Hancock, P. A., & Quilter, R. E. (1994). Age differences and changes in reaction time: The Baltimore Longitudinal Study of Aging. *Journal of Gerontology: Psychological Sciences, 49,* P179–P189.

Giniger, B., Dispenzieri, A., & Eisenberg, J. (1983). Age, experience and performance on speed and skill jobs in an applied setting. *Journal of Applied Psychology, 68,* 469–475.

Goggin, N. L., & Stelmach, G. E. (1990). Age-related deficits in cognitive-motor skills. In E. A. Lovelace (Ed.), *Aging and cognition: Mental processes, self awareness and interventions* (pp. 135–155). Amsterdam: Elsevier/North-Holland.

Gottsdanker, R. (1982). Age and simple reaction time. *Journal of Gerontology, 37,* 342–348.

Grant, E. A., Storandt, M., & Botwinick, J. (1978). Incentive and practice in the psychomotor performance of the elderly. *Journal of Gerontology, 33,* 413–415.

Greene, L. S., & Williams, H. G. (1996). Aging and coordination from the dynamic pattern perspective. In A. Ferrandez & N. Teasdale (Eds.), *Changes in sensory motor behavior in aging* (pp. 89–131). Amsterdam: Elsevier.

Haaland, K. Y., Harrington, D. L., & Grice, J. W. (1993). Effects of aging on planning and implementing arm movements. *Psychology and Aging, 8,* 617–632.

Hamerman, D. (1990). The muscle and joint systems: Aging and the musculoskeletal system. In W. R. Hazzard, R. Andres, E. L. Bierman, & J. P. Blass (Eds.), *Principles of geriatric medicine and gerontology* (2nd ed., pp. 849–860). New York: McGraw-Hill.

Henry, F. M., & Rogers, D. E. (1960). Increased response latency for complicated movements and a "memory drum" theory of neuromotor reaction. *Research Quarterly, 31,* 448–458.

Hick, W. E. (1952). On the rate of gain of information. *Quarterly Journal of Experimental Psychology, 4,* 67–77.

Hobson, D. A. (1994). Technologies for seniors' living environment: Directions for product development. *Experimental Aging Research, 20,* 291–301.

Hu, M.-H., & Woollacott, M. H. (1994a). Multisensory training of standing balance in older adults: I. Postural stability and one-leg stance balance. *Journal of Gerontology: Medical Sciences, 49,* M52–M61.

Hu, M.-H., & Woollacott, M. H. (1994b). Multisensory training of standing balance in older adults: II. Kinematic and electromyographic postural responses. *Journal of Gerontology: Medical Sciences, 49,* M62–M71.

Hultsch, D. F. , Hammer, M., & Small, B. J. (1993). Age differences in cognitive performance in later life: Relationship to self-reported health and activity life styles. *Journal of Gerontology: Psychological Sciences, 48,* P1–P11.

Ilmarinen, J., & Louhevaara, V. (1994). The FINNAGE Program: Respect for the ageing. *Proceedings of the International Ergonomics Association Congress, 6*(2), 150–152.

Jagacinski, R. J., Liao, M.-J., & Fayyad, E. A. (1995). Generalized slowing in sinusoidal tracking in older adults. *Psychology and Aging, 10,* 8–19.

Jette, A. M., Branch, L. G., & Berlin, J. (1990). Musculoskeletal impairments and physical disablement among the aged. *Journal of Gerontology: Medical Sciences, 45,* M203–M208.

Kail, R., & Salthouse, T. A. (1994). Processing speed as a mental capacity. *Acta Psychologica, 86,* 199–225.

Kaneko, M. (1990). *Fitness for the aged, disabled, and industrial worker.* Champaign, IL: Human Kinetics.

Khalil, T. M., Abdel-Moty, E., Diaz, E. L., Steele-Rosomoff, R., & Rosomoff, H. L. (1994). Efficacy of physical restoration in the elderly. *Experimental Aging Research, 20,* 189–199.

Kornblum, S. (1965). Response competition and/or inhibition in two choice reaction time. *Psychonomic Science, 2,* 55–56.

Kornblum, S., Hasbroucq, T., & Osman, A. (1990). Dimensional overlap: Cognitive basis for stimulus-response compatibility—A model and taxonomy. *Psychological Review, 97,* 253–270.

Lawton, M. P. (1990). Aging and performance of home tasks. *Human Factors, 32,* 527–536.

Luce, R. D. (1986). *Response times: Their role in inferring elementary mental organization.* New York: Oxford University Press.

Mahurin, R. K., & Pirozzolo, F. J. (1986). Chronometric analysis: Clinical application in aging and dementia. *Developmental Neuropsychology, 2,* 345–362.

Maki, B. E., Holliday, P. J., & Topper, A. K. (1994). A prospective study of postural balance and risk of falling in an ambulatory and independent elderly population. *Journal of Gerontology: Medical Sciences, 49,* M72–M84.

McDowd, J. M., & Birren, J. E. (1990). Aging and attentional processes. In J. E. Birren & K. W. Schaie (Eds.), *Handbook of the psychology of aging* (3rd ed.) (pp. 222–233). San Diego, CA: Academic Press.

McDowd, J. M., Vercruyssen, M., & Birren, J. E. (1991). Aging, divided attention, and dual-task performance. In D. L. Damos (Ed.), *Multiple-task performance* (pp. 387–414). London: Taylor & Francis.

Mortimer, J. A., Pirozzolo, F. J., & Maletta, G. J. (Ed.). (1982). *The aging motor system.* New York: Praeger.

Murrell, K. F. H., & Humphries, S. (1978). Age, experience, and short-term memory. In M. M. Gruneberg, P. E. Morris, & R. N. Sykes (Eds.), *Practical aspects of memory.* New York: Academic Press.

Murrell, K. F. H., Powesland, P. R., & Forsaith, B. A. (1962). A study of Pillar-drilling in relation to age. *Occupational Psychology, 36,* 45–52.

Myerson, J., Hale, S., Wagstaff, D., Poon, L. W., & Smith, G. A. (1990). The information-loss model: A mathematical theory of age-related cognitive slowing. *Psychological Review, 97,* 475–487.

Myerson, J., Wagstaff, D., & Hale, S. (1994). Brinley plots, explained variance, and the analysis of age differences in response latencies. *Journal of Gerontology: Psychological Sciences, 49,* P72–P80.

Nebes, R. D. (1978). Vocal and manual response as a determinant of age differences in simple reaction time. *Journal of Gerontology, 33,* 884–889.

Perfect, T. J. (1994). What can Brinley plots tell us about cognitive aging? *Journal of Gerontology: Psychological Sciences, 49,* P60–P64.

Plude, D. J., Hoyer, W. J., & Lazar, J. (1982). Age, response complexity, and target consistency in visual search. *Experimental Aging Research, 8,* 99–102.

Pratt, J., Chasteen, A. L., & Abrams, R. A. (1994). Rapid aimed limb movements: Age differences and practice effects in component submovements. *Psychology and Aging, 9,* 325–334.

Rabbitt, P. M. A. (1965). An age decrement in the ability to ignore irrelevant information. *Journal of Gerontology, 20,* 233–238.

Rogers, R. L., Meyer, J. S., & Mortel, K. F. (1990). After reaching retirement age physical activity sustains cerebral perfusion and cognition. *Journal of the American Geriatric Society, 38,* 123–128.

Rowe, J. W., & Kahn, R. L. (1987). Human aging: Usual and successful. *Science, 237,* 143–149.

Salthouse, T. A. (1984). Effects of age and skill in typing. *Journal of Experimental Psychology: General, 113,* 345–371.

Salthouse, T. A. (1985). Speed of behavior and its implications for cognition. In J. E. Birren & K. W. Schaie (Eds.), *Handbook for the psychology of aging* (2nd ed., pp. 400–426). New York: Van Nostrand-Reinhold.

Salthouse, T. A. (1988). Cognitive aspects of motor functioning. In J. A. Joseph (Ed.), *Central determinants of age-related declines in motor function* (pp. 33–41). New York: New York Academy of Sciences.

Salthouse, T. A. (1990). Influence of experience on age differences in cognitive functioning. *Human Factors, 32,* 551–569.

Salthouse, T. A., Babcock, R. L., Skovronek, E., Mitchell, D. R. D., & Palmon, R. (1989). Age and experience effects in spatial visualization. *Developmental Psychology, 26,* 128–136.

Salthouse, T. A., & Somberg, B. L. (1982a). Isolating the age deficit in speeded performance. *Journal of Gerontology, 37,* 59–63.

Salthouse, T. A., & Somberg, B. L. (1982b), Skilled performance: The effects of adult age and

experience on elementary processes. *Journal of Experimental Psychology: General, 111,* 176–207.
Salthouse, T. A., & Somberg, B. L. (1982c). Time-accuracy relationship in young and old adults. *Journal of Gerontology, 37,* 349–353.
Schmidt, R. A. (1988). *Motor control and learning* (2nd ed.). Champaign, IL: Human Kinetics.
Seidler, R., & Stelmach, G. (1996). Motor Control. In J. E. Birren (Ed.), *Encyclopedia of gerontology* (pp. 177–185). San Diego, CA: Academic Press.
Shephard, R. J. (1978). *Physical activity and aging* (2nd ed.). Rockville, MD: Aspen Publications.
Shephard, R. J. (1990). The scientific basis of exercise prescribing for the very old. *Journal of the American Geriatric Society, 38,* 62–70.
Shoyer, J. L. (1994). Recommendations for environmental design research correlating falls and the physical environment. *Experimental Aging Research, 20,* 303–309.
Smith, D. B. D. (1990). Human factors and aging: An overview of research needs and application opportunities. *Human Factors, 32,* 509–526.
Sparrow, P. R., & Davies, D. R. (1988). Effects of age, tenure, training, and job complexity on technical performance. *Psychology and Aging, 3,* 307–314.
Spirduso, W. W. (1975). Reaction and movement time as a function of age and physical activity level. *Journal of Gerontology, 30,* 435–440.
Spirduso, W. W. (1980). Physical fitness, aging, and psychomotor speed: A review. *Journal of Gerontology, 35,* 850–865.
Spirduso, W. W. (1983). Exercise and the aging brain. *Research Quarterly for Exercise and Sport, 54,* 208–218.
Spirduso, W. W. (1987). Physical activity and the prevention of premature aging. In V. Seefeldt (Ed.), *Physical activity and well-being* (pp. 142–160). Reston, VA: American Association for Health, Physical Education, Recreation, and Dance.
Spirduso, W. W. (1995a). Aging and motor control. In D. R. Lamb, C. V. Gisolfi, & E. Nadel (Eds.), *Perspectives in exercise science and sports medicine: Exercise in older adults* (pp. 53–114). Carmel, IN: Cooper Publishing Group.
Spirduso, W. W. (1995b). *Physical dimensions of aging.* Champaign, IL: Human Kinetics.
Spirduso, W. W., & Clifford, P. (1978). Replication of age and physical activity effects on reaction time and movement time. *Journal of Gerontology, 33,* 26–30.
Spirduso, W. W., & MacRae, P. G. (1990). Motor performance and aging. In J. E.Birren & K. W. Schaie (Eds.), *Handbook of the psychology of aging* (3rd ed., pp. 183–200). San Diego, CA: Academic Press.
Sprott, R. L. (1988). Age-related variability. In J. A. Joseph (Ed.), *Central determinants of age-related declines in motor function* (Vol. 515, pp. 42–51). New York: New York Academy of Sciences.
Stelmach, G. E., Amrhein, P. C., & Goggin, N. L. (1988). Age differences in bimanual coordination. *Journal of Gerontology: Psychological Sciences, 43,* P18–P23.
Stelmach, G. E., & Nahom, A. (1992). Cognitive-motor abilities of the elderly driver. *Human Factors, 34,* 53–65.
Stelmach, G. E., & Worringham, C. J. (1985). Sensorimotor deficits related to postural stability: Implications for falls in the elderly. *Clinics in Geriatric Medicine, 1,* 679–694.
Stones, M. J., & Kozma, A. (1985). Physical performance. In N. Charness (Ed.), *Aging and human performance* (pp. 261–291). New York: Wiley.
Stones, M. J., & Kozma, A. (1989). Physical activity, age and cognitive/motor performance. In M. L. Howe & C. J. Brainerd (Eds.), *Cognitive development in adulthood: Progress in cognitive development research* (pp. 273–321). New York: Springer.
Surwillo, W. W. (1968). Timing of behavior in senescence and the role of the central nervous

system. In G. A. Talland (Ed.), *Human aging and behavior: Recent advances in research and theory* (pp. 1–35). New York: Academic Press.

Thomas, J. C., Waugh, N. C., & Fozard, J. L. (1978). Age and familiarity in memory scanning. *Journal of Gerontology, 33,* 528–533.

Vercruyssen, M. (1994). Slowing of behavior with age. In R. Kastenbaum (Ed.), *Encyclopedia of adult development* (pp. 457–467). Phoenix, AZ: Oryx.

Vercruyssen, M., Brogmus, G. E., Welford, A. T., & Fozard, J. L. (in review). Longitudinal changes in speed and accuracy of hand movements.

Vercruyssen, M., Graafmans, J. A. M., Fozard, J. E., Bouma, H., & Rietsema, J. (1996). Gerontechnology. In J. E. Birren (Ed.), *Encyclopedia of gerontology* (pp. 593–603). San Diego, CA: Academic Press.

Waldman, D. A., & Avolio, B. J. (1986). A meta-analysis of age differences in job performance. *Journal of Applied Psychology, 71,* 33–38.

Welford, A. T. (1958). *Ageing and human skill.* Oxford University Press for the Nuffield Foundation. (Reprinted 1973 by Greenwood Press: Westport, CT)

Welford, A. T. (1968). *Fundamental of skill.* London: Methuen.

Welford, A. T. (1976). Motivation, capacity, learning and age. *International Journal of Aging and Human Development, 7,* 189–199.

Welford, A. T. (1977a). Causes of slowing of performance with age. *Interdisciplinary Topics in Gerontology, 11,* 43–51.

Welford, A. T. (1977b). Motor performance. In J. E. Birren & K. W. Schaie (Eds.), *Handbook of the psychology of aging* (2nd ed., pp. 450–496). New York: Van Nostrand-Reinhold.

Welford, A. T. (1977c). Serial reaction times, continuity of task, single-channel effects, and age. In S. Dornic (Ed.), *Attention and performance VI* (pp. 79–97). Hillsdale, NJ: Erlbaum.

Welford, A. T. (1978). Mental work load as a function of demand, capacity, strategy and skill. *Ergonomics, 21,* 151–167.

Welford, A. T. (Ed.). (1980a). *Reaction times.* London: Academic Press.

Welford, A. T. (1980b). Relationship between reaction time and fatigue, stress, age and sex. In A. T. Welford (Ed.), *Reaction times* (pp. 321–354). London: Academic Press.

Welford, A. T. (1981). Signal noise, performance, and age. *Human Factors, 23,* 97–109.

Welford, A. T. (1982). Motor skills and aging. In J. A. Mortimer, F. J. Pirozzolo, & G. J. Maletta (Eds.), *The aging motor system* (pp. 152–187). New York: Praeger.

Welford, A. T. (1984). Between bodily changes and performance: Some possible reasons for slowing with age. *Experimental Aging Research, 10,* 73–88.

Welford, A. T. (1985a). Changes in performance with age: An overview. In N. Charness (Ed.), *Aging and human performance* (pp. 333–369). Chichester, UK: Wiley.

Welford, A. T. (1985b). Practice effects in relation to age: A review and a theory. *Developmental Neuropsychology, 1*(2), 173–190.

Welford, A. T. (1993). Work capacity across the adult years. In R. Kastenbaum (Ed.), *Encyclopedia of adult development* (pp. 541–553). Phoenix, AZ: Oryx.

Welford, A. T., Norris, A. H., & Shock, N. W. (1969). Speed and accuracy of movement and their changes with age. *Acta Psychologica, 30,* 3–15.

Whitfield, J. W. (1954). Individual differences in accident susceptibility among coal miners. *British Journal of Industrial Medicine, 11,* 126—139.

Wickens, C. D. (1991). *Engineering psychology and human performance.* New York: Harper Collins.

Wickens, C. D., Braune, R., & Stokes, A. (1987). Age differences in speed and capacity of information processing: 1. A dual-task approach. *Psychology and Aging, 2,* 70–78.

Williams, M. E., Gaylord, S. A., & McGahie, W. C. (1990). Timed manual performance in a community elderly population. *Journal of American Geriatrics Society, 38,* 1120–1126.

Wolfson, L., Whipple, R., Berby, C. A., Amerman, P., & Nashner, L. (1994). Gender differences in balance of healthy elderly as demonstrated by dynamic posturography. *Journal of Gerontology: Medical Sciences, 49,* M160–M167.

Woollacott, M. H., & Shumway-Cook, A. (1989). *Development of posture and gait across the life span.* Columbia: University of South Carolina Press.

Chapter 5

Anthropometry and Biomechanics

K. H. E. Kroemer

INTRODUCTION

Anthropometry measures and shows the size and mobility of the human body. *Biomechanics* models and describes actions and reactions of the body in mechanical terms. Taking into account also human "signal processing" (by the nervous system), the ergonomist (also called *human factors engineer*) can use this entire knowledge to model the human acting in and interacting with the natural and technical environment. The design task is to employ this knowledge to make the environment (objects, conditions, and tasks) fitting and suitable to the user in order to achieve "ease and efficiency" for the human.

We have been designing most of our human–technology systems for the "regular" adult who is presumed to have

- "Normal" *anthropometry;* that is, with body dimensions such as stature, hand reach, or body weight within an "average" range and with no severe limitations regarding posture or mobility.
- "Normal" *biomechanic* functions, regarding muscular, metabolic, circulatory, and respiratory capacities and nervous control, whose sensory capabilities and intelligence are fully functional.

Handbook of Human Factors and the Older Adult

In fact, some ergonomic texts, implicitly or even explicitly, use as their model the "average male" of North America. Therefore, by habit or for reasons, the normative sterotype of many human factors engineers is the "regular adult" woman or man who is physically and psychologically healthy, who is able and willing to perform.

The following text (in parts adapted from Kroemer, Kroemer, & Kroemer-Elbert, 1994) describes first characteristic of that normative adult. This serves as reference for the following discussion of how older persons may be different in their features and attributes, especially in terms of anthropometry and biomechanics, and how this leads to special concepts and purposes of ergonomic accommodation.

THE NORMATIVE MODEL OF THE "REGULAR ADULT"

How the Body Works

The anthropometric–biomechanical model of the human body consists of *links* (long bones), connected in *articulations* (body joints), each segment embellished with properties of volume and mass. The segments are moved against each other and in relation to an outside reference system by *engines* (muscles) that span the articulations. The body is energized by its *metabolic system,* which transports chemically stored energy (supplied as food and drink) to the muscles where it is transformed into physically useful energy, muscular work (and heat). The body's *circulatory system* distributes energy, oxygen, and metabolic by-products. It is powered by the heart. The functioning of these body systems can be assessed via physiological measures.

The "stick person" of articulated powered links is the 17th century concept of Giovanni Alfonso Borelli, taken up two centuries later by Weber and Weber in their discussion of the mechanics of the legs, by Harless and von Meyer in their considerations of body mass properties, and by Braune and Fischer for the analysis of the biomechanics of a gun-firing infantryman. In 1873, von Meyer modeled body segments as ellipsoids and spheres. This biomechanical model was refined and expanded by Dempster in the 1950s. The 1960 model of Simons and Gardner still depicted body segments as uniform geometric shapes: cylinders for the appendages, neck, and torso, and a sphere for the head. Using equations developed by Barter in 1957, inertial parameters were computed for the geometric forms and the moments of inertia of body segments, and the total body (see Kroemer, Snook, Meadows, & Deutsch, 1988, for more historical details). This elementary work still is the basis for much of the present biodynamic modeling of the human body.

Åstrand and Rodahl (1977) compared the body, in terms of how it generates and transforms energy, with a combustion engine: fuel is combusted with oxygen, yielding mechanical energy to move body parts against resistance. Blood brings fuel (oxygen and carbohydrate and fat derivatives) to the combustion sites (muscles and other organs), and it removes metabolic by-produces (particularly carbon dioxide, water, heat) for dissipation (at lung and skin surfaces). Thus, the processes that convert chemically stored energy into mechanically useful work depend on close interaction of the metabolic, circulatory, and respiratory systems.

The *ability to perform physical work* is different from person to person. It depends on many components and their interactions including body size, health, motivation, and the environment. These relations are sketched in Figure 1.

Only when all systems work well together, can the human body function as an strong energy generator. With changes in age and health, or during pregnancy, one system or several of these vital systems may become less capable. This alone leads to a decrease in work capacity that, however, is often accompanied by anthropometric and biomechanical changes, usually detrimental (such as reduced muscle mass due to less use).

Borelli's model applies to all people, but link lengths, joint mobilities, as well as muscular, metabolic and circulatory capabilities change systematically from infancy into agedness. Furthermore, persons with impairments (age or injury related) have specific limitations that make them different from the common biomechanical model.

How Body Control Works

The human body has two parallel control systems, the hormonal (endocrine) and the nervous systems, which have similar functions. Yet, in ergonomic terms, little is known at present about human engineering use of the hormonal system, while neuromuscular functions are rather well researched; hence, primarily these are discussed in the following text.

Functionally, one may divide the *nervous system* into three sections. The *sensory* (afferent) part receives information from internal body sensors and from peripheral sensors and transmits the information to the *central* part. Here, the signals are processed, decisions are made, and control signals generated. These control commands are transmitted to body organs, including muscles, in the *motor* (efferent) part.

Anatomically, one divides the nervous system into three major subdivi-

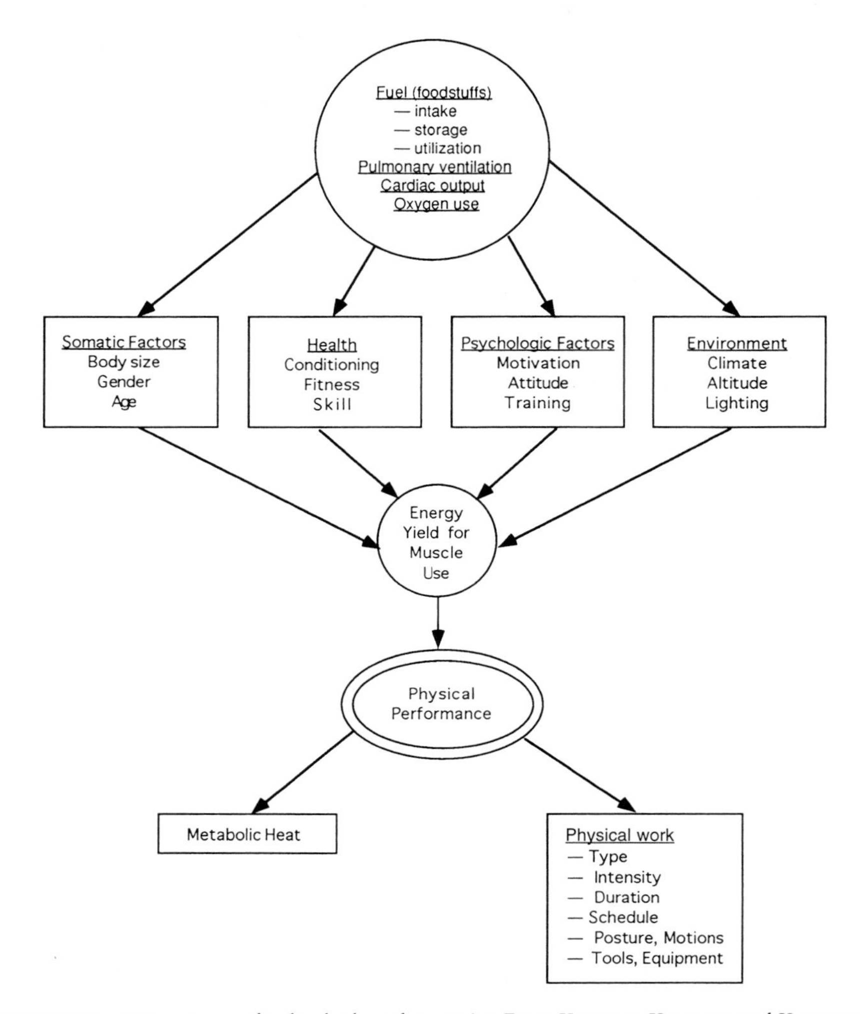

FIGURE 1 Determiners of individual work capacity. From Kroemer, Kroemer, and Kroemer-Elbert (1994), *Ergonomics—How to Design for Ease and Efficiency*, with permission by the publisher, Prentice-Hall. All rights reserved.

sions: the *central* nervous system (CNS) includes brain and spinal cord; it has primarily control functions. The *peripheral* nervous system (PNS) includes the cranial and spinal nerves and their extensions to all body parts; it transmits signals to and from the center, but usually does not control. The *autonomic* nervous system consists of the sympathetic and the parasympathetic subsystems that regulate, among other involuntary functions, those of smooth and cardiac muscle and of blood vessels, digestion, and glucose release in the liver. (The autonomic system is not under conscious control.)

The *spinal cord* is an extension of the brain. The uppermost section of the spinal cord contains the 12 pairs of *cranial nerves,* which serve structures in the head and neck, as well as the lungs, heart, pharynx and larynx, and many abdominal organs. Thirty-one pairs of *spinal nerves* pass out between the appropriate vertebrae and serve defined sectors of the rest of the body. Nerves are mixed sensory and motor pathways. Figure 2 shows how the spinal nerves emanating from sections of the spinal column innervate de-

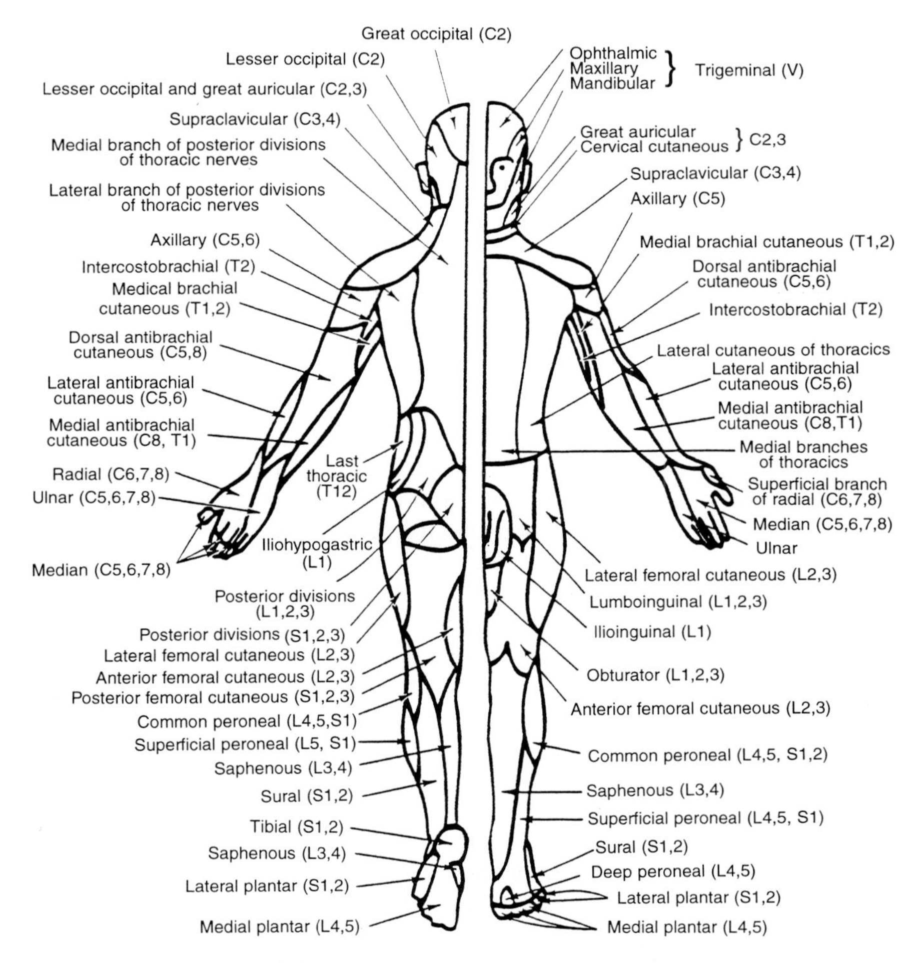

FIGURE 2 Territories of the major nerves. From Kroemer, Kroemer, and Kroemer-Elbert (1994), *Ergonomics—How to Design for Ease and Efficiency,* with permission of the publisher, Prentice-Hall.

fined areas of the body. Damages to these nerves can cut sensory feedback from these parts and their efficient motor and autonomic control.

The central nervous system receives information from internal receptors, *interoceptors,* that report on conditions within the body: digestion, circulation, excretion, hunger, thirst, sexual arousal, and feeling well or sick. *Exteroceptors* respond to light, sound, touch, temperature, electricity, and chemicals. Since all of these sensations come from various parts of the body, external and internal receptors together are also called *somesthetic sensors.*

Internal receptors include the *proprioceptors.* Among these are the muscle spindles, nerve filaments wrapped around muscle fibers that detect the amount of stretch of the muscle. Golgi organs are associated with muscle tendons and detect their tension. Ruffini organs are kinesthetic receptors that respond to angulation of the joints. The sensors in the vestibulum report the position of the head.

Exteroceptors provide information about the interaction between the body and the outside: sight (vision), sound (audition), taste (gustation), smell (olfaction), temperature, electricity, and touch (taction)—see later. Free nerve endings, Meissner's and Pacinian corpuscles, and other receptors are located throughout the skin of the body, however, in different densities. They transmit the sensations of touch, pressure, and pain. Since the nerve pathways from the free endings interconnect extensively, the sensations reported are not always specific to a modality; for example, very hot or cold sensations can be associated with pain, which may also be caused by hard pressure on the skin.

Signals from internal and external sensors are of particular importance for the control of everyday life: the sensations of touch, pressure, and pain can be used as feedback to the body regarding the direction and intensity of muscular activities transmitted to an outside object.

Traditionally, the human as a sequential processor of signals has been modeled in some detail, shown in Figure 3. Information (in some form of energy) is received by a sensor and impulses sent along the *afferent* pathways of the PNS to the CNS. Here, the signals are processed and an action chosen. Appropriate feedforward impulses are generated and transmitted along the *efferent* pathways of the PNS to the *effectors* (voice, hand, etc.). Of course, many feedback loops exist although only a few are shown in the model.

Both sides of the processor model can be analyzed further. Figure 4 illustrates the input side; it shows how *distal stimuli* provide information, usually visual, auditory, or tactile. To be sensed, the stimulus must appear in a form to which human sensors can respond; it must have suitable qualities and quantities of electromagnetic, mechanical, electrical, or chemical energy. If the distal events do not generate *proximal stimuli* that can be sensed

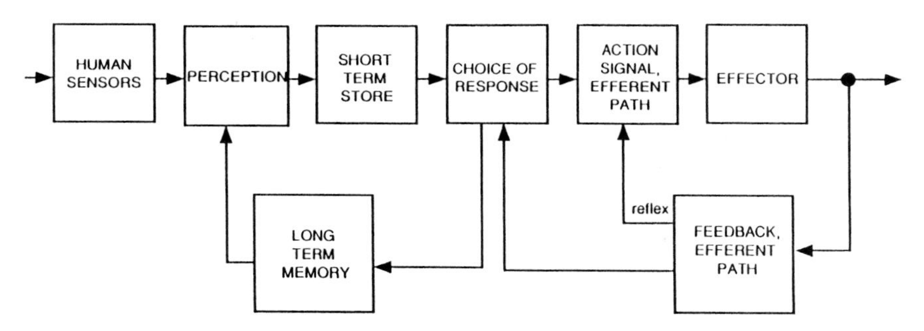

FIGURE 3 The human processor. From Kroemer, Kroemer, and Kroemer-Elbert (1994), *Ergonomics—How to Design for Ease and Efficiency,* with permission of the publisher, Prentice-Hall.

directly, the distal events must be transformed into energies that can trigger human sensations. For this, (input) *transducers* are designed by the ergonomist; for example, a "display" of some kind, such as a computer screen, dial, or a light or sound can serve as transducer.

Provision of suitable proximal stimuli (if needed through transducers, often amplified) is of particular importance for persons whose sensory capabilities are different from the normative adult. This important ergonomic task also concerns the provision of suitable outputs, especially to assist impaired persons.

On the output side, the actions of a human *effector* (such as hand or foot) may directly control the "machine" or one may need another (output) transducer; for example, movement of a steering wheel by the human hand may be amplified by auxillary energy ("power steering"). Figure 5 portrays the model. Recognizing the need for a transducer and providing information for its suitable design is among the primary tasks of the ergonomist or human factors engineer.

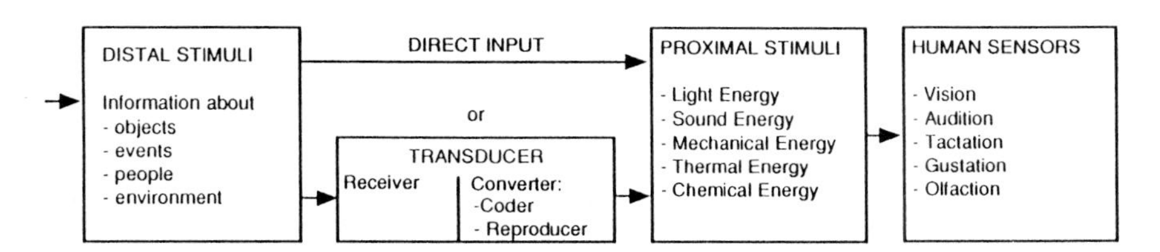

FIGURE 4 Energy input side. From Kroemer, Kroemer, and Kroemer-Elbert (1994), *Ergonomics—How to Design for Ease and Efficiency,* with permission of the publisher, Prentice-Hall.

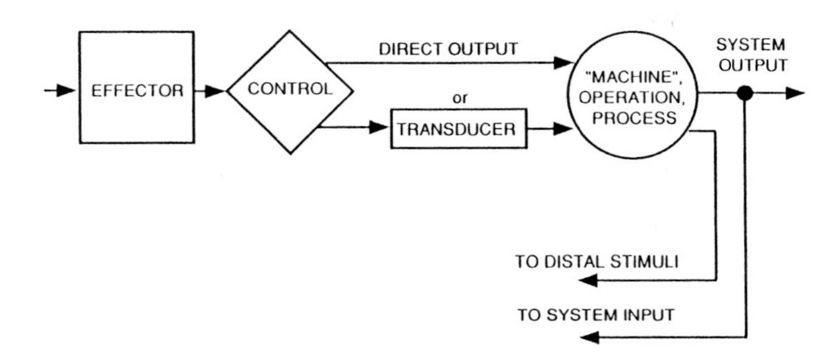

FIGURE 5 Energy output side. From Kroemer, Kroemer, and Kroemer-Elbert (1994), *Ergonomics—How to Design for Ease and Efficiency,* with permission of the publisher, Prentice-Hall.

Note that the traditional model of a sequential signal processing system may be too simplistic to describe the complex simultaneous "ecological" interactions. Still, nearly all current ergonomic information assumes the singular step-by-step sequence.

An aging (or impaired) person often has changed (usually reduced) control capabilities in sensory input; afferent signal transmission; signal processing, decision making, and generation of output signals; motor signal transmission; and efferent execution.

ANTHROMECHANIC (ANTHROPOMETRIC AND BIOMECHANIC) CHANGES WITH AGING

Most designs are for the normative adult population in the age range of about 20 to 50 years. This is the group of most interest to industry and society as movers and contributors to the gross national product. Although the anthropometry, biomechanics, physiology, and psychology of adults in Europe and North America are fairly well known, large subgroups of this population—pregnant women, children, the aging and the disabled—have not been studied extensively enough for complete ergonomic design. In the early 1970s, the first conference on ethnic variables in human factors engineering provided a compilation of worldwide ergonomic information (Chapanis, 1975), but even today too little information of direct human engineering relevance is known about populations outside Europe and North America (Kroemer et al., 1994) although a 1994 symposium on Productive Aging has provided more insight (Kumashiro, 1995).

FITTING BODY AND MIND

While the statistical "average" is a descriptor of the central properties of a Gaussian data distribution, people do not come assembled of parts that are all average nor in any other given single percentile value; instead, every individual has dimensions, physiological characteristics, and psychological traits at different percentile ranges. Taking into account human variability is the hallmark of ergonomics.

Body dimensions of people change slowly at first with aging, then become more and more apparent in most persons. There are usually gradual decreases but occasionally sharp declines in strength and work capabilities; the losses become more pronounced in the years of old age.

Muscle strength is determined not only by the bulk of available muscle mass, which can change through training or lack thereof, but also depends on the skill and willingness to exert the inherent capabilities. There is close interaction between types of muscular exertion (such as one-time strength versus endurance work) and the demands on the metabolic, circulatory, and respiratory systems, as discussed before.

The *metabolism* of a teenager and of an old person are likely to be rather different, as are their subjective judgments of the external climate or of their "efforts" in performing the same physical task. The *thermoregulation* of the body in children, pregnant women, and the elderly is apparently quite different, although neither systematically nor completely researched yet.

The *respiratory system* absorbs oxygen from the inhaled air into the bloodstream, extracts from it carbon dioxide, water, and heat, and expels these into the air to be exhaled. The *circulatory system* transports oxygen and energy carriers to the consuming organs (such as muscles) and removes metabolic by-products (CO_2, water, heat) to the lungs and the skin for dispersion. The heart pumps the blood through the system. The number of heart beats per minute provides a convenient and rather accurate assessment for most circulatory efforts and for the physical effort of the body in general. In healthy persons, oxygen consumption correlates well with heart rate.

The body is a generator of heat, the dissipation of which must be diminished in a cold environment and facilitated in a hot environment. Knowing the interaction between climate and body, the ergonomist can take specific measures to control the environment and the work requirements.

Given current understanding of the human mind, it is still futuristic to expect that devices can be controlled by thinking about them. Yet, some success based on empirical knowledge has been made, for example, in rehabilitation engineering: one may electrically stimulate paralyzed muscles for feedforward or use stimulation of skin sensors for feedback control of prostheses.

As mentioned earlier, it is the ergonomist's task to provide information about outside events as input for the user in such modalities and quantities that the information can be perceived unambiguously and quickly; for this, transducers may be necessary, such as visible lights indicating otherwise insensible radiation. Human output may have to be amplified, as by a power-assist device for automobile brakes and steering. Suitable selection of stimuli can reduce response time, but the same external stimuli may trigger different, even unpredictable, response in children, aging persons, or impaired individuals.

Human *vision* is known exactly, including how it changes with age, illness, or injury. The same is true about *hearing*, particularly regarding its changes hearing loss due to aging together or noise induced. While the sensations related to *taction* (namely, touch, pain, temperature, and electricity) as well as smell and taste have been researched for nearly two centuries, they are still not well defined and not quantitatively measured. They appear to be interconnected, depending on prevailing conditions, and are quite different from person to person.

Hence, with respect to seeing and hearing we can design technical systems and assistive devices so that they meet the sensory needs of most persons (unless the nervous system is dysfunctional). Yet, as regards the other senses, general and specific uncertainties prevail even for "regular" adults. The changes in these experienced from childhood to advanced age or associated with illness or injury are difficult to define and measure; this explains the rather imprecise, tentative, and often contradictory statements in the literature. Much basic research needs to be done, and the specific needs of special groups, such as the aging or impaired individuals, must be specifically assessed so that they then can be met by proper ergonomic designs.

An example of such assessment of needs and a derived ergonomic solution is that of signaling when it is safe for a pedestrian to cross a busy road at an intersection. The normal solution is to provide a light system to the walker, with green meaning "go" and red meaning "stay." For people who cannot see or cannot distinguish red and green, acoustical indicators can be added, such as a chirping sound for "go" and a cuckooing sound for "stay." This redundancy has proven to be very advantageous even for "regular" persons, as well as for children and elderly people. But it does not help people who are blind and deaf, or those who have difficulties ambulating.

Describing Variability

Ergonomic descriptors of the human, especially anthropometric, biomechanical, and physiological data show variability stemming mainly from

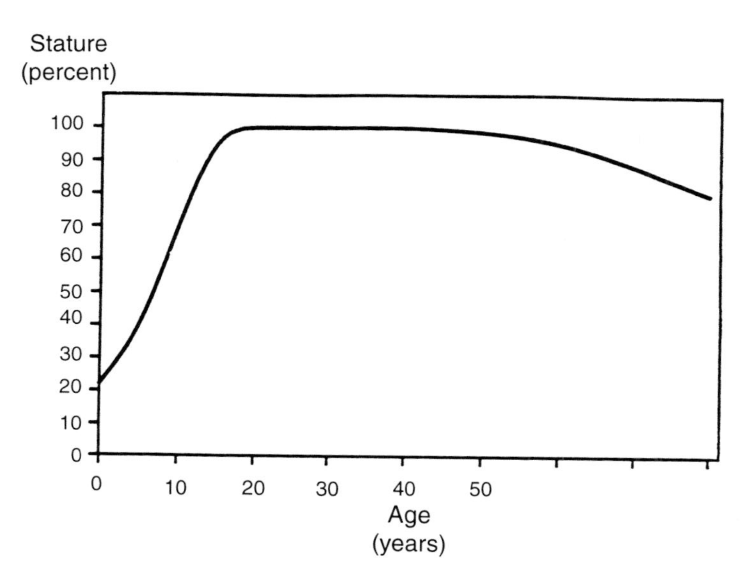

FIGURE 6 Approximate changes in stature with age. From Kroemer, Kroemer, and Kroemer-Elbert (1994), *Ergonomics—How to Design for Ease and Efficiency*, with permission of the publisher, Prentice-Hall.

four sources: intraindividual variability, interindividual variability, secular variability, and measurement variability.

Intraindividual Variability

The size of the same body segment of a given person or that person's strength changes with age, depending also on nutrition, exercise, and health. Such alterations become apparent in a longitudinal (as opposed to cross-sectional) study, in which an individual is observed over years and decades. Most (but not all) such variations from youth to age follow the scheme shown in Figure 6. During childhood and adolescence, body dimensions such as stature, muscle strength, and endurance change rapidly. From the early 20s into the 50s, little change occurs in general, with stature declining slightly. From the 60s on, many dimensions decline, while others—for example, weight or bone circumference—often increase.

Interindividual Variability

Individuals differ from each other in many respects. Data describing a population sample are usually collected in a cross-sectional study, in which every subject is measured at the same moment in time, meaning that people of different age, health, and fitness are included in the sample set. The anthropometric and biomechanical data are found in most textbooks are gathered in cross-sectional studies.

Secular Variability
There is some factual and much anecdotal evidence that European, North Americans, and Japanese people nowadays are larger (although possibly neither stronger nor more able to do demanding physical work), on average, than their ancestors. Also, older people tend to live longer; thus, the portion of aged people in the work force and especially among those retired from work is rapidly increasing, at least in Europe and North America. Probably, improved nutrition, hygiene, and health care have allowed persons to achieve more of their genetically determined potential.

Measurement Variability
Measurements can be done with differing levels of care in selecting population samples, using measurement instruments, storing the measured data, and applying statistical treatments.

Normal (Gaussian) distributions of data can be fully described by the statistics of *average* (mean), *standard deviation* (SD), and *sample size* (N). Fortunately, ergonomic data are usually distributed in a reasonably normal distribution (with exceptions, such as with some muscle strength and physiological data). One easy way to check on data diversity of a normal distribution is to divide the standard deviation in question by its average to get the *coefficient of variation,* CV. In most cross-sectional studies of adult body dimensions, the CV is in the neighborhood of 5%, in most strength data around 10%. Even if the distribution is not normal, percentile values can be established, if needed, by simply counting or estimating.

The *coefficient of determination,* R^2, measures the proportion of variation in the dependent variable (often designated y) associated with the independent variable (x). R^2 is the square of the correlation coefficient r between the two variables used in a bivariate regression equation or among more variables in multiple regression equations.

DESIGNING FOR REAL PEOPLE INSTEAD OF FOR PHANTOMS, GHOSTS, AND THE "AVERAGE PERSON"

Given the varying correlations among body measures, the attempt is futile to express "all" body characteristics as related to one "basic" denominator. Yet, many designers used a scheme that misleadingly expressed body heights, body breadths, and segment lengths in terms of percent of stature; for instance, hip breadth supposedly was "19.1% of stature"—deceptive nonsense, of course, because hip breadth varies widely between men and women as groups and among individuals, furthermore nothing can be fittingly designed for a fixed "average" hip breadth.

In spite of the obvious fallacy of the "single percentile model," too many such constructs have been generated, assuming that homunculi exist whose body segments are all of the same percentile value. Not only the 50th-percentile phantom (the "average person") has been used as a design template, but other ghostly figures have been created that have; for example, all 5th or 95th percentile values. Of course, designs for these figments hardly fit actual users.

Yet, some ergonomists, physiologists, and physicians still express body attributes in terms of stature (probably because body height is easily measured), disregarding the lack of logical or statistical correlation. For example, body weight currently is often expressed in relation to stature, even though the correlation between these two variables is usually only about 0.4. Other indices use stature squared, even cubed!

If the data distribution is known for which design should be achieved, the appropriate procedure is first to determine the range or spread of data that needs to be considered for proper fit. In many cases, at least the 5th to the 95th percentile of the appropriate data range needs to be considered, subsections often put together into sizing groups (tariffs) such as in clothing, or the product can be made adjustable, such as the height of work chairs.

Given percentile values can be determined from any known distribution, most easily for a normal (Gaussian) distribution, where one simply multiplies the standard deviation by known factors, with the results either added to or subtracted from the mean. (For more information about this procedure, see ergonomic textbooks, such as Kroemer et al., 1994; Roebuck, 1995).

Table 1 contains an overview of the trends of changes in these functions, discussed previously, that are of main concern to the ergonomist. However, it must be recognized that these changes are individually quite different in their temporal development, magnitude, and importance.

There is a curious use of "aging terminology" in the United States: a "middle-aged" person becomes "older" at 45 years of age; "elderly" at 65 years; "old" as one reaches 75 years; and "very old" or "old old" if one lives beyond 85 years of age. Habitually, anthropometric and most demographic and capability-related information is collected in five-year intervals until the age of 65, and then just lumped together for the remaining years, with only occasionally a time marker set at 75 years of age.

The majority of "adults of working age" can be statistically treated as a

TABLE 1
Changes in Function as Compared to "Regular Adults"

	During pregnancy	During childhood	During aging	Permanent disability
Energetic capabilities (metabolism, circulation, respiration)	Less and decreasing	Less but improving	Less and decreasing	No general statement possible, depends on individual case
Biomechanical capabilities (strength, mobility, endurance)	Less and decreasing	Less but improving	Less and decreasing	No general statement possible, depends on individual case
Capability to endure and function in heat and cold	Somewhat less and decreasing	Less but improving	Less and decreasing	No general statement possible, depends on individual case
Stress tolerance	Somewhat less and decreasing	Unknown	Depends on individual and circumstances	No general statement possible, depends on individual case
Sensations, perception, decision making, controlling actions	No change (except in taste and smell)	Not systematically known	Less and decreasing	No general statement possible, depends on individual case

"set" that may be divided into "subsets" according to physical criteria, such as size, strength, endurance, or related to psychological or cognitive traits. Usually these (sub)sets include sufficiently large numbers to apply common statistical procedures to describe their design-relevant characteristics (such as body size) by ranges, percentiles, averages, and standard deviations, which in turn allow the use of group design approaches, such as "tariffing" of clothes. Not so for the aging. Their descriptors (of features and capabilities) change with aging, and their needs are usually individually unique and so require specific ergonomic solutions.

CHANGES IN ANTHROPOMETRIC CHARACTERISTICS

A thorough collection of anthropometric data available in the mid-1970s was contained in the NASA/Webb sourcebook published in 1978. Juergens, Aune, and Pieper (1990) attempted to classify the total population of the earth into 20 area groups and estimate their main anthropometric dimensions. Because of many voids, they had to "guesstimate" and leave out certain subgroups (e.g., pygmies). Publications describing national and ethnic populations have been compiled, for example, by Kroemer et al. (1994), Pheasant (1986), and especially by Roebuck (1995).

The most reliable observations of secular anthropometric trends are from military surveys; for example, measurements of U.S. soldiers have been minutely recorded since the Civil War. Soldiers are certainly a subsample of the general population, but they are selected to be youngish, healthy, and neither extremely small nor big. Thus, their body dimensions may not exactly represent the adult civilian population, although it appears that there are no major differences in head, hand, and foot sizes (McConville, Robinette, & Churchill, 1981). An analysis of 22 body dimensions of white, black, Hispanic, and Asian, female and male U.S. Army soldiers, taken in 1988, showed that secular increases in stature and sitting height seem to be slowing down: it now takes about 20 years before the gains are measurable (with current techniques), by which time they are approximately another centimeter. Leg length is not changing appreciably, but body weight is still increasing by two to three kilograms per decade. Shoulder breadth and chest circumference are increasing at rates of about one centimeter per decade. Altogether, white, black, and Hispanic U.S. Army soldiers show similar changes, while soldiers of Asian extraction exhibit quite different trends, which may be explained by recent immigration to the United States (Greiner & Gordon, 1990). Data from Japan indicated initially a much faster growth

TABLE 2

U.S. Adults' Body Dimensions, Female/Male, in cm.

	Percentiles			Standard Deviation
	Female 5th Male	Female 50th Male	Female 95th Male	Female S Male
Heights				
(*f* above floor, *s* above seat)				
Standing				
Stature ("height")^f	152.78 / 164.69	162.94 / 175.58	173.73 / 186.65	6.36 / 6.68
Eye height^f	141.52 / 152.82	151.61 / 163.39	162.13 / 174.29	6.25 / 6.57
Shoulder (acromial) height^f	124.09 / 134.16	133.36 / 144.25	143.20 / 154.56	5.79 / 6.20
Elbow height^f	92.63 / 99.52	99.79 / 107.25	107.40 / 115.28	4.48 / 4.81
Wrist height^f	72.79 / 77.79	79.03 / 84.65	85.51 / 91.52	3.86 / 4.15
Crotch height^f	70.02 / 76.44	77.14 / 83.72	84.58 / 91.64	4.41 / 4.62
Sitting				
Height (sitting)^s	79.53 / 85.45	85.20 / 91.39	91.02 / 97.19	3.49 / 3.56
Eye height^s	68.46 / 73.50	73.87 / 79.20	79.43 / 84.80	3.32 / 3.42
Shoulder (acromial) height^s	50.91 / 54.85	55.55 / 59.78	60.36 / 64.63	2.86 / 2.96
Elbow height^s	17.57 / 18.41	22.05 / 23.06	26.44 / 27.37	2.68 / 2.72
Thigh height^s	14.04 / 14.86	15.89 / 16.82	18.02 / 18.99	1.21 / 1.26
Knee height^f	47.40 / 51.44	51.54 / 55.88	56.02 / 60.57	2.63 / 2.79
Popliteal height^f	35.13 / 39.46	38.94 / 43.41	42.94 / 47.63	2.37 / 2.49
Depths				
Forward (thumbtip) reach	67.67 / 73.92	73.46 / 80.08	79.67 / 86.70	3.64 / 3.92
Buttock–knee distance (sitting)	54.21 / 56.90	58.89 / 61.64	63.98 / 66.74	2.96 / 2.99
Buttock–popliteal distance (sitting)	44.00 / 45.81	48.17 / 50.04	52.77 / 54.55	2.66 / 2.66
Elbow–fingertip distance	40.62 / 44.79	44.29 / 48.40	48.25 / 52.42	2.34 / 2.33
Chest depth	20.86 / 20.96	23.94 / 24.32	27.78 / 28.04	2.11 / 2.15

Breadths				
Forearm–forearm breadth	41.47 / 47.74	46.85 / 54.61	52.84 / 62.06	3.47 / 4.36
Hip breadth (sitting)	34.25 / 32.87	38.45 / 36.68	43.22 / 41.16	2.72 / 2.52
Head dimensions				
Head circumference	52.25 / 54.27	54.62 / 56.77	57.05 / 59.35	1.46 / 1.54
Head breadth	13.66 / 14.31	14.44 / 15.17	15.27 / 16.08	0.49 / 0.54
Interpupillary breadth	5.66 / 5.88	6.23 / 6.47	6.85 / 7.10	0.36 / 0.37
Foot dimensions				
Foot length	22.44 / 24.88	24.44 / 26.97	26.46 / 29.20	1.22 / 1.31
Foot breadth	8.16 / 9.23	8.97 / 10.06	9.78 / 10.95	0.49 / 0.53
Lateral malleolus height[f]	5.23 / 5.84	6.06 / 6.71	6.97 / 7.64	0.53 / 0.55
Hand dimensions				
Circumference, metacarpale	17.25 / 19.85	18.62 / 21.38	20.03 / 23.03	0.85 / 0.97
Hand length	16.50 / 17.87	18.05 / 19.38	19.69 / 21.06	0.97 / 0.98
Hand breadth, metacarpale	7.34 / 8.36	7.94 / 9.04	8.56 / 9.76	0.38 / 0.42
Thumb breadth, interphalangeal	1.86 / 2.19	2.07 / 2.41	2.29 / 2.65	0.13 / 0.14
Weight (in kg)	39.2[a] / 57.7[a]	62.01 / 78.49	84.8[a] / 99.3[a]	13.8[a] / 12.6[a]

Note: In this table, the entries in the 50th percentile column are actually "mean" (average) values. The 5th and 95th percentile values are from measured data, not calculated (except for weight). Thus, the values given may be slightly different from those obtained by subtracting 1.65 S from the mean (50th percentile) or by adding 1.65 S to it.

[a] Estimated by Kroemer.

Source: Adapted from Gordon et al. (1989); Greiner (1991).

TABLE 3
Anthropometric Data on the Elderly: Means and Standard Deviations

Age range: Sample size:	50–100[a] 822	60–69[b] 43	60–69[c] 72	65–69[d] 24	65–74[e] 72	65–90[f] 184	66–70[a] 169	70+[b] 12	70+[d] 20	70+[c] 28	72–91[e] 130	75–94[e] 40
Stature, against wall		172.8 (6.6)		171.9 (6.6)				171.5 (9.0)	170.4 (7.5)			
Stature, free standing	175.1 (8.9)		172.6 (6.4)	171.2 (6.6)		169.0			169.6 (7.6)	171.9 (8.4)	168.4 (5.3)	
Sitting height	79.9 (5.3)	90.8 (3.0)	90.8 (2.9)	90.0 (2.9)				89.5 (3.5)	89.0 (3.4)	89.8 (3.9)	88.3 (3.1)	
Knee height		53.9 (2.5)	53.6 (2.5)					53.5 (3.4)	53.2 (2.9)	53.7 (3.2)	53.8 (2.1)	
Popliteal height	42.1 (3.5)		42.1 (2.3)							42.1 (3.0)	44.0 (2.1)	
Thigh clearance height			19.7 (1.4)							14.8 (1.2)		
Hip breadth	37.4 (3.9)			36.0 (2.3)					35.8 (1.7)	37.8 (2.4)		
Bideltoid breadth			45.3 (2.4)	45.1 (2.1)					44.7 (1.6)	45.0 (1.7)	43.4 (2.3)	
Biacromial breadth			38.9 (1.7)							39.2 (1.8)	37.8 (1.6)	
Hand breadth	7.7 (0.6)		8.5 (0.4)	8.5 (0.4)					8.5 (0.4)	8.6 (0.4)	8.4 (0.4)	
Head breadth			15.5 (0.5)	15.5 (0.5)					15.5 (0.5)	15.5 (0.4)	15.4 (0.5)	
Foot breadth			9.8 (0.6)							9.9 (0.5)	10.0 (0.5)	
Head circumference			57.1 (1.4)	57.1 (1.3)					58.0 (1.4)	57.4 (1.6)	56.9 (1.8)	
Calf circumference			35.9 (2.5)	36.0 (2.9)					34.7 (2.1)	34.3 (2.2)	34.3 (2.7)	
Chest circ., resting			99.6 (7.1)	99.9 (6.3)					99.6 (5.5)	99.7 (5.9)	96.2 (7.6)	
Chest circ., maximum			101.8 (6.9)	101.7 (6.1)					101.5 (5.4)	101.7 (5.7)	98.7 (7.4)	

Chest circ., minimum		97.6 (7.2)	97.5 (6.5)				97.8 (5.6)	97.9 (6.0)	94.5 (7.6)	
Upper arm circumference		30.9 (2.7)	30.5 (2.6)				30.0 (2.4)	28.7 (2.8)		
Waist circumference		95.5 (9.3)	97.4 (8.9)				97.1 (8.0)	97.0 (7.6)		
Head length		19.6 (0.6)	19.6 (0.6)				19.5 (0.6)	19.7 (0.7)	19.7 (0.6)	
Hand length	175.5 (1.2)	18.9 (0.9)	18.9 (0.9)				18.8 (0.9)	19.0 (1.0)	18.8 (0.8)	
Buttock-knee length		58.6 (3.0)						58.4 (3.2)	59.1 (2.4)	
Buttock-popliteal length	46.3 (3.6)	48.2 (2.8)						48.1 (3.1)	47.2 (2.5)	
Elbow to middle finger length	44.2 (2.8)	46.8 (2.0)	46.8 (1.9)				46.6 (2.5)	46.9 (2.8)	46.4 (1.8)	
Shoulder to elbow length		37.3 (1.8)	37.4 (1.7)				37.0 (2.1)	37.4 (2.2)	36.9 (1.7)	
Forward reach		84.2 (3.7)						85.9 (5.4)	86.9 (3.8)	
Span		178.7 (7.5)	178.8 (7.5)				177.6 (9.0)	179.2 (9.9)	174.0 (7.0)	
Skinfold (triceps)(right)			1.1 (0.4)		1.2 (0.3)			0.9 (0.4)	1.1 (0.4)	
Skinfold (subscap.)(right)			1.7 (0.8)					1.5 (0.7)	1.6 (0.7)	
Foot height			26.3 (1.2)	26.4 (1.2)			26.5 (1.3)	26.8 (1.4)	26.0 (1.0)	
Weight (kg)	63.7	76.6 (1.1)	76.4 (1.0)	65.6 (11.6)	63.7		74.3 (0.9)	75.3 (9.0)	69.0 (10.5)	63.7 (11.7)
Grip strength (left)(N)		432 (88)				323 (58)		352 (88)	262 (80)	
Grip strength (right)(N)		461 (88)				370 (68)		412 (88)	283 (78)	

Note: All measures in centimeters unless otherwise noted. Letters *a–f* indicate different surveys; see the 1990 article by Kelly and Kroemer for details.
Source: Excerpted from Kelly and Kroemer (1990).

than found among Caucasians, but it seems to slow down now (Roebuck, 1995; Roebuck, Smith, & Raggio, 1988). An excerpt from the U.S. Army data appears in Table 2.

Anthropometric information reported in the literature on sufficiently large samples is, as a rule, the result of cross-sectional surveys. The apparently most recent compilation of available data is listed in Table 3. It exemplifies the current problems with anthropometric information: most of the samples are exceedingly small; surveys are done for a few age ranges only; there are no distinctions between ethnic origins, regions, socioeconomic status, health, or other attributes that are codeterminers of anthropometry. Given the limitation, in fact paucity, of these data from the United States, one anticipates even poorer and less complete data from other regions of the earth.

The apparent *height loss with age* (of about 1 cm per decade) starting in the 30s may be a result of (1) flattening of the cartilaginous disks between the vertebrae; (2) a flattening or thinning of the bodies of the vertebrae; (3) a general thinning of all weight-carrying cartilages; (4) a change in the S-shape of the spinal column in the side view, particularly an increased kyphosis in the thoracic area (humpback); (5) in some cases, scoliosis, a lateral deviation from the straight line displayed by the spinal column in the frontal view; and (6) possibly bowing of the legs and flattening of the feet (Barlow, Braid, & Jayson, 1990; Stoudt, 1981). As groups, American men usually have their *largest body weights* in their 30s, then lose weight with aging; American women are relatively light in their 20s, but then increase their weight with age, becoming heaviest, on average, at about 60 years (Annis, Case, Clauser, & Bradtmiller, 1991).

Life expectancy of humans has increased dramatically. The average life span was about 20 years in "prehistory" (until about 1000 B.C.) and reached only the low 20s in Ancient Greece and Rome. In the Middle Ages (about 1000 A.D.), the life span had increased in Western Europe to the 30s and included the low 40s late in the 19th century. In Colonial America, until about 1700, the average life span was 35 years. It increased to about 50 years by 1900, and to about 75 around 1990 in the United States (Committee on an Aging Society, 1988; Kermis, 1984). The expected life span depends on genetic heritage, gender, climate, hygiene, nutrition, diseases, wars, and accidents. American demographic aspects regarding both current and future aging cohorts have been discussed by Annis et al. (1991), Czaja (1990a, 1990b, 1991), National Institutes on Aging (1982); Serow and Sly (1988), Soldo and Longino (1988), Verbrugge (1989), and by Coleman (1993) for the United Kingdom.

The aging subpopulation rapidly increases in the U.S. population in terms of absolute numbers and percentages. Older employees now constitute a large portion of the work force. Daily living requirements of the retired population must be met, whether they live independently or in care facilities. Habitat, furniture, transportation, workstations, tools, controls, and displays, all must be designed (or redesigned) to fully utilize functional capabilities and help overcome age-related deficiencies.

Measurement of body dimensions is done habitually in a cross-sectional approach: one measures all available people and then lumps together their measurements, commonly within certain age brackets. Usually this does not create a problem in describing the "young adult" population, because attributes do not change very much in its age span. However, his is a major problem in the description of the aging (as well as of children) for two reasons:

- Among the aging, some persons change dimensions rapidly within a few years; for example, in stature because of posture and shrinking thickness of spinal disks or in weight because of changes in nutrition, metabolism, and health; and in measurements of musculature and strength because of changes in activity levels, habits, and health. Other aging people, in contrast, show little change over long periods of time.
- The age brackets used for surveys are rather wide, usually encompassing decades or even longer time spans, as opposed to the common five years in younger cohorts. Thus, people with very different dimensions are contained in each observation sample.

Therefore, chronological age is not a good classifying criterion for the aging (or for children). They would be better described by a longitudinal procedure in which changes in body dimensions and capacities are observed within one individual over many years; yet, few such data are available.

CHANGES IN BIOMECHANICAL CHARACTERISTICS

Together with the anthropometric changes, there are numerous alternations with increasing age in musculoskeletal, biomechanical, and control features.

Particularly the long *bones* become larger in outer diameter, and larger in inner diameter (hollower), and larger pores appear; total bone mass decreases. The mineral content changes. These are the major components in age-related osteoporosis. Biomechanically, the bones become stiffer and more brittle (Osthere & Gold, 1991). Women and persons who exercise little are more exposed to this development than men and active people. The changes in bone structure are associated with an increased likelihood of breakage as a result of falls or other accidents in which sudden forces and impulses are exerted on the body. Injuries to the pelvic girdle, hip joint, or femur are particularly frequent in older women, followed by bone injuries to the shoulder and arms.

Smoothness of the bony surfaces in joints, the thickness of joint linings, the supply of synovial fluids, the elasticity and resilience of joint capsules and ligaments all diminish. This leads to reduced mobility in the joints, to arthrosis and painful arthritis. The spinal column is often affected in terms of mobility, curvature, and strength (Olczyk, 1993; Spence, 1989).

Well-used *muscles* can retain their capabilities into old age, but disuse, often accompanied by decreased circulatory supply, leads to a degenerative loss of musculature (as reduction of diameter and number of fibers) and ensuing permanent loss of strength capabilities.

Respiration capabilities reduce with increasing age, mostly because the alveoli in the lungs are less able to perform the exchanges of gases, that is, oxygen and carbon dioxide. Furthermore, the intercoastal muscles and the chest diaphragm lose some of their ability to generate "breathing space" in the chest, hence vital capacity reduces. This is coupled with reduced blood flow and possibly emphysema, often resulting from smoking.

Blood supply may be diminished by a decrease in elasticity of blood vessels. Resistance to blood passage in vessels may be increased due to deposits along their walls. Blood cell production in the bone marrow is decreased. Thin aging people may have reduced volumes of body fluids.

Heart functions also change. The size of the heart may be reduced. Cardiac output is lower. Heart rate takes longer to return to resting level after the rate had been increased. Neural control of the heart may be impaired (Spence, 1989).

The ability to cope with the environment depends on detecting, interpreting, and then responding appropriately to sensory information. The numbers of sensor cells in the skin (dermis and epidermis) decrease, together with collagen and elastic fibers. The reduction of sensors and afferent fibers may be combined with reduced nerve conduction velocity. Thus, both *sensation* (the reception of stimuli at sensors and the resulting neural inpulses in the afferent part of the neurons system) and *perception* (the interpretation of the stimuli) change with age, with the information processing particularly slowed (Larish, Kramer, DeAntona, & Strayer, 1993; Manivannan, Czaja, Drury, & Ip, 1993; Rogers, Gilbert, & Fisk, 1993). A reduction and alteration of cells, together with diminished arterial and venous flow in the blood vessels, changes the stimulation and conduction activities in the nervous system. This may lead to increased variability in reception and integration of, and hence varying responses to, external and internal stimuli (Hayslip & Panek, 1989).

In the *brain,* many anatomical changes occur during aging, first observable in healthy persons in their 50s and 60s, becoming often more pronounced in the 70s and very obvious in many people in the 80s. Certain molecules and cells become increasingly impaired or disappear, but these changes are heterogeneous, like the brain itself. Almost 90% of all persons older than 65 years are free of dementia, but about 20% of persons aged 75–84 years show that symptom, and the number jumps to about 50% in people older than 85 years (Selkoe, 1992).

There are various changes in *taste* and *smell,* but they are rather different from person to person, variable over time, and difficult to quantity. The number of taste buds and the production of saliva in the mouth is often reduced. Fissuring of the tongue may occur. The sense of smell is often diminished (Belsky, 1990; Birren & Schaie, 1990; Hayslip & Panek, 1989; Kermis, 1984). The reduction in sensitivity to smells and tastes may simply make the environment less stimulating and hence more boring, but adding more taste ingredients to food and drink, and more intensive smells to the environment, may make up for lost sensitivity.

Changes in *visual functions* are tied to many concurrent anatomical, physiological and psychological processes that develop with age (Committee on Vision, 1987; Cowen, 1988; Fozard, 1990; Sekuler, Kline, & Dismukes, 1982). Using the analogy of the camera, the human eye as a photographic device loses precision. Structures change that bend, guide, and transform light, which reduces the amount of light reaching the retina, and defocuses the image projected to the retina. It becomes difficult to focus on near objects, particularly if they are elevated or move fast (Heuer, Bruewer, Roemer, Kroeger, & Knapp, 1991; Rabbitt, 1991; Tyrell and Leibowitz, 1990). Visual acuity, contrast sensitivity, and related spatial vision capabilities, especially in a "busy" background or "dim" lighting, decline with age. Some problems, such as myopia and hyperopia, can be fairly easily corrected by either contact lenses or eyeglasses; others require more involved chemical or surgical treatment; some are currently untreatable.

Many vision difficulties can be overcome, or at least alleviated, by proper human factors engineering. For example, several ergonomic design principles facilitate exact binocular eye fixation: the first is that the binocular accommodation and vergence positions, to which the eyes return at rest, are quite different from individual to individual, but a given for each person. Hence, one should allow and encourage each person to adjust a target that must be visually fixated to her or his "personal distance." The second practical important finding is that a similar effect on the natural vergence distance is brought about by tilting either the eyes or the head. This explains why people find it more comfortable to lean back in a chair while tilting the head forward/down to look at a close object (at about eye height) than to sit upright: this reduces the natural vergence distance. The third principle is that targets at or near "reading distance" should be distinctly below eye level, particularly if the viewer is elderly, when the head is held erect (Kroemer et al., 1994).

Hearing ability decreases in most persons quite dramatically in the course of adulthood and aging, first at the high frequencies between below 20 kHz to about 10 kHz, then down to about 8000 Hz, an impairment typically recognized as "age-related hearing loss" (presbycusis). Yet, difficulties in hearing may extend into the lower frequencies, and they are often coupled with noise-induced hearing loss.

The changes start at the pinna, the outer ear, which becomes hard, inflexible, and may change in size and shape. Wax buildup is frequent in the ear canal. Often, the Eustachian tube becomes obstructed, leading to an accumulation of fluid in the middle ear. There may also be arthrosic changes in the joints of the bones (anvil, hammer, stirrup) of the middle ear, but these do not usually impair sound transmission to the oval window of the inner ear; however, atrophy and degeneration of hair cells in the basilar membrane of the cochlea occur commonly. Deficiencies in the bioelectric and biomechanical properties of the inner ear fluid and mechanical degeneration of the cochlear partition also appear, often together with a loss of auditory neurons. These degenerations cause either frequency-specific or more general deficiencies in hearing capabilities.

Loss of hearing ability in the higher frequencies of the speech range especially reduces the understanding of consonants that have such high frequency components. This explains why older persons often are unable to discriminate between phonetically similar words, which may make it difficult to follow conversations in a noisy environment (Stine, Wingfield, & Poone, 1989). Severe hearing disorders may lead to speech disorders that, to some extent, may be psychologically founded; for example, if others have to speak loudly for you to hear, they may not want to interact with you to avoid embarrassment. There may be hesitance to speak if it is uncertain what level of loudness is required and that one understands what is said.

Changes in the *somesthetic* (*kinesthetic*) *senses* (those related to touch, pain, vibration, temperature, and motion) are anecdotally well known, but too little reliable quantitative information is available (Boff, Kaufman, & Thomas, 1986). Apparently, absolute thresholds increase, which may be associated with a loss of touch receptors, but that phenomenon and its explanation are still rather unresearched. The same is true for pain sensitivity, which appears much reduced as one gets older. There is a well-observed change in vibratory sensitivity, particularly in the lower extremities. This effect is used in the diagnosis of disorders of the nervous system. Decrease in information from kinesthetic receptors or decrease in the use of that information in the central nervous system may contribute to the higher incidence of falls: with increasing age, one seems to be less able to perceive that one is being moved (such as in an automobile or airplane) or that one moves body parts. Again, surprisingly little is known in a systematic fashion. Possible explanations are reduction in the number of Meissner's corpuscles and other receptor organs in the skin, in the number of myelinated fibers in the peripheral nervous system, and in blood supply (Committee on an Aging Society, 1988; Hayslip & Panek, 1989). Dietary deficiencies might also play a role.

The observed differences in "temperature behavior" may be associated with a decline in the ability of the body's temperature regulation system. Temperature sensitivity also seems to decline, but this may be partially offset by the often observed desire of elderly persons to be in warmer temperatures, outside or within a building. In a colder climate, old persons may be in severe danger if they do not recognize their falling body temperature. Yet, even although a review of the literature on tolerance to cold and heat suggests declines with age, these effects (if true) may be more correlated with health, fitness, and acclimatization than with aging per se (Pandolf, 1991; Young, 1991).

Apparently inevitably, the aging human body and mind lose many capabilities (Belsky, 1990; Birren & Schaie, 1990; Kermis, 1984; Shephard, 1995; Spence, 1989). The most obvious changes are in size and appearance but these anthropometric features interact with (and may be signs of) other alterations, biomechanical and attitudinal in nature.

Associated with the changes in musculoskeletal, respiratory, circulatory, and nervous functions is a general decrease in the capability to maintain postural stability and perform physical work in terms of *strength,* that is, short-time efforts, and *endurance,* that is lasting efforts (Åstrand & Rodahl, 1977; Prieto, Myklebust, & Myklebust, 1993). Hand strength, for example, declines steeply from the 50s on (Haigh, 1993). These declines are often accompanied by increased propensities for acute or cumulative injuries (Chaffin & Ashton-Miller, 1991; Garg, 1991). Yet, the overall capacity to "do physical work" is composed of so many components, both physical and attitudinal, that a wide spread prevails among aging individuals from strong to weak. Jackson, Beard, Wier, and Stuteville (1992) have shown, for example, that, in a cross-sectional sample of more than 1600 men of ages 25–70 years, the physical work capacity (expressed as maximal oxygen uptake capability) was more correlated with changes in body composition (body fat content) and exercise habits than with age. Similarly, tolerance of heat (Pandolf, 1991) or cold (Young, 1991) was related more to "fitness" than age.

Manipulation capability can be considered a special subgroup of skill: it requires strength, mobility, and sensory control. Even though manipulation skills are very important for many tasks (on the job, at home, or during leisure), unified and standardized measuring techniques are not available, although progress is being made (Scott & Marcus, 1991). Thus, little reliable information on hand capability exists for adults in general, and information on aging persons is piecemeal. Yet, obviously, severe declines in manipulation capability are frequent, often associated with arthritic joint diseases.

EXAMPLES OF ERGONOMIC HELP FOR THE OLDER WORKER

The U.S. Age Discrimination Acts have defined the "older" person as someone 40–45 years or older. While one cannot set one given age year as the beginning of aging, there is no doubt that certain work tasks become more difficult as one approaches retirement: this includes strenuous physical exertion, such as moving heavy loads; tasks that require high mobility, particularly of the trunk and back; and tasks that require high visual acuity and close focusing. On the other hand, at least "anecdotal evidence" shows tasks demanding patient and experience-generated skill may be performed better by at least some older workers than by young persons.

For the older worker, nearly all age-related difficulties can be reduced or overcome by proper workplace and tool design and selection, by arrangement of work procedures and tasks, by provision of working aids such as power-assisted tools or magnifying lenses, or by managerial measures such as assignment of work tasks and provision of work breaks (Czaja, 1991; Graafmans & Bouma, 1993; Kelly & Kroemer, 1990; Kroemer et al., 1994; Rice & Kemmerling, 1990; Shephard, 1995; Small, 1987). Manipulation tasks are facilitated by providing proper work height, support for arms and elbows, and provision of special handtools that might be power assisted. Postural aids include providing proper work height coupled with a seat of appropriate dimensions and good adjustability: in essence the same recommendations for chair design exist whether used in the shop or office, but the shop seat must be especially sturdy and protected against soiling. For work with computers, tasks that require strong involvement of short-term memory may be facilitated by proper software or other provisions to reduce the load on the memory (Boyer, Pollack, & Eggemeier, 1992; Czaja, 1988; Czaja, Hammond, Blascovich, & Swede, 1989; Czaja & Sharit, 1993; Jay & Willis, 1992; Shephard, 1995). Several researchers have dealt with the aging (arthritic) hand, and recommended accommodations, including special designs of hand-operated controls (Czaja, 1984; Jones, Unsworth, & Haslock, 1987; Kanis, 1993; Metz, Isle, Denno, & Li, 1990; H. B. Smith, 1973).

Many sensory problems also can be overcome by ergonomic interventions. For example, vision deficiencies can be counteracted by provision of corrective eye lenses, by intense and well-directed illumination, and by avoiding direct or indirect glare. If text must be read, on either paper or a dial or on a computer screen, proper character size and contrast as well as carefully selected color schemes should be used (for example, avoid difficult visual discriminations of similar hues, particularly in the blue–green range). The auditory environment should be controlled to keep background noise at a minimum, to provide sufficient "penetration" of auditory signals that must be heard, by selecting appropriate intensities and frequencies (avoid frequencies above 4000 Hz). One can try to improve a person's ability to hear by providing "hearing aids" that amplify sounds for which hearing deficiencies exist. This, however, is difficult if the deficient areas are not known exactly (for example, because a person has not taken a hearing test recently), and the amplification of sounds might also enforce unwanted background noise. Improvement is very difficult if the hearing loss is due to destruction of structures of the middle and inner ear, and with current technology nearly impossible if the auditory nerves have been damaged. Further technical development may bring better help in the future. Ergonomic measures can improve the "clarity of the message" (as discussed by Kroemer et al., 1994): provision of sound signals that are easily distinguishable, that are of sufficient intensity, and avoidance of masking background sounds ("noise"). Another solution is to provide, at least some, information through other sensory channels, such as vision (e.g., present illustrations and written texts to accompany an auditory message) or to employ the taction sense, such as when using Braille.

Regarding "public" transportation (planes, trains, subways, buses, trams, lifts, elevators, moving walkways, etc.), aging persons report (among others) the following problems.

- *Information* (cues and signs) indicating use, direction, and location, such as these: How do I buy a ticket? Where does the bus go that I see coming? Where does the tram stop? Where is the exit to Brown Street? Where are we? Many of these problems can be overcome by applying common "human engineering principles" such as using signs with good lettering (contrast, size, symbols), proper illuminance and avoidance of glare, auditory announcements that are timely and understandable, and redundant information such as showing the floor number in an elevator in large numerals and announcing it early over a public address system.

• *Ingress and egress, and body posture,* while using the transport system. Entrance and exit passages and steps are often difficult to maneuver and may require forceful and complex stepping, typically so in trams, trains, buses, or moving walkways. Uneven floors, damaged or misplaced floor coverings often pose problems, in vehicles or hallways. Handholds used to be a problem in buses and trams, but most now provide a variety of hooks, columns, and hand grips.

• *Use of walking aids and wheelchairs.* Many aged people use canes, walkers, and some need wheelchairs. While a cane usually does not pose a problem in public transportation (in fact, it may alert other passengers to be considerate and helpful), walking aids and specifically wheelchairs are often not easily accommodated and may be a serious deterrent to use of public transportation.

In essence, use of proper ergonomic measures, carefully selected and applied, is just "good human engineering" that would help workers of all age groups but that is of particular importance for the older person. Examples of the efficiency of ergonomic practice are selection of proper "signal" words for signs and labels (Silver, Gammella, Barlow, & Wogalter, 1993) and design features of and use instructions for bank teller machines (Adams & Thieben, 1991) that help older persons, non-native English speakers, and everyone else.

CASE STUDY: THE HOME FOR THE AGING

A 50-year-old who purchases a home (or durable product) will be a rather different individual but may still be using it 10, 20, or 30 years later. Whether a person can reside alone, can live in the home with some outside help, may be cared for at home, or must be in a care environment is a complex function of various abilities, or disabilities, and ergonomic condition of the "designed environment." Figure 7 presents an overview of common disorders among the aged adapted from Kemmerling (1991), based in part on information compiled by Faste in 1977. Many of the problems can be alleviated, at least to some degree, by proper ergonomic measures.

Functional ability, or its opposite, dependency, is commonly assessed in terms of clusters of activities: "instrumental activities of daily living" (IADL) or the less specific "activities of daily living" (ADL) shown in Table 4. Numerous surveys of elderly persons have been done using these two

DISORDERS

PROBLEMS/ MANIFESTATIONS	Senescence	Arteriosclerosis	Hypertension	Parkinson's disease	Peripheral neuropathy	Drowsiness	Cataracts/glaucoma	Arthritis	Paget's disease	Osteoporosis	Low back pain	Bronchitis/emphysema	Pneumonia	Diabetes	Senile dementia
General debility	☆		☆	☆	☆			☆	☆	☆	☆	☆	☆	☆	
Mobility	☆	☆		☆	☆		☆	☆	☆		☆				
Posture	☆			☆			☆	☆	☆	☆	☆				
Pain		☆		☆	☆			☆	☆		☆				
Incoordination		☆		☆	☆		☆	☆							
Reduced sensory input	☆	☆			☆	☆	☆								
Loss of balance	☆	☆		☆			☆								
Reduced joint mobility								☆	☆	☆	☆				
Weakness in muscles	☆			☆	☆			☆							
Auditory disorders	☆					☆		☆						☆	☆
Locating body in space		☆					☆	☆							
Shortness of breath		☆		☆								☆	☆		
Deformity								☆	☆	☆					
Memory impairment		☆													☆
Visual problems	☆	☆					☆							☆	
Disorientation		☆		☆											☆
Loss of sensation	☆				☆	☆									
Cognition disturbance		☆		☆											
Incontinence		☆													☆
Speech disorders				☆		☆	☆								
Touch disabilities	☆				☆			☆						☆	

FIGURE 7 Problems arising from common age-related disorders. From Kroemer, Kroemer, and Kroemer-Elbert (1994), *Ergonomics—How to Design for Ease and Efficiency,* with permission of the publisher, Prentice-Hall. All rights reserved.

listings. The results have served to classify persons into groups that require help and specifically designed environments (see, for example, Committee on an Aging Society, 1988; Lawton, 1990; Smith, 1990). While IADLs are practical and self-explanatory, they lack specificity, objectivity, and are not

TABLE 4
Measures of "Daily Living"

Instrumental activities of daily living (IADL)	Activities of daily living (ADL)
Managing money	Living
Shopping	Bed/chair transference
Light housework	Indoor and outdoor mobility
Laundry	Dressing
Meal preparation	Bathing
Making a phone call	Toileting
Taking medication	

easily scaled. One attempt to improve them was to subdivide ADLs into more specific tasks such as lifting/lowering, pushing/pulling, bending/stooping, and reaching (Clark, Czaja, & Weber, 1990). Further work in this direction could result in a list of basic demands and activities similar to the "motion elements" used in industrial engineering for method studies.

Severely curtailed functional abilities are at the core of our fears about growing old. In the United States, currently only one of four people of 65 years has any problems negotiating life, but there is the likelihood that impairments are in progress. As more functional disabilities occur, the elderly person needs first more help in his or her own home. Initially, that care may be privately secured either through friends and relatives or through a hired person. For many, this is the beginning of a path that leads to a nursing home.

Residents who need ongoing assistance in functioning but not intensive care are in "intermediate" care facilities. Thus, the architectural and other ergonomic recommendations for the private home also apply to intermediate care facilities in so far as they facilitate the residents' efforts to look after themselves. However, in addition, the caregiver must be considered in design and organizational means to facilitate such activities as easy access, cleaning, provision of immediate help requirements, and emergency.

Little control over their life, activities, and environment exists for patients in what is usually called in the United States *skilled nursing care facilities*. Their resident tend to be very old and in continual need of help and care. Owing to gender differences in longevity and types of illnesses and injuries, women are more likely than men to be disabled but not to have a life-threatening illness. Since nursing home care is largely financed by Medicaid in the United States, most residents are poor; furthermore, many are single, divorced, or widowed (Belsky, 1990). Regarding the architecture and interior design of nursing homes for people who need intensive care, some of the common ergonomic recommendations for designs still apply; but now the aspects of providing 24-hour supervision and care, and possibly intensive medical treatment, prevail. (Committee on Aging Society, 1988; Czaja, 1990b; Meadows, 1988).

To be in one's home has the major advantage of being in a "familiar" setting with all its physical and emotional implications. Unless by happenstance or foresight designed to be ergonomic, private homes usually need some adjustments to allow the aging inhabitant to perform all necessary activities even with somewhat reduced sensory, motoric, and decision-making capabilities. In addition to passage areas, several rooms are of particular concern.

The Kitchen

In the kitchen, one stores, prepares, and serves food. Often, it is also a phone-in message center. In the past, the kitchen was the woman's territory, however this is now no longer true. The first "scientific" study of kitchens was completed by Lillian Gilbreth in the 1920s. Her classical study relied mainly on work flow and the time and motion study methods that she pioneered with her husband. Her redesigned kitchen reduced motion by nearly 50%.

"Seven principles" derived from time and motion studies, augmented by ergonomic findings, apply to the kitchen:

1. One shall design for a small "work triangle," the corners of which are the refrigerator, sink, and the stove.
2. The "work flow" for food preparation is to remove food from the refrigerator or cabinet, mix or otherwise prepare ingredients near the sink, cook on the range or in the oven, and serve. Kitchen components should facilitate that flow.
3. If there is "traffic flow" by others, it should not cut through the patterns of work triangle and work flow.
4. Items should be stored at the "point of first use," as determined by work triangle and flow.
5. The work space for the hands should be at about elbow height or slightly below. This facilitates manipulation and visual control. Counter and sink heights are derived from elbow height. Note that it might be advisable to consider walking aids, and that stools or chairs might be used.

6. The reach to items stored in the kitchen should be at or slightly below eye height to allow for visual control and easy arm and shoulder motion.
7. The motion and working space should not be reduced or interrupted by doors of appliances and cabinets, hence they should open "outward" from the working person.

The Bathroom

Other areas of major ergonomic concern are the bedroom (Parsons, 1972) and especially the bathroom. The bath is one of the busiest and unfortunately most dangerous rooms in the house. Basic equipment includes a bathtub or shower or both, toilet, and lavatory. Furthermore, there are usually storage facilities for toiletries, towels, and the like. Current bathroom designs in the United States are difficult to use, for both aging and disabled persons (Malassigne & Amerson, 1992).

The bathtub and shower are the two common areas for cleansing the whole body, and these are common accident sites. Their major danger stems from slipperiness between bare skin and floor or walls. The more dangerous of the two is the bathtub because of its commonly slanted surfaces are combined with high sides, above which one has to step, a procedure not easy for most people and particularly difficult for the elderly who have balance and mobility deficiencies. Kira (1976) described several techniques employed by most users getting in and out of a tub. They involve shifts in body weight: from the legs to arms and legs used together, and finally to the buttocks while entering the tub; in leaving, these shifts occur in the reverse order. There is much potential for loss of balance and the hazard of a slip and ensuing fall. While resting in the tub, the angle of the backrest and its slipperiness is the most critical design aspect. Proper handrails and grab bars, within easy reach both for sitting and getting in and out, are of importance. The shower stall may also have a slippery floor to step on, but its lower enclosure rim makes it easier to move in and out.

Use of the control handles for hot and cold water is quite often difficult for aged persons, particularly when they are not at their familiar home and have to cope with different handle designs, movement directions, and varying resistances (Meindl & Freivalds, 1992). Better design principles and their standardization would be helpful; for example, in the mode and direction of control movement to regulate water temperature.

The washbasin may be difficult to use if it is too far away, for example, if inserted in a cabinet, so that one cannot step close to it. The faucet often reduces the usable opening area of the washbasin. Proper height is important, as are the water controls.

The toilet is, obviously, of great importance for relieving oneself of body wastes and keeping the body openings and close anatomical areas clean. Kira's classical study has provided much information about proper design, sizing, shaping, and location, with further recommendations supplied by McClelland and Ward (1982).

For Western-style private homes, a variety of publications contains valuable ergonomic design recommendations (see, for example, Graeff & Singer, 1994; Singer & Graeff, 1988). Yet, in other civilizations and other parts of the earth quite different customs and conditions exist, for which at present little ergonomic information appears available.

SUMMARY AND CONCLUSIONS

The aging of one's friends and relatives and our own aging are of perpetual interest and concern. More than two decades ago, Chapanis suggested developing a "Human Engineering Guide of Design for the Elderly" (Chapanis, 1974), but the first draft for such guidelines was published only in 1992 (Denno et al., 1992); in 1993 the American Association of Retired Persons and in 1994 Pirkl published guides for architects.

Anecdotal observations and case studies abound but the results of systematic research findings do not provide yet a complete picture. This is largely because cross-sectional research is nearly meaningless: comparing the anthropometry or performance of persons of similar age just provides very limited information, chronological age is not a meaningful classifier. Better classification systems need to be established: the so-called biological age is one attempt in that direction, but its definition is rather difficult. It is typical that, in most studies, younger persons are divided into 5- or 10-year age brackets, while the elderly and aged are lumped together as those 65 years or older, regardless of differences in capability or deficiencies among them. Thus, a basic research task is to establish a suitable reference system, or reference systems, with proper scales and anchoring points.

Although the aging are recognized as a distinct population, they are insufficiently represented in anthropometric, biomechanical, and physiological/psychological studies. Even the common chronological starting year for retirement because of aging, 65, appears to be set by industry and retirement policies but not by data distinguishing this age group functionally from other age groups (D. B. D. Smith, 1990), particularly with respect to on-the-job performance and regarding demands on the design of the living environment.

It is obvious that many or almost all physical, perceptual, cognitive, and decision-making capabilities decline with age. Some of those losses are slow and not easily observed. Other capabilities and facilities decline fast, or they may deteriorate slowly at first and then quickly at some point in time, perhaps again stabilizing for a while. Some of these changes are independent from each other, but many are linked, directly or indirectly; for example, failing physical health may have effects on attitude and intentfulness, or failing eyesight might lead to a fall and serious injury with ensuing illness.

- *Anthropometric and biomechanical changes among aging persons are not highly correlated with chronological age but exhibit variance, and the variance among aged persons tends to increase with age.*
- *Similar changes among aging people are not manifest as a simple linear decline but show a variety of rates; change may even be arrested.*
- *Changes in function may produce varying effects in different persons.*
- *The rate of change can proceed along some dimensions relatively independent of change in others, but the serious loss or compromise of functional capacity in one area can accelerate the rate of decline in others.*
- *A supportive social or physical environment, or positive change, can retard the rate of functional loss.*

People have different coping strategies. One's failing ability to recall names, for example, may be overcome to some extent and for some time by developing mnemonic strategies. An aging person may reduce activity boundaries by maintaining only those with which he or she is comfortable and can competently handle. Maintaining physical or mental activities, possibly purposely so, can counteract reductions in facility significantly and for long periods of time.

Therefore, in our current framework scaled by chronological age, one finds an immense variety of maintained, perhaps in some respect even increased facilities, of decreasing capabilities, and of either slow or fast changes with time. As the absolute numbers of aging persons and their percentage in the American population become larger, the need for complete, reliable, quantitative, valid information about this population increases.

Basic to the design of even the simplest handtool, or a complex habitat, is information about the user's body size, motion capabilities, strength, endurance, sensorimotor control; information traditionally subsumed in anthropometry, biomechanics, physiology, psychology, now compiled in ergonomics and human factors engineering.

Ergonomic knowledge and ergonomic procedures can be of aid from infancy through adulthood into old age. The ergonomic principles and techniques for architectural and interior layout, for design of workplace, equipment and tools are the same for anybody; they are just more critical and important for persons different from the "normal adult" model.

References

Adams, A. S., & Thieben, K. A. (1991). Automatic teller machines and the older population. *Applied Ergonomics, 22,* 85–90.

American Association of Retired Persons. (1993). *Life-span design of residential environments for an aging population.* Washington, DC: Author.

Annis, J. F., Case, H. W., Clauser, C. E., & Bradtmiller, B. (1991). Anthropometry of an aging work force. *Experimental Aging Research, 17,* 157–176.

Åstrand, P. O., & Rodahl, K. (1977). *Textbook of work physiology* (2nd ed.). New York: McGraw-Hill.

Barlow, A. M., Braid, S. J., & Jayson, W. (1990). Foot problems in the elderly. *Clinical Rehabilitation, 4,* 217–222.

Belsky, J. K. (1990). *The psychology of aging. Theory, research, and interventions.* Pacific Grove, CA: Brooks/Cole.

Birren, J. E., & Schaie, K. W. (Eds.). (1990). *Handbook of the psychology of aging* (3rd ed.). New York: Van Nostrand-Reinhold.

Boff, K. R., Kaufman, L., & Thomas, J. P. (Eds.). (1986). *Handbook of perception and human performance.* New York: Wiley.

Boyer, D. L., Pollack, J. G., & Eggemeier, F. T. (1992). Effects of aging on subjective workload and performance. In *Proceedings of the Human Factors Society 36th annual meeting* (pp. 156–159.). Santa Monica, CA: Human Factors Society.

Chaffin, D. B., & Ashton-Miller, J. A. (1991). Biomechanical aspects of low-back pain in the older worker. *Experimental Research, 17,* 177–187.

Chapanis, A. (1974). Human engineering environments for the aged. *Applied Ergonomics, 5,* 72–80.

Chapanis, A. (Ed.) (1975). *Ethnic variables in human factors engineering.* Baltimore, MD: John Hopkins University Press.

Clark, M. C., Czaja, S. J., & Weber, R. A. (1990). Older adults and daily living task profiles. *Human Factors, 32,* 537–549.

Coleman, R. (1993). A demographic overview of the aging of first world populations. *Applied Ergonomics, 24,* 5–8.

Committee on an Aging Society (Ed.). (1988). *The social and built environment in an older society.* Washington, DC: National Academy Press.

Committee on Vision (Ed.). (1987). *Work, aging, and vision.* Washington, DC: National Academy Press.

Cowen, R. (1988). *Eyes on the workplace.* Washington, DC: National Academy Press.

Czaja, S. J. (1984). *Hand anthropometrics.* Washington, DC: U.S. Architectural and Transportation Barriers Compliance Board.

Czaja, S. J. (1988). Microcomputers and the elderly. In M. Helander (Ed.), *Handbook of human-computer interaction* (pp. 581–598). Amsterdam: Elsevier.

Czaja, S. J. (Ed.). (1990a). Aging. *Human Factors* (Special Issue). *32,* 505–622.

Czaja, S. J. (Ed.). (1990b). *Human factors research needs for an aging population.* Washington, DC: National Academy Press.

Czaja, S. J. (1991). Work design for older adults. In A. Mital & W. Karwowski (Eds.), *Workspace, equipment, and tool design* (pp. 345–369). Amsterdam: Elsevier.

Czaja, S. J., Hammond, K., Blascovich, J. J., & Swede, H. (1989). Age related differences in learning to use a text-editing system. *Behaviour and Information Technology, 8,* 309–319.

Czaja, S. J., & Sharit, J. (1993). Age differences in the performance of computer-based work. *Psychology and Aging, 8,* 59–67.

Denno, S., Isle, B. A., Ju, G., Koch, C. G., Metz, S. V., Penner, R., Wang, L., & Ward, J. (1992).

Human factors design guidelines for the elderly and people with disabilities (Revision 3, Draft). Minneapolis, MI: Honeywell.

Faste, R. A. (1977). New system propels design for the handicapped. *Industrial Design, pp. 51–55.*

Fozard, J. L. (1990). Vision and hearing in aging. In J. E. Birren & K. W. Schaie (Eds.), Handbook of the psychology of aging (3rd ed. pp. 150–170). New York: Academic Press.

Garg, A. (1991). Ergonomics and the older worker: An overview. *Experimental Aging Research, 17,* 143–155.

Gordon, C. C., Churchill, T., Clauser, C. E., Bradtmiller, B., McConville, J. T., Tebbetts, I., & Walker, R. A. (1989). *1988 Anthropometric Survey of U.S. Army Personnel: Summary Statistics Interim Report* (Technical Report NATICK/TR-89-027). Natick, MA: United States Army Natick Research, Development and Engineering Center.

Graafmans, J. A. M., & Bouma, H. (1993). Gerontechnology, fitting task and environment to the elderly. In *Proceedings of the Human Factors and Ergonomics Society 37th annual meeting* (pp. 182–186). Santa Monica, CA: Human Factors and Ergonomics Society.

Graef, R. F., & Singer, L. D. (1994). A bathroom for the elderly. In J. J. Pirkl (Ed.), *Design products for an aging population* (pp. 192–215). New York: Van Nostrand-Reinhold.

Greiner, T. M. (1991). *Hand Anthropometry of U.S. Army Personnel* (Technical Report TR-92/011) Natick, MA: U.S. Army Natick Research, Development and Engineering Center.

Greiner, T. M., & Gordon, C. C. (1990). *An assessment of long-term changes in anthropometric dimensions: Secular trends of U.S. Army males* (Natick/TR-91/006). Natick, MA: U.S. Army Natick Research, Development and Engineering Center.

Haigh, R. (1993). The aging process: A challenge for design. *Applied Ergonomics, 24,* 9–14.

Hayslip, B., & Panek, P. (1989). *Adult development and aging.* New York: Harper-Row.

Heuer, H., Bruewer, M., Roemer, T., Kroeger, H., & Knapp, H. (1991). Preferred vertical gaze direction and observation distance. *Ergonomics, 34,* 379–392.

Jackson, A. S., Beard, E. F., Wier, L. T., & Stuteville, J. E. (1992). Multivariate model for defining changes in maximal physical working capacity of men, ages 25 to 70 Years. In *Proceedings of the Human Factors Society 36th annual meeting* (pp. 171–174). Santa Monica, CA: Human Factors Society.

Jay, G. M., & Willis, S. L. (1992). Influence of direct computer experience on older adults' attitudes toward computers. *Journal of Gerontology, 47,* 250–257.

Jones, A. R., Unsworth, A., & Haslock, I. (1987). Functional measurements in the hands of patients with rheumatoid arthritis. *International Journal of Rehabilitation Research, 10,* 62–72.

Juergens, H. W., Aune, I. A, & Pieper, U. (1990). International data on Anthropometry. *Occupational Safety and Health Series #65.* Geneva, Switzerland: International Labour Office.

Kanis, H. (1993). Operation of controls on consumer products by physically impaired users. *Human Factors, 35,* 305–328.

Kelly, P. L., & Kroemer, K. H. E. (1990). Anthropometry of the elderly: Status and recommendations. *Human Factors, 32,* 571–595.

Kemmerling, P. T. (1991). *Human factors engineering for the disabled and aging* (Class Notes, ISE 5654, Fall Semester). Blacksburg, VA: Virginia Tech (VPI&SU).

Kermis, M. D. (1984). *Psychology of human aging.* Boston, MA: Allyn & Bacon.

Kira, A. (1976). *The bathroom.* New York: Viking.

Kroemer, K. H. E., Kroemer, H. B., & Kroemer-Elbert, K. E. (1994). *Ergonomics: How to design for ease and efficiency.* Englewood Cliffs, NJ: Prentice-Hall.

Kroemer, K. H. E., Snook, S. H., Meadows, S. K., & Deutsch, S. (Eds.). (1988). *Ergonomic models of anthropometry, human biomechanics, and operator–equipment interfaces.* Washington, DC: National Academy Press.

Kumashiro, M. (Ed.). (1995). *The paths for productive aging.* Bristol, PA: Taylor & Francis.

Larish, J., Kramer, A., DeAntona, J. & Strayer, D. (1993). Aging and dual-task training. In *Proceedings of the Human Factors and Ergonomics Society 37th Annual Meeting* (pp. 162–166). Santa Monica, CA: Human Factors and Ergonomics Society.

Lawton, M. P. (1990). Aging and performance of home tasks. *Human Factors, 32,* 527–536.

Malassigne, P., & Amerson, T. L. (1992). In the era of ADA do we really have accessible bathrooms: A survey. In *Proceedings of the Human Factors Society 36th annual meeting* (pp. 578–581). Santa Monica, CA: Human Factors Society.

Manivannan, P., Czaja, S., Drury, C., & Ip, C. M. (1993). The impact of age on visual search performance. In *Proceedings of the Human Factors and Ergonomics Society 37th Annual Meeting* (pp. 172–176). Santa Monica, CA: Human Factors and Ergonomics Society.

McClelland, I. L., & Ward, J. S. (1982). The ergonomists of toilet seats. *Human Factors, 24,* 713–725.

McConville, J. T., Robinette, K. M., & Churchill, T. (1981). *An anthropometric data base for commercial design applications* (Final Report, NSF-DAR-80 09 861). Yellow Springs, OH: Anthropology Research Project, Inc.

Meadows, S. (1988). The wave of innovation for an aging society: Enhancing independent living. In *Proceedings of the Human Factors Society 32nd annual meeting* (p. 184). Santa Monica, CA: Human Factors Society.

Meindl, B. A., & Freivalds, A. (1992). Shape and placement of faucet handles for the elderly. In *Proceedings of the Human Factors Society 36th annual meeting* (pp. 811–815). Santa Monica, CA: Human Factors Society.

Metz, S., Isle, B., Denno, S., & Li, W. (1990). Small rotary controls: Limitations for people with arthritis. In *Proceedings of the Human Factors Society 34th annual meeting* (pp. 137–140). Santa Monica, CA: Human Factors Society.

National Institutes on Aging (Ed.). (1982). *Behavioral and social research, retrospects and prospects.* (Administrative Document, March 1992). Bethesda, MD: Author.

Olczyk, K. (1993). Age-related changes in collagen of human intervertebral disks. *Gerontology, 38,* 196–204.

Osthere, S. J., & Gold, R. H. (1991). Osteoporosis and bone density measurement methods. *Clinical Orthopaedics, 271,* 149–163.

Pandolf, K. B. (1991). Aging and heat tolerance at rest or during work. *Experimental Aging Research, 17,* 189–204.

Parsons, H. M. (1972). The bedroom. *Human Factors, 14,* 421–450.

Pheasant, S. (1986). *Bodyspace.* London: Taylor & Francis.

Pirkl, J. J. (Ed.). (1994). *Design products for an aging population.* New York: Van Nostrand-Reinhold.

Prieto, E., Myklebust, J. B., & Myklebust, B. M. (1993). Characteristics and modeling of postural steadiness in the elderly: A review. *IEEE Transactions on Rehabilitation Engineering, 1,* 26–34.

Rabbitt, P. (1991). Management of the working population. *Ergonomics, 34,* 775–790.

Rice, V. B., & Kemmerling, P. T. (1990). The impact of the aging U.S. population on the workforce and on workplace design. In *Proceedings of the International Ergonomics Association Conference on Human Factors in Design for Manufacturability and Process Planning* (pp. 347–354). Buffalo, NY: Helander, Department of IE, SUNYAB.

Roebuck, J. A. (1995). *Anthropometric methods—Designing to fit the human body.* Santa Monica, CA: Human Factors and Ergonomics Society.

Roebuck, J. A., Smith, K., & Raggio, L. (1988). *Forecasting crew anthropometry for shuttle and space station* (STS 88-0717). Downey, CA: Rockwell International.

Rogers, W. A., Gilbert, D. K., & Fisk, A. D. (1993, October). Ability-performance relationships in memory skill tasks for young and old adults. In *Proceedings of Factors and Ergonomics Society 37th annual meeting* (pp. 167–171). Santa Monica, CA: Human Factors and Ergonomics Society.

Scott, D., & Marcus, S. (1991). *Hand impairment assessment: Some suggestions. Applied Ergonomics, 22,* 263–269.

Sekuler, R., Kline, D., & Dismukes, K. (Eds.). (1982). *Aging and human visual function.* New York: Alan R. Liss.

Selkoe, D. J. (1992). Aging brain, aging mind. *Scientific American, 267,* 135–142.

Serow, W. J., & Sly, D. F. (1988). The demography of current and future aging cohorts. In *Committee on an Aging Society (Ed.), America's aging—The social and built environment in an older society* (pp. 42–102). Washington, DC: National Academy Press.

Shephard, R. J. (1995). A personal perspective on aging and productivity, with particular reference to physically demanding work. *Ergonomics, 38,* 617–636.

Silver, N. C., Gammella, D. S., Barlow, A. S., & Wogalter, M. S. (1993). Connoted strength of signal words by elderly and non-native English speakers. In *Proceedings of the Human Factors and Ergonomics Society 37th annual meeting* (pp. 516–519). Santa Monica, CA: Human Factors and Ergonomics Society.

Singer, L. D., & Graeff, R. F. (1988). *A bathroom for the elderly* (Report on Grants 230-11-110H-150-8903081 and CAE-86-005-01). Blacksburg, VA: Virginia Polytechnic Institute and State University, College of Architecture and Urban Studies.

Small, A. M. (1987). Design for older people. In G. Salvendy (Ed.), *Handbook of human factors* (pp. 495–504). New York: Wiley.

Smith, D. B. D. (1990). Human factors and aging: An overview of research needs and application opportunities. *Human Factors, 32,* 509–526.

Smith, H. B. (1973). Hand function evaluation. *American Journal of Occupational Therapy, 27,* 244–251.

Soldo, B. J., & Longino, C. F. (1988). Social and physical environments for the vulnerable aged. In Committee on an Aging Society (Ed.), *America's aging—The social and built environment in an older society* (pp. 103–133). Washington, DC: National Academy Press.

Spence, A. P. (1989). *Biology of human aging.* Englewood Cliffs, NJ: Prentice-Hall.

Stine, E. L., Wingfield, A., & Poon, L. W. (1989). Speech comprehension and memory through adulthood: The roles of time and strategy. In L. W. Poon, D. C. Rubin, & B. A. Wilson (Eds.), *Everyday cognition in adulthood and later years* (pp. 195–221). Cambridge, UK: Cambridge University Press.

Stoudt, H. W. (1981). The anthropometry of the elderly. *Human Factors, 23,* 29–37.

Tyrrell, R. A., & Leibowitz, H. W. (1990). The relation of vergence effort to reports of visual fatigue following prolonged near work. *Human Factors, 32,* 341–357.

Verbrugge, L. M. (1989). Recent, present, and future health of American adults. *Annual Review of Public Health, 10,* 333–361.

Young, A. J. (1991). Effects of aging on human cold tolerance. *Experimental Aging Research, 17,* 205–213.

Chapter 6

Language and Communication: Fundamentals of Speech Communication and Language Processing in Old Age

Patricia A. Tun
Arthur Wingfield

INTRODUCTION

Of the various abilities necessary for the independent functioning of the individual across the life span and into old age, one of the most essential is the ability to comprehend and use information from language. To maintain an independent lifestyle, an elderly person must be able to understand, remember, and utilize the information that is communicated daily. For example, it is not possible to live independently unless one can understand and remember instructions regarding diet, medications and self-care, personal appointments, and communications from everyday contacts.

Handbook of Human Factors and the Older Adult

It is interesting to note that this ability has become increasingly more important, rather than less so, in the "information age" in which we live. With each advance of modern technology, the ability to process spoken language becomes more crucial to survival in our society. Consider the barrage of automated spoken and written instructions that we encounter daily, from banking machines, to automated instructions in shopping, to phone services of all sorts. Just one example is the branching-option instructions that have become common in phone contacts with airline reservations, banks, and government agencies (e.g., "Push 1 if you have a touch-tone phone. Push 2 if you know your party's extension . . ."). They work well, but they place a heavy processing burden on attention to speech and memory for the particulars of the spoken message.

In this chapter we will review some of the most salient issues regarding speech processing in old age, with special attention to how age-related changes in processing rates and capacity for speech can affect many of the activities covered in this book. We will describe some aspects of language processing that are well-preserved with age, and other features that show age-related declines. Language processing affords a view of several naturally occurring compensatory mechanisms by which older adults can offset deficits in component processes, and these compensations can serve as a model by which the worker in human factors can design the environment and make appropriate interventions to optimize communication with the elderly. With the demographic shift toward larger numbers of older adults and longer life expectancies, this becomes a matter of increasing concern.

THE IMPORTANCE OF SPEECH COMMUNICATION IN A TECHNOLOGICAL SOCIETY: READING AND LISTENING

The bulk of early research on older adults' memory for language focused on written materials and nearly ignored speech. Text is an important source of information, but in fact, the elderly in particular rely much more on spoken communication, including radio and TV, for news of family, friends, and the world around them (Rubin, 1986).

Although understanding and remembering speech is an everyday activity that healthy people tend to take for granted, in fact, it is one of the most complex of cognitive activities. First, consider the very rapid rate of information input. Speech rates in ordinary conversations average between 100 to 180 words per minute (wpm), while a newscaster reading a prepared script can easily exceed 210 wpm (J. L. Miller, Grosjean, & Lomanto, 1984). Moreover, in spoken communication, unlike reading, the speed at which new information arrives is not easily controlled by the listener. In conversations a listener has some ability to signal a speaker to slow down, but one cannot moderate speech rates in radio or TV broadcasts or in group situations. In addition, words in spoken discourse are often underarticulated. Indeed, many words in spoken discourse would be unrecognizable if they were spliced from a recorded sentence and heard in isolation (Pollack & Pickett, 1963; Wingfield, Alexander, & Cavigelli, 1994).

Thus, the successful listener's task requires a continuous on-line analysis of a rapid (and often impoverished) speech stream, that involves (1) segmenting the speech signal into words, (2) accessing word meaning, (3) parsing the message into syntactic and semantic units, and (4) linking together the idea units (or "propositions") to form a coherent macrostructure so that the communication as a whole has meaning (Flores d'Arcais & Scheuder, 1983; Marslen-Wilson & Tyler, 1980; van Dijk & Kintsch, 1983). Most important, unlike reading, one lacks the ability to backtrack and review when one falls behind.

A consideration that will be discussed in a later section is the burden discourse processing places on working memory. Although we shall see that the exact form of memory involved is in dispute, it is clear that, to give speech coherence, one must hold important idea units in temporary storage to connect new information with what came before (van Dijk & Kintsch, 1983). An important characteristic of speech is that it is typically less structured than written material; speakers do not always speak in complete sentences but may wander and repair an utterance along the way. Finally, although speech is usually simpler in syntax and organization than written language, it is also less precise, with more ambiguous referents and generalized terms such as *you know* (Brown & Yule, 1983).

Given current theories of cognitive aging, most of these characteristics—rapid rate, lack of control by the listener of pacing, on-line sequential processing demands, and lack of precision—might be expected to work against good speech comprehension by the elderly. We will now turn to the question of how older adults' handling of spoken language actually fares under this challenge.

FACTORS THAT AFFECT SPEECH PROCESSING

Hearing Loss

There is no question that aging is associated with declines in the sensitivity of peripheral auditory processing (Olsho, Harkins, & Lenhardt, 1985), details of which will be covered in the accompanying chapter on sensory processes (Chapter 3). However, the actual numbers of elderly suffering from serious hearing loss are smaller than many people imagine. Some estimates report an incidence of approximately 12% hearing impairment in adults from 45 to 64 years of age, 24% in adults from 65 to 74, and 39% in adults 75 years and older. Only about 2–4% of the elderly are actually deaf (U.S. Congress, Office of Technology Assessment, 1986). These figures may prove surprising to those who tend to assume that any elderly person with whom they converse must be deaf and that they must therefore speak at an exaggeratedly loud level (Ryan, Giles, Bartolucci, & Henwood, 1986).

Presbycusis is the term given to the typical pattern of geriatric hearing loss, which is characterized by decreased auditory sensitivity, especially in the high-frequency range, over 3000 Hz (Bergman, 1980). High-frequency loss can have effects on comprehending speech. Speech is heavily weighted toward frequencies lower than 3000 Hz but losses at 4000 Hz can produce difficulties for high frequency sounds such as *s, k, f,* and *t.*

Age is also associated with an increased probability of recruitment, or an abrupt increase in the perceived loudness of a sound with an increase in the intensity of the stimulus. More important to our understanding of aging speech perception is *phonemic regression,* in which an individual's understanding of speech (or other complex signals) is poorer than would be predicted on the basis of his or her sensitivity for pure tones. This means that even when speech is amplified to a level at which pure tones can be clearly heard, the individual may still have reduced comprehension.

Speech presented under conditions of background noise, such as those common to everyday listening, can add special difficulty for many elderly adults. (Ambient noise levels have been estimated to average about 45 dBA in suburban homes, 54 dBA for department stores, and 77 dBA for transportation systems; Pearsons, Bennett, & Fidell, 1977).

Even when young and elderly adults have been matched for equivalent thresholds for pure tones and for speech presented in quiet, older adults may show deficits in recognizing speech masked by noise (Dubno, Dirks, & Morgan, 1982; Duquesnoy, 1983; Gordon-Salant, 1987). This can be demonstrated using the Speech Perception in Noise (SPIN) test, in which subjects are asked to repeat words in simple sentences presented over a background of multiple talkers ("babble") with a range of signal-to-noise ratios (Kalikow, Stevens, & Elliott, 1977).

Elderly listeners' speech comprehension is sensitive to a variety of other everyday suboptimal conditions, which include reverberation patterns that simulate listening in a hall with unfavorable acoustics and speech filtered through different bandwidths, such as occurs during telephone conversations (Bergman, 1980; Bergman et al., 1976). Available evidence suggests that the difficulty in understanding speech in noise reflects deficits at not only peripheral but cognitive levels (Working Group on Speech Understanding and Aging, 1988). It seems probable that background noise increases the processing load in many tasks; and studies have shown poorer memory performance for materials presented in noise, even when subjects had accurately shadowed the stimuli, ruling out the possibility of peripheral sensory problems (Pichora-Fuller, Schneider, & Daneman, in press; Rabbitt, 1968, 1991).

Therefore, a variety of factors have important practical consequences for those who need to design communication systems that are effective for elderly adults. Clearly, they must be prepared for a wide range of auditory sensitivity across individuals. Moreover, it is important to assess sensitivity not merely by traditional pure-tone audiometric screening but for speech comprehension as well. As we have seen, these abilities can differ. Finally, it is important to take into consideration the characteristics of the environment in which the communication will take place, particularly the level of background noise.

Slowing

One of the most common observations in the literature is that aging is associated with a reduction in processing speed (Birren, 1964; Salthouse, 1991; Welford, 1958). Several current theories of cognitive aging are based on the premise that a central slowing of information processing underlies the age-related changes shown for a wide range of cognitive behaviors including attention, learning, and memory (e.g., Cerella, 1985, 1990). This premise has given rise to the "complexity hypothesis" (Cerella, Poon, & Williams, 1980), which suggests that the magnitude of age differences increases with greater task complexity. More recently, however, it has become apparent that slowing of verbal processes is less severe and has a different slowing function than nonverbal processing skills (Lima, Hale, & Myerson, 1991). While perceptual and cognitive slowing is clearly associated with adult aging, it is less clear whether a single slowing function can serve as an adequate account for age differences in cognitive performance (cf. Cerella & Hale, 1994; Fisk & Fisher, 1994).

If age-related slowing is as ubiquitous as it is thought to be, it might seem surprising that elderly adults are so adept at processing a stimulus stream as complex as linguistic input that arrives at the relatively rapid rates of everyday speech. One way to probe this question is to use a technique that pushes the limits of speech processing to discover at what point it begins to break down. In a number of studies we have electronically accelerated speech by first digitizing it on a computer, then removing very small segments (e.g., 20 ms) at regular intervals from both spoken words and pauses between words.

This time-compression method results in speech that retains the same pitch contour and relative temporal pattern of normal speech but is presented in a fraction of the normal time. To the extent that age is associated with cognitive slowing, depriving listeners of processing time in this way should have a differentially greater effect on comprehension and recall for the spoken materials in elderly adults relative to young adults. In fact, this is a result we have consistently found (Riggs, Wingfield, & Tun, 1993; Stine, Wingfield, & Poon, 1986; Tun, Wingfield, Stine, & Mecsas, 1992; Wingfield, Poon, Lombardi, & Lowe, 1985).

In a typical rapid speech study (Tun et al., 1992) young and elderly adults listened to sentences that were presented at three speech rates: a normal speech rate (140 wpm), a medium rate that compressed the speech to 77% of the normal time (182 wpm), and a fast rate that compressed the speech to 50% of the normal time (280 wpm). The subjects' task was to recall each sentence immediately after hearing it, as accurately as possible. Figure 1

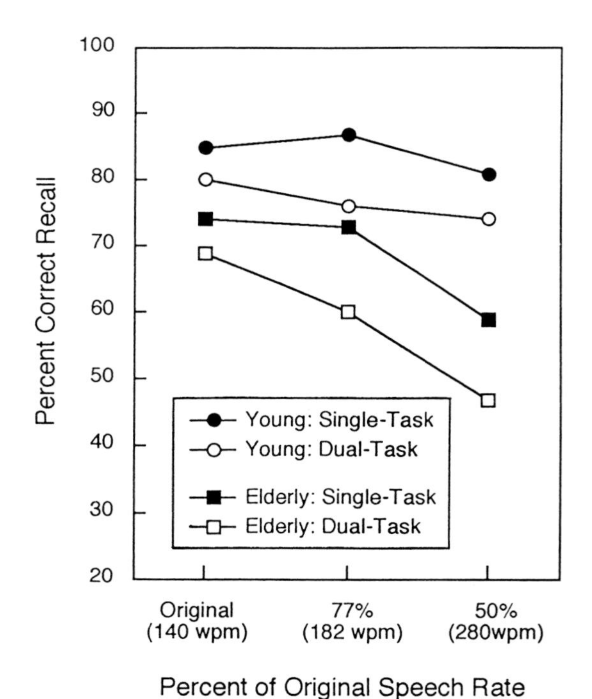

FIGURE 1 Percentage of words correctly recalled from sentences by young and elderly adults in single- and dual-task conditions for three speech rates controlled by computer time compression. (Data from Tun, Wingfield, Stine, & Mecsas, 1992).

shows results taken from this study. The ordinate shows the proportion of words correctly recalled from the sentences by the young and elderly subjects and the abscissa shows the three speech rates in which the speech was heard. (This study had both a single-task and a dual-task condition, which will be discussed further in the next section.)

The pattern shown in Figure 1 is typical of that seen in such studies: older adults show a sharper drop in recall than young adults as speech rates are increased. The age difference for the fast speech is twice as large as it is for the speech presented at the normal rate. It is important to note that this differential effect of time compression on the elderly listener is known to appear independent of any peripheral sensory impairment the elderly subjects might have. That is, elderly adults continue to show special vulnerability to time compression of speech even when young adults are selected who have a hearing loss that matches that of an elderly group, or when normally hearing young adults are compared with elderly adults who have no audiometric signs of presbycusis (Gordon-Salant & Fitzgibbons, 1993; Konkle, Beasley, & Bess, 1977; Luterman, Welsh, & Melrose, 1966; Sticht & Gray, 1969).

Although some of the effect of rapid speech may be due to a loss of richness of the speech signal (Heiman, Leo, Leighbody, & Bowler, 1986), most investigators attribute the primary effect of speech compression to the loss of processing time (Chodorow, 1979). Our data supports others' showing that this loss is particularly disruptive for elderly adults, consistent with claims for an age-related cognitive slowing.

Generalized slowing, however, cannot completely account for these data. The "complexity hypothesis" would predict that age differences at fast speech rates should be magnified as the speech task is made more difficult. As we shall see in the next section, however, this predicted pattern of interactions is not found in many studies of divided attention, nor when other manipulations of processing load are used, such as manipulating the amount of information packed into the speech messages (Stine et al., 1986), or manipulating the average interword predictability in the passages (Tun, Wingfield, & Stine, 1991). While the content difficulty of the speech makes recall more difficult, it does not interact with speech rate for either young or elderly adults (Riggs et al., 1993; Wingfield & Lindfield, 1995). Thus, although the age-related susceptibility to disruption by fast speech rates provides evidence for slowing of language processing, further manipulations of processing load have independent effects that do not necessarily exacerbate this limitation in the elderly.

The practical implications of age-related slowing in speech processing are clear. Speech rate is an important variable that should be considered in designing communications, and care must be taken that elderly listeners are afforded ample processing time at each stage of a message for optimal comprehension and recall of the material. Age-related differences in processing rapid speech may be of particular importance in situations such as aircraft pilots communicating with air traffic controllers, where the amount of information transmitted in brief intervals may lead to problems with "speed feed" (Taylor et al., 1994).

Resource Limitations

While some theorists have focused on age-related slowing, others have postulated age-related reductions in processing resources that are available to carry out mental tasks (Craik & Byrd, 1982). The central presumption is that of a general pool of resources that must be allocated to various tasks based on cognitive needs and task priorities (Kahneman, 1973). These models suggest that if age is associated with a reduction in resource capacity, then age differences in cognitive performance should become more pronounced as the difficulty of the task situation increases. This should be especially so under conditions of divided attention.

However, findings from studies of divided attention and aging have not been consistent in showing age-related increases in the cost of divided attention. Some studies have reported differentially greater effects of divided attention for elderly relative to young adults (Craik & McDowd, 1987; Macht & Buschke, 1983; Park, Smith, Dudley & Lafronza, 1989; Somberg & Salthouse, 1982), while others have found the effects to be similar for young and older adults (Gick, Craik, & Morris, 1988; Morris, Gick, & Craik, 1988; Tun, 1989; Tun & Wingfield, 1994; Tun et al., 1991; Wickens, Braune, & Stokes, 1987).

A key factor in this diversity of findings is the nature of the tasks studied. In general, tests involving visual attention and reaction time have tended to report the elderly to be differentially penalized by the need to divide attention, while those studying meaningful speech have not. Our own survey of the literature on dual-task studies has shown that studies using digit lists or lists of unrelated words as stimuli tend to show differentially greater dual-task deficits for elderly than for young adults, while differential age differences are absent in dual-task studies that have used meaningful connected speech (Tun & Wingfield, 1993).

To illustrate this point we can return to the Tun et al. (1992) study discussed in the previous section (Figure 1). Under the condition of this experiment previously described, young and elderly subjects simply listened to sentences for immediate recall (the single-task condition). As indicated in Figure 1, however, there was also a dual-task condition. Under this condition, the subjects had to listen to spoken sentences for immediate recall while simultaneously having to carry out a continuous recognition test for pictures that were presented on a computer screen. (As each picture was presented the subject had to press a key to indicate whether or not that picture had been presented previously in the study.) Processing load was varied both by the speech rate at which sentences were presented and by whether the task involved divided attention.

If older adults suffer from a generalized reduction in processing resources, age differences in performance should be magnified in the dual-task condition relative to single-task performance. As we see in Figure 1, however, this is not the case. Figure 1 shows very similar declines in sentence recall performance for the young and elderly adults when going from the single-task to the dual-task conditions. In other words, although the young adults generally recalled more from the sentences than did the older adults, and both groups recalled less in the dual-task condition than with just a single task, the cost of dividing attention was not differentially greater for the elderly relative to the young subjects. (A similar pattern also held for the findings from the picture recognition task. The older adults recognized slightly fewer pictures overall than the young adults, but they were not differentially impaired, relative to the young subjects, by the combination of the picture task and the speech recall task.)

In summary, we see that the elderly adults in this study were not *differentially* impaired by the dual-task requirement, although they, like the young adults, showed a significant lowering of performance in the dual-task condition relative to their single-task baselines. While speech comprehension can sometimes appear to be a protected function in human cognition, other tasks with different information processing characteristics may be more vulnerable to overload. Comprehending written text can sometimes be such a case (Britton, Graesser, Glynn, Hamilton, & Penland, 1983; Graesser, 1981; Inhoff & Fleming, 1989; Stine, 1990a; see Stine, 1990b, for a good review of differences between reading and listening in discourse processing).

Working Memory

As an alternative to the central resource model, some theorists have argued for the modularity, or independence, of memory associated with different cognitive functions, and particularly of speech abilities (Fodor, 1983). Support for this position comes from studies with brain-damaged patients with very poor short-term memory ability on traditional memory span tests (e.g., digit span) but who are nevertheless able to comprehend relatively complex sentences, even those with embedded clause constructions (Caplan & Waters, 1990; Martin, 1993). These finding suggest that the memory system required for language processing may be distinct from the sort of memory that would subserve, for example, numerical or spatial abilities (see also Daneman & Tardiff, 1987; Monsell, 1984).

One model that posits a reduction in the capacity of specific components of the cognitive architecture is Baddeley's (1986) model of working memory. While short-term memory is usually characterized as a temporary buffer store to hold information for immediate use or transfer to long-term memory, working memory represents a more dynamic construct. Specifically, working memory is characterized as having the simultaneous functions of both holding and processing (or manipulating) information. The model includes two peripheral storage systems, an articulatory loop for verbal material, and a visuo–spatial "scratchpad" for visual input not easily verbalized. These are monitored by a central executive that oversees the operations and scheduling of both systems. A test of working memory span developed by Daneman and Carpenter (1980) has been shown to be predictive of several performance measures related to verbal ability (Daneman & Carpenter, 1983), including verbal SAT scores and comprehension scores.

In contrast to tests of short-term memory such as the digit span, which typically show minimal age effects, tests of working memory have been shown to be sensitive to the effects of age (Light, 1991; Poon, 1985). This contrast can be seen clearly in Figure 2, which shows data from a study that compared three different measure of memory span in the same group of young and elderly adults (Wingfield, Stine, Lahar, & Aberdeen, 1988). As is often found, the young and older adults did not differ on a traditional measure of digit span, in which the subject simply heard a series of digits and repeated them back. Doing the same with a list of words (simple word span) showed a small but significant age difference. By contrast, a large age difference was found on a "loaded" word span test, which required both storage and organization of the materials. (Subjects had to listen to and comprehend a series of sentences and then recall the last word of each sentence.) These finding suggest that although short-term maintenance of information is not necessarily a problem for older adults, the manipulative aspect of working memory is especially sensitive to changes with age. It remains to be demonstrated whether this holds true for working memory as a general system (Engle, Cantor, & Carullo, 1992) or as a number of subsystems for temporary storage that serve different domains (Monsell, 1984).

In either case, the implications of these findings are clear. In situations that risk processing overload, such as TV news or weather reports, or situations that require the simultaneous maintenance and manipulation of incoming spoken information, care must be taken that older adults' working memory systems are not overloaded (Stine, Wingfield, & Myers, 1990). This is especially important in discourse processing, where age differences in

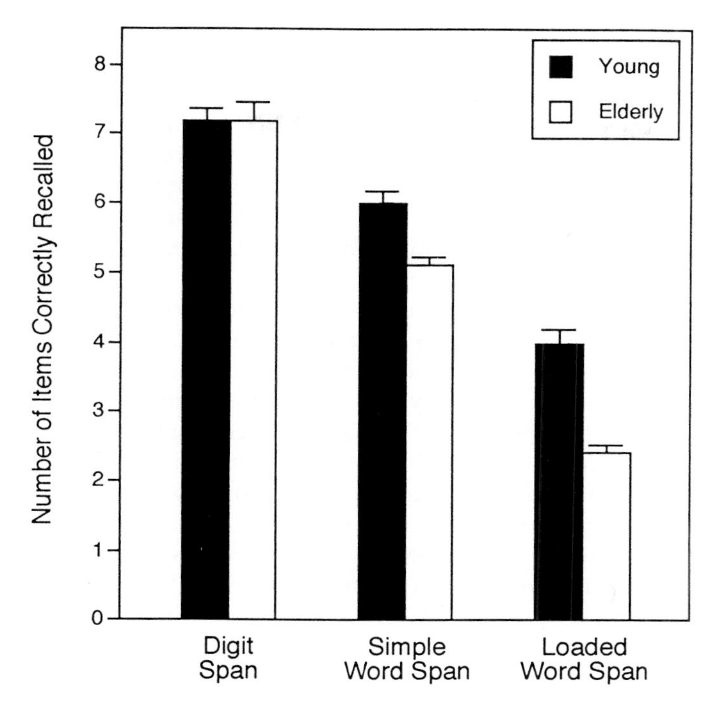

FIGURE 2 Mean number of items correctly recalled by young and elderly adults using three span measures. (From Figure 1 of *Experimental Aging Research, 14,* 103–107. Wingfield, Stine, Lahar & Aberdeen, Taylor & Francis, Inc., Washington, D.C. Reproduced with permission. All rights reserved. Wingfield, Stine, Lahar, & Aberdeen, 1988).

recall have been attributed to limitations in working memory capacity (Light, 1991). A reduced span of working memory may make it harder to integrate syntactic and pragmatic information, or to maintain multiple interpretations of potentially ambiguous areas of text (Just & Carpenter, 1992). Particularly, in elderly adults' reading of text, syntactic complexity may overload an already reduced working memory (Kemper, Jackson, Cheung, & Anagnopoulos, 1993).

In medical compliance it is easy to overburden the memory capacity of the elderly with information. Studies have shown that young as well as older adults show poor memory for prescription instructions, even when the number of medications is relatively small compared to what many elderly individuals use in the course of medical treatment (Morrell, Park, & Poon, 1989; Rice & Okun, 1994). Similarly, computer software use is an area where working memory can easily become overtaxed with the need to memorize multiple commands while carrying out operations simultaneously (e.g., press "control-K-D" to save a file).

An important area in human factors work is the way in which expertise can interact with declining working memory function in the elderly. Numerous studies have shown that testing material drawn from an elderly adult's repertoire of highly practice skills or knowledge base, typically shows smaller age differences than performance using less familiar material (Charness, 1985; Morrow, Leirer, & Altieri, 1992; Morrow, Leirer, Altieri, & Fitzsimmons, 1994).

In spoken language communication the need to recognize working memory limitations in elderly adults is especially important. Sentences with especially complex syntax, such as those with left-branching constructions, can cause the elderly listener difficulty (Kemper, 1988; Norman, Kemper, Kynette, Cheung, & Anagnopoulus, 1991). Other effects can be even more subtle. For example, while we shall show in a subsequent section that speech recognition and memory in elderly listeners is aided by linguistic context, this is less true for the use of context that *follows* a poorly perceived piece of information. These cases are limited by age differences in the ability to hold in memory the ambiguous speech awaiting the arrival of potentially clarifying information (Wingfield et al., 1994). The branching-option systems of touch-tone phone instructions can also place a heavy burden on working memory, especially if a listener is not familiar with a particular program of instructions. These often require holding in store several pieces of information while one listens to the next option and waits to decide which is the most appropriate course of action (e.g., "If you know your party's extension push 1; if this is an inquiry about an existing account push 2; if you have a question about new programs push 3 . . ."). As systems similar to this proliferate, it is important to take into account the limits of the aging memory.

Speech Processing and Cognitive Inhibition

An active area in cognitive aging research stems from the proposal by Hasher and Zacks (1988) that age effects may lie in the contents, rather than the absolute capacity, of working memory. According to this formulation, older adults have a reduced ability to inhibit irrelevant stimuli, such as material that is not oriented toward the goal path of a task at hand. This results in crosstalk between streams of information, producing an inefficient allocation of attentional resources. The result will be a deficit in comprehension and memory for the target information.

Converging support for the inhibition framework comes from several lines of experimental work related to language processing and memory for language. Connelly, Hasher, and Zacks (1991) presented subjects with written passages in which distracting text (in a standard font) was interpolated between sections of target text printed in italics. Older adults' comprehension and reading times for the materials with distracters were compromised differentially more than that of young adults. Particularly interesting were increased age differences when the distracter text was semantically related to the content of the target material. Although young adults did not find this case especially difficult, the elderly were less able to ignore this kind of material.

Older adults also tend to keep what turns out to be irrelevant material activated longer than young adults (Hamm & Hasher, 1992). Hartman and Hasher (1991) reported that, when subjects made inferences about the endings of sentences and some of those inferences were later disconfirmed, older adults but not young adults continued to remember the disconfirmed endings. Finally, other studies have shown that older adults produce more personal comments and material that is off-goal-path in narratives than young adults (Arbuckle & Gold, 1993), as well as showing an increased number of intrusions in free recall of prose materials (Stine & Wingfield, 1987b; Tun, 1989).

The general conclusion from this work is that the elderly have more difficulty in inhibiting irrelevant information than young adults and that this failure of inhibition results in increased activation of material that is not goal-path oriented. It remains to be seen whether age-related inhibitory failures are domain specific rather than general in nature, as some researchers have claimed (Kramer, Humphrey, Larish, Logan, & Strayer, 1994; Stine & Wingfield, 1994).

COMPENSATORY PROCESSES AND REAL-WORLD PERFORMANCE

Use of Linguistic Structure and Prosody

Although older adults' memory for language may be taxed when processing demands are high, the work we have discussed up to this point demonstrates that language-processing abilities are well-preserved into old age relative to many other cognitive skills. A key factor in the elderly's linguistic competence lies in the richness of the natural structure of speech, and the elderly subject's ability to use this structure to provide compensatory support against potential declines in memory or sensory capability. For example, it is well known that, at the acoustic level, up to 50% of the speech signal can be deleted without a complete loss of intelligibility (Wingfield et al., 1985). At the sentence level, as much as 50% of the words from text can be removed and the message can still be comprehended (Chapanis, 1954). This level of comprehension and associated recall is made possible by the support from the natural structure of language, with constraints at the phonetic, syntactic, semantic, and pragmatic levels as well as from acoustic features of speech prosody. (*Prosody* is a general term that includes the pitch contour, stress patter, and timing of natural speech.)

Studies of spoken word recognition have demonstrated that older adults benefit at least as much, if not more, than young adults from hearing words in a sentence context, particularly under conditions of noise or with degraded stimuli (Cohen & Faulkner, 1983; Hutchinson, 1989; Perry & Wingfield, 1994; Wingfield, Aberdeen, & Stine, 1991). Similar findings have been reported for visual recognition of degraded printed words (Madden, 1988).

These studies suggest that older adults may benefit, relative to their own baselines, even more than young adults from the linguistic structure provided by natural syntactic and semantic constraints. In one study, subjects listened to strings of words that were either normal sentences, strings that were syntactically correct but semantically anomalous (e.g., "colorless green ideas sleep furiously"), or simple random word strings (Wingfield et al., 1985). Processing load was varied by the length of the strings and the presentation rate, which ranged from normal to rapid speech rates of up to 425 wpm. The recall data for these materials indicated that age differences in the effect of rapid speech rates on memory were dramatically reduced when normal syntactic structure was present and even somewhat reduced for the semantically anomalous "sentences" that resembled real sentences in their structure. This sensitivity of elderly adults to the linguistic structure of speech, especially when the listening conditions are difficult, is a robust phenomenon that can be demonstrated under a variety of conditions (Wingfield, Tun, & Rosen, 1995).

The prosodic pattern of spoken language (i.e., intonation pattern, word stress, loudness, and pauses between words) can serve many functions in spoken communication. These include aiding syntactic parsing, giving the semantic focus of a sentence, indicating the mood of the speaker, or clarifying ambiguities in sentences. Studies have shown that older adults are more likely than young adults to remember information that received prosodic stress (Cohen & Faulkner, 1986), and the disruption of normal prosodic pattern is more detrimental to immediate recall in the elderly than in young adults (Stine & Wingfield, 1987b). Also, under conditions of rapid speech rates older adults are more reliant than young adults on normal prosody as an aid in comprehension (Wingfield, Wayland, & Stine, 1992). These findings would suggest that the elderly adult may be at a serious disadvantage in communication in speech systems deprived of normal prosody, such as the robotic, monotonic computerized messages that give transportation information in some airports and subway systems. Speech deprived of normal prosody also occurs in some voice mail systems and in telephone information systems that use concatenated digits, often with an attempt to simulate natural prosody ("The number is three . . . four . . . six . . ."). Age-related changes in memory processing must be considered in designing systems that rely on synthesized speech, especially in view of the ever-increasing numbers of older adults that will use these services.

At the other extreme, the term *elderspeak* has been coined to refer to the style of speech that many young adults adopt when speaking to an elderly adult (Cohen & Faulkner, 1986). Elderspeak mimics the highly exaggerated prosodic patterns and simplification of language found in "motherese" or speech to young children (Snow, 1972). This speech style reflects more a patronizing attitude toward the elderly than that of a functionally effective strategy. It is a speech style that can be demeaning to older adults and hence counterproductive (Ryan et al., 1986).

Predictability

Another means by which older adults compensate for declining sensory abilities, or degraded "bottom-up" input, is by relying heavily on the predictability of discourse to provide "top-down" cues for comprehension and memory. One can illustrate this effect by testing memory for speech that varies in its *redundancy.* We use the term here in its classical information theory sense, in which redundancy refers to the average predictability of stimuli within a specified context (Shannon & Weaver, 1949). Predictability can be determined using the *cloze* procedure, in which subjects are asked to guess the identity of words that have been removed at specified intervals from a passage (G. R. Miller & Coleman, 1967).

In one experiment, young adults and older adults heard spoken passages that had previously been determined to be high, medium, or low in average word predictability within the passages. After listening to each passage subjects attempted to recall it as completely as possible (Tun & Wingfield, 1994). Within a general finding that both young and older subjects showed superior recall for more predictable passages, subjects' recall also showed a "levels" effect. The levels effect refers to the common observation that propositions higher in an importance hierarchy in a narrative are better recalled than lower level details. It is also typically found that age differences are smaller for central elements of a story than for story details (Stine & Wingfield, 1987a; Zelinski, Light, & Gilewski, 1984).

This experiment replicated these findings, but also showed that, when passages were difficult to process (low predictability passages), the elderly subject's recall of details from those passages was especially impaired. For major ideas, older adults showed a pattern of recall similar to the young regardless of whether the passages were high, medium, or low in predictability. By contrast, the older adults' recall of detailed information was far below that of the young adults when the passages were low in predictability. That is, the largest age differences in memory began to appear at the level of detailed information when the processing load was great. This should be a consideration in applied settings in which the details of the communication are important, such as medical information, instructions in filling out forms, or emergency weather instructions.

THE THRESHOLD OF FUNCTIONAL ADEQUACY

A difficulty in dividing attention is commonly cited in the aging literature as a hallmark of the aging process (e.g., Craik, 1977; Welford, 1958). In fact, in self-ratings, elderly adults report increasing difficulty in dividing attention with age, especially for activities that require monitoring complex or novel information (e.g., driving while reading road signs). By contrast, self-perceived difficulty of performing combinations of activities that include routine activities (e.g., household chores) and those that involved speech (e.g., planning your reply while listening to someone talk) remain relatively stable in old age, with little change across an age range running from age 60 to age 90 (Tun & Wingfield, 1995).

This latter point may not be surprising given that language processing is a highly overlearned activity in which older adults may be considered to be "expert" listeners who are able to utilize the many types of support that occur in natural speech (Wingfield & Stine, 1991). However, making simple predictions about elderly adults' willingness to undertake high-load tasks, we believe, is complicated by what we refer to as a *threshold of functional adequacy.*

Imagine, for example, that we were to conduct an experiment in which performance drops equally for young and elderly subjects when going from single-task to dual-task performance. For example, both age groups might drop in recall accuracy by 20 percentage points or they both might get slower in their responses by, for example, 200 ms. We have illustrated such an imaginary outcome in Figure 3, which shows hypothetical performance for young and elderly adults on a particular task, first when the task is performed alone (single task) and then when the same task is performed while the subject is engaged in a concurrent secondary activity (dual task). For the purposes of this illustration, the performance measure on the *y*-axis could be either speed or accuracy. Were we to conduct a traditional analysis

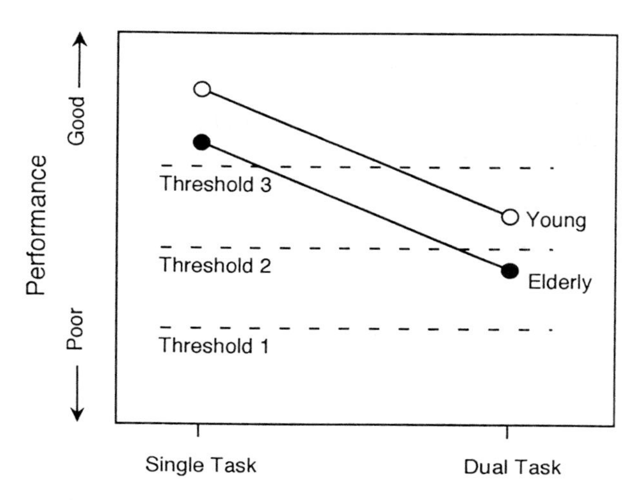

FIGURE 3 Hypothetical single- and dual-task performance data for young and elderly adults with three different thresholds of functional adequacy.

of variance on these data, we would most probably get significant main effects of age, and of single versus dual-task activity. Although the main effect of age would be present, the parallel lines for the young and elderly subjects make it unlikely we would see a significant age by dual-task interaction. From this we would reasonably conclude that the elderly subjects were no more debilitated by the imposition of a secondary task than were the young.

In many regards, however, this is a pass–fail word in which minimum levels of performance signify adequate function for a particular task. Let us say that under a cognitive load both young and elderly adults' reaction times increase by 100 ms; going from a baseline average of 450 ms to 550 for a young subject and from, say, 550 to 650 ms for an elderly subject. The young subject's reaction speed of 550 ms may still be fast enough to avert an accident while driving a car if the car in front suddenly stopped. But a slowing of reaction speed by the same 100 ms for the elderly subjects could put their reaction times just over the reaction threshold needed to stop the vehicle within the necessary distance. In this case, the physics of stopping distances will determine the threshold of functional adequacy: the older person may end up bumping the tailgate of the car in front.

As we have indicated, in many cases in the aging literature, one does not see a statistical age by dual-task interaction of the sort that would be evidence for the elderly being *differentially* impaired by dual-task conditions. However, in these same experiments one almost always sees highly significant main effects of age. If these main effects were large enough to tip the elderly over a situationally defined threshold of functional adequacy, this could produce a real-world differential deficit. This would be true even though, statistically speaking, the elderly were performing no worse in the face of dual-task load than the young relative to their own baselines. That is, the theoretical interests in the research literature that have focused on age interactions, rather than on main effects, may have tended to obscure the importance of the simple main effects of age that almost invariably occur.

We have illustrated this point with the hypothetical data in Figure 3, where we show such a parallel drop in performance for young and elderly adults when a secondary task is added. Although the dual-task condition does not lower the elderly subjects' performance to a greater degree than the young, if adequate performance is defined by Threshold levels 2 or 3, the elderly would drop below an acceptable level of performance. That is, a performance drop that keeps the young above a threshold of functional adequacy may drop the elderly subject below that critical performance level. (Note that the young are not immune from detrimental effects of dual-task interference, as would be the case for a task whose level of minimally acceptable performance was at Threshold 3. Similarly, in a situation where a level of performance indicated by Threshold level 1 is adequate for success, the elderly subject might be functionally unimpaired by a dual-task load even though a significant drop in performance has occurred.)

The question of what is adequate performance on a task will obviously vary with the specifics of the situation. For example, forgetting to buy a single ingredient for a cake you intend to make can represent total failure if the single ingredient is a critical one. Remembering to mail an application form one day after deadline does not make the grade nor does remembering a grandchild's birthday after the party. The same is true when one attempts to introduce a person but for the moment is unable to remember that person's name. Remembering the name later (e.g., in the middle of the night) is just too late.

In many cases, one can fail at some proportion of a task and still function adequately. A momentary inability to retrieve a desired word in the midst of a conversation can go unnoticed if we can make do with another, similar word. Similarly, although it is frustrating to see an exit sign just as one passes it on the highway, in most cases one can turn off at the next exit and go back. There will be some loss of time, but it is not an irreparable error.

We have considered here objective, external criteria for setting a threshold of functional adequacy. Subjective judgments of what counts as adequate performance may also change with age. Older subjects' adequacy judgments are likely to be influenced by their sense of their own past performance when they were younger and their perceptions of the abilities of other people. There may, in fact, be a developmental shift in the type of awareness of memory performance from a more systematic knowledge of facts about memory in youth, to a heightened awareness of one's ongoing cognitive activities in old age (Cavanaugh, 1991). This heightened awareness may contribute to the elderly's increased dissatisfaction with their performance on tasks and reports of memory failures. Such "failures" are often reported even in the absence of age-differences in objectively measured memory performance (Hertzog, Dixon, & Hultsch, 1990; Zelinski, Gilewski, & Thompson, 1980). Age differences in the extent of awareness of deficiencies in ongoing performance means that the threshold of functional adequacy will be affected not only by objective circumstances but by subjective standards that may differ at different points in the life span.

CONCLUSION

In this chapter we have outlined a number of important issues in aging and language processing. As we have shown, comprehension and memory for speech are typically well maintained into old age even under the challenges of divided attention. This is so, we believe, because older adults are able to compensate for deficits in lower level sensory and memory processes by means of an increased reliance on top-down processing aided by contextual cues and the linguistic support provided by natural speech.

It is true that age-related declines in performance do occur when language abilities are overburdened, as in the case of very rapid speech. However, even as the studies we have cited have demonstrated age-related processing limitations, they have also suggested sources of compensation for those deficits. The speech-processing system can thus serve as an excellent model of how elderly adults are able to adapt to changing cognitive capabilities by means of compensation and effective use of structure, context, and environmental support. It remains our continuing challenge to design the environment in such a fashion that it provides appropriate support for communication to be optimized across the life span for the ever-increasing numbers of older adults.

We have highlighted in this chapter a number of important principles that should be taken into account by the human factors scientist. Among these is the importance of controlling speech rate in spoken communication and respecting working memory limitations in the elderly. This latter goal can be accomplished by using syntax that is not overly complex, maintaining normal prosody as an aid to comprehension, and limiting the amount of rapidly arriving detail in a message.

A final point to be considered in any applied setting is the concept of functional adequacy for a particular ask or situation. That is, the real-world impact of a decline in performance is often situationally defined, so that the same performance decline that has only minimal consequences in one case can prove devastating in another. We have referred to this important principle as the *threshold of functional adequacy.*

Acknowledgments

We gratefully acknowledge support from NIH grant AG04517 from the National Institute on Aging and support from the W. M. Keck Foundation.

References

Arbuckle, T. Y., & Gold, D. P. (1993). Aging, inhibition, and verbosity. *Journal of Gerontology: Psychological Sciences, 48,* 225–232.

Baddeley, A. (1986). *Working memory.* New York: Oxford University Press.

Bergman, M. (1980). *Aging and the perception of speech.* Baltimore: University Park Press.

Bergman, M., Blumenfeld, V. G., Cascardo, D., Dash, B., Levitt, H., & Margulies, M. K. (1976). Age-related decrements in hearing for speech. *Journal of Gerontology, 31,* 533–538.

Birren, J. E. (1964). *The psychology of aging.* Englewood Cliffs, NJ: Prentice-Hall.

Britton, B. K., Graesser, A. C., Glynn, S. M., Hamilton, T., & Penland, M. (1983). Use of cognitive capacity in reading: Effects of some content features of text. *Discourse Processes, 6,* 39–57.

Brown, G., & Yule, G. (1983). *Discourse analysis.* Cambridge, UK: Cambridge University Press.

Caplan, D., & Waters, G. (1990). Short-term memory and language comprehension: A critical review of the neuropsychological literature. In G. Vallar & T. Shallice (Eds.), *Neuropsychological impairments of short-term memory* (pp. 337–389). Cambridge, UK: Cambridge University Press.

Cavanaugh, J. C. (1991). The importance of awareness in memory aging. In L. W. Poon, D. C. Rubin, & B. A. Wilson (Eds.), *Everyday cognition in adulthood and old age* (pp. 416–436). New York: Cambridge University Press.

Cerella, J. (1985). Information processing rates in the elderly. *Psychological Bulletin, 98,* 67–83.

Cerella, J. (1990). Aging and information-processing rate. In J. E. Birren & K. W. Schaie (Eds.), *Handbook of the psychology of aging* (3rd ed., pp. 201–221). San Diego, CA: Academic Press.

Cerella, J., & Hale, S. (1994). The rise and fall in information-processing rates over the life span. *Acta Psychologica, 86,* 109–197.

Cerella, J., Poon, L. W., & Williams, D. M. (1980). Age and the complexity hypothesis. In L. W. Poon (Ed.), *Aging in the 1980s: Psychological Issues* (pp. 332–340). Washington, DC: American Psychological Association.

Chapanis, A. (1954). The reconstruction of abbreviated printed messages. *Journal of Experimental Psychology, 48,* 496–510.

Charness, N. (1985). Aging and problem-solving performance. In N. Charness (Ed.), *Aging and human performance* (pp. 225–259). New York: Wiley.

Chodorow, M. S. (1979). Time-compressed speech and the study of lexical and syntactic processing. In W. E. Cooper & E. C. T. Walker (Eds.), *Sentence processing: Psycholinguistic studies presented to Merrill Garrett* (pp. 87–111). Hillsdale, NJ: Erlbaum.

Cohen, G., & Faulkner, D. (1983). Word recognition: Age differences in contextual facilitation effects. *British Journal of Psychology, 74,* 239–251.

Cohen, G., & Faulkner, D. (1986). Does "Elderspeak" work? The effect of intonation and stress on comprehension and recall of spoken discourse in old age. *Language and Communication, 6,* 91–98.

Connelly, S. L., Hasher, L., & Zacks, R. T. (1991). Age and reading: The impact of distraction. *Psychology and Aging, 4,* 533–541.

Craik, F. I. M. (1977). Age differences in human memory. In J. E. Birren & K. W. Schaie (Eds.), *Handbook of the psychology of aging* (pp. 384–420). New York: Van Nostrand-Reinhold.

Craik, F. I. M., & Byrd, M. (1982). Aging and cognitive deficits: The role of attentional resources. In F. I. M. Craik & S. Trehub (Eds.), *Aging and cognitive processes* (pp. 191–211). New York: Plenum.

Craik, F. I. M., & McDowd, J. (1987). Age differences in recall and recognition. *Journal of Experimental Psychology: Learning, Memory and Cognition, 13,* 474–479.

Daneman, M., & Carpenter, P. A. (1980). Individual differences in working memory and reading. *Journal of Verbal Learning and Verbal Behavior, 19,* 450–466.

Daneman, M., & Carpenter, P. A. (1983). Individual differences in integrating information between and within sentences. *Journal of Experimental Psychology: Learning, Memory, and Cognition, 9,* 561–583.

Daneman, M., & Tardiff, T. (1987). Working memory and reading skill re-examined. In M. Coltheart (Ed.), *Attention and Performance XII: The Psychology of Reading* (pp. 491–508). Hillsdale, NJ: Erlbaum.

Dubno, J. R., Dirks, D. D., & Morgan, D. E. (1982). Effects of mild hearing loss and age on speech recognition in noise. *Journal of the Acoustical Society of America, Supplement, 72,* S34–S35.

Duquesnoy, A. J. (1983). The intelligibility of sentences in quiet and noise in aged listeners. *Journal of the Acoustical Society of America, 74,* 1136–1144.

Engle, R. W., Cantor, J., & Carullo, J. J. (1992). Individual differences in working memory and comprehension: A test of four hypotheses. *Journal of Experimental Psychology: Learning, Memory, and Cognition, 18,* 972–992.

Fisk, A. D., & Fisher, D. L. (1994). Brinley plots and theories of aging: The explicit, muddled, and implicit debates. *Journal of Gerontology: Psychological Sciences, 49,* P81–P89.

Flores D' Arcais, G. B., & Scheuder, R. (1983). The process of language understanding: A few issues in contemporary psycholonguistics. In G. B. Flores D'Arcais, & K. J. Jarvella (Eds.), *The process of language understanding* (pp. 1–41). New York: Wiley.

Fodor, J. A. (1983). *The modularity of mind.* Cambridge, MA: MIT Press.

Gick, M. L., Craik, F. I. M., & Morris, R. G. (1988). Task complexity and age differences in working memory. *Memory & Cognition, 16,* 353–361.

Gordon-Salant, S. (1987). Age-related differences in speech recognition performance as a function of test format and paradigm. *Ear and Hearing, 8,* 227–282.

Gordon-Salant, S., & Fitzgibbons, P. J. (1993). Temporal factors and speech recognition performance in young and elderly listeners. *Journal of Speech and Hearing Research, 36,* 1276–1285.

Graesser, A. C. (1981). *Prose comprehension beyond the word.* New York: Springer-Verlag.

Hamm, V. P., & Hasher, L. (1992). Age and the availability of inference. *Psychology and Aging, 7,* 56–64.

Hartman, M., & Hasher, L. (1991). Aging and suppression: Memory for previously relevant information. *Psychology and Aging, 6,* 587–594.

Hasher, L., & Zacks, R. T. (1988). Working memory, comprehension, and aging: A review and a new view. In G. H. Bower (Ed.), *The psychology of learning and motivation* (Vol. 22, pp. 193–225). San Diego, CA: Academic Press.

Heiman, G. W., Leo, R. J., Leighbody, G., & Bowler, K. (1986). Word intelligibility decrements and the comprehension of time-compressed speech. *Perception and Psychophysics, 40,* 407–411.

Hertzog, C., Dixon, R. A., & Hultsch, D. F. (1990). Metamemory in adulthood: Differentiating knowledge, belief, and behavior. In T. M. Hess (Ed.), *Aging and cognition: Knowledge organization and utilization* (pp. 161–212). New York: Elsevier.

Hutchinson, K. M. (1989). Influence of sentence context on speech perception in young and older adults. *Journal of Gerontology, 44,* 36–44.

Inhoff, A. W., & Fleming, K. (1989). Probe-detection times during the reading of easy and difficult text. *Journal of Experimental Psychology: Learning, Memory, and Cognition, 15,* 339–351.

Just, M. A., & Carpenter, P. A. (1992). A capacity theory of comprehension: Individual differences in working memory. *Psychology and Aging, 99,* 122–149.

Kahneman, D. (1973). *Attention and effort.* Englewood Cliffs, NJ: Prentice-Hall.

Kalikow, D. N., Stevens, K. N., & Elliott, L. L. (1977). Development of a test of speech intelligibility in noise using sentence materials with controlled word predictability. *Journal of the Acoustical Society of America, 61,* 1337–1351.

Kemper, S. (1988). Geriatric psycholinguistics: Syntactic limitations of oral and written language. In L. L. Light & D. M. Burke (Eds.), *Language, memory, and aging* (pp. 58–76). New York: Cambridge University Press.

Kemper, S., Jackson, J. D., Cheung, H., & Anagnopoulos, C. A. (1993). Enhancing older adults' reading comprehension. *Discourse Processes, 16,* 405–428.

Konkle, D. F., Beasley, D. S., & Bess, F. H. (1977). Intelligibility of time-altered speech in relation to chronological aging. *Journal of Speech and Hearing Research, 20,* 108–115.

Kramer, A. F., Humphrey, D. G., Larish, J. F., Logan, G. D., & Strayer, D. L. (1994). Aging and inhibition: Beyond a unitary view of inhibitory processing in attention. *Psychology and Aging, 9,* 491–512.

Light, L. L. (1991). Memory and aging: Four hypotheses in search of data. *Annual Review of Psychology, 42,* 333–376.

Lima, S. D., Hale, S., & Myerson, J. (1991). How general is general slowing? Evidence from the lexical domain. *Psychology and Aging, 6,* 416–425.

Luterman, D. M., Welsh, O. L., & Melrose, J. (1966). Responses of aged males to time-altered speech stimuli. *Journal of Speech and Hearing Research, 9,* 226–230.

Macht, M. L., & Buschke, H. (1983). Age differences in cognitive effort in recall. *Journal of Gerontology, 38,* 695–700.

Madden, D. J. (1988). Adult age differences in the effects of sentence context and stimulus degradation during visual word recognition. *Psychology and Aging, 3,* 167–172.

Marslen-Wilson, W. D., & Tyler, L. K. (1980). The temporal structure of spoken language understanding. *Cognition, 8,* 1–71.

Martin, R. C. (1993). Short-term memory and sentence processing: Evidence from neuropsychology. *Memory & Cognition, 21,* 176–183.

Miller, G. R., & Coleman, E. B. (1967). A set of thirty-six prose passages calibrated for complexity. *Journal of Verbal Learning and Verbal Behavior, 6,* 851–854.

Miller, J. L., Grosjean, F., & Lomanto, C. (1984). Articulation rate and its variability in spontaneous speech: A reanalysis and some implications. *Phonetica, 41,* 215–225.

Monsell, S. (1984). Components of working memory underlying verbal skills: A "distributed capacities" view. In H. Bouma & D. G. Bouwhuis (Eds.), *Attention and Performance X. Control of language processes* (pp. 327–350). Hillsdale, NJ: Erlbaum.

Morrell, R. W., Park, D. C., & Poon, L. W. (1989). Quality of instructions on prescription drug labels: Effects on memory and comprehension in young and old adults. *Gerontologist, 29,* 345–354.

Morris, R. G., Gick, M. L., & Craik, F. I. M. (1988). Processing resources and age differences in working memory. *Memory & Cognition, 16,* 362–366.

Morrow, D. G., Leirer, V. O., & Altieri, P. A. (1992). Aging, expertise, and narrative processing. *Psychology and Aging, 7,* 376–388.

Morrow, D. G., Leirer, V. O., Altieri, P. A., & Fitzsimmons, C. (1994). When expertise reduces age differences in performance. *Psychology and Aging, 9,* 134–148.

Norman, S., Kemper, S., Kynette, D., Cheung, H., & Anagnopoulus, C. (1991). Syntactic complexity and adults' running memory span. *Journal of Gerontology: Psychological Sciences, 46,* P346–P351.

Olsho, L. W., Harkins, S. W., & Lenhardt, M. L. (1985). Aging and the auditory system. In J. E. Birren & K. W. Schaie (Eds.), *Handbook of the psychology of aging* (2nd ed., pp. 332–377). New York: Van Nostrand-Reinhold.

Park, D., Smith, A. D., Dudley, W., & Lafronza, V. N. (1989). Effects of age and a divided attention task presented during encoding and retrieval on memory. *Journal of Experimental Psychology: Learning, Memory, and Cognition, 15,* 1185–1191.

Pearsons, K. D., Bennett, R. L., & Fidell, S. (1977). *Speech levels in various noise environments* (EPA 600/1-77-025). Washington, DC: Office of Health & Ecological Effects.

Perry, A. R., & Wingfield, A. (1994). Contextual encoding by young and elderly adults as revealed by cued and free recall. *Aging and Cognition, 1,* 120–139.

Pichora-Fuller, M. K., Schneider, B. A., & Daneman, M. (in press). How young and old adults listen to and remember speech in noise. *Journal of the Acoustical Society of America.*

Pollack, I., & Pickett, J. M. (1963). Intelligibility of excerpts from conversation. *Language and Speech, 28,* 97–102.

Poon, L. W. (1985). Differences in human memory with aging: Nature, causes, and clinical implications. In J. E. Birren & K. W. Schaie (Eds.), *Handbook of the psychology of aging* (2d ed., pp. 427–462). New York: Van Nostrand-Reinhold.

Rabbitt, P. M. A. (1968). Channel capacity, intelligibility, and immediate memory. *Quarterly Journal of Experimental Psychology, 20,* 241–248.

Rabbitt, P. M. A. (1991). Mild hearing loss can cause apparent memory failures which increase with age and reduce with IQ. *Acta Oto-Laryngologica, 476,* 167–176.

Rice, G. E., & Okun, M. A. (1994). Older readers' processing of medical information that contradicts their beliefs. *Journal of Gerontology: Psychological Sciences, 49,* P119–P128.

Riggs, K. M., Wingfield, A., & Tun, P. A. (1993). Passage difficulty, speech rate, and age differences in memory for spoken text: Speech recall and the complexity hypothesis. *Experimental Aging Research, 19,* 111–128.

Rubin, A. M. (1986). Television, aging, and information seeking. *Language and Communication, 6,* 125–137.

Ryan, E. B., Giles, H., Bartolucci, G., & Henwood, K. (1986). Psycholinguistics and social psychological components of communication by and with the elderly. *Language and Communication, 6,* 1–24.

Salthouse, T. A. (1991). *Theoretical perspectives on cognitive aging.* Hillsdale, NJ: Erlbaum.

Shannon, C. E., & Weaver, W. (1949). *The mathematical theory of communication.* Urbana: University of Illinois Press.

Snow, C. E. (1972). Mother's speech to children in language learning. *Child Development, 43,* 549–565.

Somberg, B. L., & Salthouse, T. A. (1982). Divided attention abilities in young and old adults. *Journal of Experimental Psychology: Human Perception and Performance, 8,* 651–663.

Sticht, T. G., & Gray, B. B. (1969). The intelligibility of time compressed words as a function of age and hearing loss. *Journal of Speech and Hearing Research, 12,* 443–448.

Stine, E. A. L. (1990a). On-line processing of written text by younger and older adults. *Psychology and Aging, 5,* 68–78.

Stine, E. A. L. (1990b). The way reading and listening work: A tutorial review of discourse processing and aging. In E. A. Lovelace (Ed.), *Aging and cognition: Mental processes, self awareness and interventions* (pp. 301–327). North-Holland: Elsevier.

Stine, E. A. L., & Wingfield, A. (1987a). Levels upon levels: Predicting age differences in text recall. *Experimental Aging Research, 13,* 179–183.

Stine, E. A. L., & Wingfield, A. (1987b). Process and strategy in memory for speech among younger and older adults. *Psychology and Aging, 2,* 272–279.

Stine, E. A. L., & Wingfield, A. (1994). Older adults can inhibit high-probability competitors in speech recognition. *Aging and Cognition, 1,* 152–157.

Stine, E. A. L., Wingfield, A., & Myers, S. D. (1990). Age differences in processing information from television news: The effects of bisensory augmentation. *Journal of Gerontology: Psychological Sciences, 45,* P1–P8.

Stine, E. A. L., Wingfield, A., & Poon, L. W. (1986). How much and how fast: Rapid speech processing of spoken language in later adulthood. *Psychology and Aging, 1,* 303–311.

Taylor, J. L., Yesavage, J. A., Morrow, D. G., Dolhert, N., Brooks, J. O., & Poon, L. W. (1994). The effects of information load and speech rate on younger and older aircraft pilot's ability to execute simulated air-traffic controller instructions. *Journal of Gerontology: Psychological Sciences, 49,* P191–P200.

Tun, P. A. (1989). Age differences in processing expository and narrative text. *Journal of Gerontology, 44,* 9–15.

Tun, P. A., & Wingfield, A. (1993). Is speech special? Perception and recall of spoken language in complex environments. In J. Cerella, W. Hoyer, J. Rybash, & M. L. Commons (Eds.), *Adult information processing: Limits on loss* (pp. 425–457). San Diego, CA: Academic Press.

Tun, P. A., & Wingfield, A. (1994). Speech recall under heavy load conditions: Age, predictability, and limits on dual-task interference. *Aging and Cognition, 1,* 29–44.

Tun, P. A., & Wingfield, A. (1995). Does dividing attention become harder with age? Findings from the Divided Attention Questionnaire. *Aging and Cognition, 2,* 39–66.

Tun, P. A., Wingfield, A., & Stine, E. A. L. (1991). Speech processing capacity in young and old adults: A dual-task study. *Psychology and Aging, 6,* 3–9.

Tun, P. A., Wingfield, A., Stine, E. A. L., & Mecsas, C. (1992). Rapid speech processing and divided attention: Processing rate versus processing resources as an explanation of age effects. *Psychology and Aging, 7,* 546–550.

U.S. Congress, Office of Technology Assessment. (1986, May). *Hearing impairment and elderly people—A background paper* (OTA-BP-30). Washington, DC: U.S. Government Printing Office.

van Dijk, T. A., & Kintsch, W. (1983). *Strategies of discourse comprehension.* New York: Academic Press.

Welford, A. T. (1958). *Ageing and human skill.* London: Oxford University Press.

Wickens, C. D., Braune, R., & Stokes, A. (1987). Age differences in the speed and capacity of information processing. 1. A dual-task approach. *Psychology and Aging, 2,* 70–78.

Wingfield, A., Aberdeen, J. S., & Stine, E. A. L. (1991). Word onset gating and linguistic context in spoken word recognition by young and elderly adults. *Journal of Gerontology: Psychological Sciences, 46,* P127–P129.

Wingfield, A., Alexander, A. H., & Cavigelli, S. (1994). Does memory constrain the utilization of top-down information in spoken word recognition? Evidence from normal aging. *Language and Speech, 37,* 221–235.

Wingfield, A., & Lindfield, K. C. (1995). Multiple memory systems in the processing of speech: Evidence from aging. *Experimental Aging Research, 21,* 101–121.

Wingfield, A., Poon, L. W., Lombardi, L., & Lowe, D. (1985). Speed of processing in normal aging: Effects of speech rate, linguistic structure, and processing time. *Journal of Gerontology, 40, 579–585.*

Wingfield, A., & Stine, E. A. L. (1991). Expert systems in nature: Spoken language processing and adult aging. In J. D. Sinnott & J. C. Cavanaugh (Eds.), *Bridging paradigms: Positive cognitive development in adulthood and aging* (pp. 237–258). New York: Praeger.

Wingfield, A., Stine, E. A. L., Lahar, C. J., & Aberdeen, J. S. (1988). Does the capacity of working memory change with age? *Experimental Aging Research, 14,* 103–107.

Wingfield, A., Tun, P. A., & Rosen, M. (1995). Age differences in veridical and reconstructive recall of syntactically and randomly segmented speech. *Journal of Gerontology: Psychological Sciences, 50B,* P257–P266.

Wingfield, A., Wayland, S. C., & Stine, E. A. L. (1992). Adult age differences in the use of prosody for syntactic parsing and recall of spoken sentences. *Journal of Gerontology: Psychological Sciences, 47,* P350–P356.

Working Group on Speech Understanding and Aging. (1988). Speech understanding and aging. *Journal of the Acoustical Society of America, 83,* 859–895.

Zelinski, E. M., Gilewski, M. J., & Thompson, L. W. (1980). Do laboratory tests relate to self-assessments of memory ability in the young and old? In L. W. Poon, J. L. Fozard, L. S. Cermak, D. Arenberg, & L. W. Thompson (Eds.), *New directions in memory and aging. Proceedings of the George A. Talland Memorial Conference* (pp. 519–544). Hillsdale, NJ: Erlbaum.

Zelinski, E. M., Light, L. L., & Gilewski, M. J. (1984). Adult age differences in memory for prose: The question of sensitivity to passage structure. *Developmental Psychology, 20,* 1181–1192.

Chapter 7

Individual Differences, Aging, and Human Factors: An Overview

Wendy A. Rogers

INTRODUCTION

The Human Factors and Ergonomics Society (HFES) is the primary organization for human factors scientists and professionals in the United States with over 5200 members. The society defines *human factors** as "the knowledge concerning the characteristics of human beings that are applicable to the design of systems and devices of all kinds . . . and the use of such knowledge to achieve compatibility in the design of interactive systems of people, machines, and environments to ensure their effectiveness, safety, and ease of performance" (Human Factors and Ergonomics Society, 1996, p. 1). Therefore, one of the goals of human factors research is to discover general "laws" that govern the relationships between people and systems.

*The term *human factors* will be used here as inclusive of human factors and ergonomics.

Handbook of Human Factors and the Older Adult

This is a lofty goal, made even more complex because there are differences between systems as well as between people. Consequently, while there may be identifiable relationships between people and systems, such relationships may be altered for specific systems and specific people.

Suppose we are trying to understand person–computer interactions, a popular and important topic in human factors (Nickerson, 1992). Our knowledge of such interactions may be dependent on whether the system is menu driven or command based (a system characteristic) as well as whether the user is a novice or an expert (a person characteristic). The focus of the present chapter is on the person characteristics (i.e., individual differences) that must be considered by human factors researchers and practitioners.

A wide range of individual differences may mediate system performance. For example, personality variables such as motivation, locus of control, introversion or extroversion, and risk taking or cautiousness have been investigated in the context of learning and instruction (Jonassen & Grabowski, 1993). Other individual difference variables that may be determinants of successful performance on a system or utilization of a device include general cognitive abilities, prior knowledge, field dependence or independence, cognitive styles, and learning styles.

Also considered to be individual difference variables are group classifications such as sex, race, or age. While racial and sex differences are important variables of study, they are not the focus of the present chapter. For age differences, our interest lies with the effects of age on the individual difference variables mentioned previously. That is, do mental abilities or motivation change with age, is one's predominant learning style likely to change as one grows older, and so on. To illustrate, Jonassen and Grabowski (1993) report that people classified as field independent learn more from individualized, self-paced instruction. However, the research they reviewed was conducted with young adults. It is unknown whether the field independent or dependent variable is similarly related to instructional preference for older adults.

The goals of the chapter are (1) to review the importance of personality and other individual differences to the field of human factors, (2) to determine whether these variables change as a function of age, and (3) to determine whether the relationships between the individual difference variables and performance are the same for young and older adults. All three goals will be aspired to for each individual difference variable discussed in the chapter. In some cases, there has been little research with older adults. The reader will thus be informed of areas in which more research is needed to understand individual difference variables in the context of aging and human factors.

THE AGE VARIABLE

Prior to embarking on our review of various individual difference variables, it is important to first specify what we mean by *aging* and *older adults*. In the present context, an older adult is an individual over age 60. Aging refers to the processes that accompany growing older. Chronological age serves only as an index for biological, psychological, and sociological changes that occur, and older adults are not a homogeneous population. Nickerson (1992) suggest that "we need also some new ways to think about aging and especially a greater recognition of the very great range of individual differences among elderly and aging people" (p. 354). There is some controversy about whether the performance of the older adult population tends to be more variable than younger populations (see Devolder, 1991, and Rabbitt, 1990, for contrasting views on this issue). However, the performance variability of older adults as a group is at least as variable as young adult groups, and this must be recognized.

INDIVIDUAL DIFFERENCES AND HUMAN FACTORS

A perusal of the different technical groups of HFES (listed in Table 1) reveals the range of systems and devices for which individual differences must be considered: aerospace systems, communications, computer systems, consumer products, medical systems, and visual performance. Moreover, individual difference variables must be considered by educators, trainers, and system developers.

Although individual differences may not come to mind immediately when one considers the study of human factors, the answer to the question of why we study individual differences was well stated by Adams:

> Performance on tasks without concern for individual differences would reflect the processes that define general laws of behavior. Measures from individuals in these same tasks would give human variation in the processes, and this would lead to general laws that include the prediction of individual behavior, which should be the goal of psychology. (1989a, p. 16)

Substitute *human factors* for *psychology* and we have answered the question. Our knowledge is incomplete if we ignore the irrefutable fact of individual differences.

TABLE 1
Technical Groups of the Human Factors and Ergonomics Society

Aerospace Systems—application of human factors to the development, design, operation, and maintenance of human-machine systems in aviation and space environments.

Aging—human factors applications appropriate to meeting the needs of older people and other special populations in a wide variety of life settings.

Cognitive Engineering and Decision Making—research on human cognition and decision making and the application of this knowledge to the design of systems and training programs.

Communications—human factors of the design, evaluation, operation, maintenance, and use of communications products; determination of user needs; service/system and user interface design; installation, maintenance, and use of systems; field evaluation; training.

Consumer Products—applying human factors and industrial design to the development and design of products used by consumers, including publicly sold goods, office equipment, and related items (excluding military and industrial production equipment).

Educators' Professional—education and training of human factors and ergonomics specialists in academia, industry, and government; accreditation of graduate programs and professional certification.

Environmental Design—all aspects of human interaction with the constructed environment, including architectural and interior design aspects of home, office, and industrial settings.

Forensics Professional—application of human factors knowledge and techniques to "standards of care" and accountability established within legislative, regulatory, and judicial systems; providing a scientific basis to issues being interpreted by legal theory.

Individual Differences in Performance—interested in personality and individual difference characteristics that influence the understanding and prediction of performance in any area of human factors research or application.

Industrial Ergonomics—application of ergonomic data and principles in the civilian industrial setting; focus is on service and manufacturing processes, not the design of the resulting product.

Medical Systems and Rehabilitation—interested in maximizing the contributions of human factors to the effectiveness of medical systems and quality of life for people who are functionally impaired.

Organizational Design and Management—improving productivity and the quality of work life by an integration of psychosocial, cultural, and technological factors with human-machine performance interface factors in the design of jobs, workstations, organizations, and related management systems.

Safety—research and applications concerning human factors for safety in all settings and attendant populations, including transportation, military, office, public buildings, recreation, and home environments.

Surface Transportation—focus on passenger, commercial, and military vehicles; mass transit; rail transit; maritime transportation; and their associated infrastructure systems (including ITS, or Intelligent Transportation Systems).

System Development—Defining human factors activities and integrating them into the system development process in order to ensure systems that meet user requirements.

(*continues*)

TABLE 1—*Continued*

Test and Evaluation—methodologies and techniques of test and evaluation (would include personality testing, ability testing, aptitude testing, and evaluation of work performance).

Training—instructional design, development, implementation and evaluation, and integration of training into overall system design.

Virtual Environments—concerned with human factors issues associated with human-virtual environment interaction (e.g., maximizing performance efficiency, minimizing health and safety problems, and circumventing potential social issues).

Visual Performance—the nature, content, and quantification of visual information and the context in which it is displayed; the physics and psychophysics of information display; perceptual and cognitive representation and interpretation of displayed information; assessment of workload using visual tasks; actions and behaviors that are consequences of visually displayed information.

Source: Human Factors and Ergonomics Society Directory and Yearbook (1996).

LOCUS OF CONTROL

The construct of locus of control represents the degree to which individuals believe that they have control over the events of their lives (internals) or that forces outside of their control determine the course of events (externals). This construct has typically been thought of as a continuum whereby individuals are classified as either internals or externals (for a review, see Jonassen & Grabowski, 1993).

Locus of control has proved to be predictive of instructional benefits. For example, children classified as internals tend to benefit more from intrinsic feedback such as self-discovery, whereas those classified as externals benefit from extrinsic feedback such as praise (Minton & Schneider, 1985). In their review of the extant literature on the relationships between locus of control and instruction, Jonassen and Grabowski (1993) reached the following conclusions. Externals will benefit most from structured instructional situations, provision of detailed cues, and postresponse rewards and praise. Internals, on the other hand, will benefit most from instructional designs that allow for individualized, self-paced learning and the opportunity to evaluate their own successes or failures.

A good deal of research has been conducted on the locus of control variable and whether it changes as people grow older. The results of this research are inconsistent; some data show that older adults are more internal, whereas other data suggest older adults are more external or no different than younger adults (for a review, see Lachman, 1986). The inconsistency of the results appears to have been due to the representation of the locus of control variable as well as to the way in which it was assessed.

The first measurement instrument for assessing locus of control was developed by Rotter (1966). His Internal–External Locus of Control Scale was designed to measure locus of control across a range of areas (e.g., government, work, social situations). However, this conceptualization of locus of control may have been too limited. Levenson (1974) developed a measurement tool with three separate scales: (1) internal, (2) powerful others, and (3) chance. This measurement technique was designed to separate the external dimension into control by others or just lack of control. Thus, instead of locus of control being on a continuum, Levenson's conceptualization broadens the construct and allows a more sensitive assessment of age-related differences. For example, Lachman (1986) demonstrated that age-related differences were least likely to be observed for the internal scale but were found for the powerful others and chance scales. She suggests the possibility that "with aging one becomes more sensitive to the forces of powerful others and chance, without changing one's sense of internal control" (p. 36).

An additional development in recent research on the construct of locus of control is the idea that it may be domain specific. To illustrate, you may believe in your own control over your personal life but in the control of powerful others in the work environment. The instantiation of the locus of control construct as a multidimensional variable has important implications for understanding age-related differences in various domains. The domain of health care will be used to illustrate.

The Multidimensional Health Locus of Control (MHLOC) measurement tool was developed for use with young adults by Wallston, Wallston, and DeVellis (1978) but has been used extensively with older adults (e.g., Lachman, 1986; Robinson-Whelan & Storandt, 1992; Roome & Humphrey, 1992). Like Levenson's (1974) multidimensional measure, the MHLOC has three scales: internal, powerful others, and chance. However, all of the items are health-related to assess locus of control orientation for the domain of health. A high internal would believe in self-control of health whereas a high powerful others would believe that health was controlled by others.

Other adults tend to have high chance and powerful others scores on the MHLOC (Lachman, 1986; Robinson-Whelan & Storandt, 1992). Moreover, scores on the MHLOC are predictive of health-related behaviors. For example, individuals who score high on the powerful others scale are more likely to go to the doctor (Bundek, Marks, & Richardson, 1993; Lachman, 1986), less likely to request information about their health (Robinson-Whelan & Storandt, 1992), and more likely to take analgesics for pain (Roome & Humphrey, 1992). High internals are more likely to perform breast self-examination (Bundek et al., 1993) whereas low internals are less likely to even get their prescriptions filled (Bazargan, Barbre, & Hamm, 1993).

A domain-specific assessment for intellectual behaviors has also been developed. The Personality-in-Intellectual-Aging Contexts (PIC; Lachman, 1983) was designed to provide the three scales (internal, powerful others, and chance) for control beliefs about everyday intellectual activities. The internal scale has been shown to decline with old age (Grover & Hertzog, 1991; Lachman, 1986, Study 1; but see Lachman Studies 2 and 3). Both of the external scales (powerful others and chance) show age-related increases (Grover & Hertzog, 1991; Lachman, 1986). Hence, with respect to intellectual activities, older adults appear to believe less in their own control and more in the control of (or need for) others. Perhaps most important, the PIC is predictive of performance on vocabulary and fluid intelligence tasks (Lachman, 1986) as well as with a composite intelligence measure (Grover & Hertzog, 1991). The powerful others scale shows the highest relationship to intellectual performance.

An important question to ask is whether intellectual decline leads to an increase in the belief of powerful others or vice versa. According to Grover and Hertzog (1991) "the direction of influence appears to be from intelligence to perceived control" (p. 113), which is also consistent with Lachman and Leff's (1989) longitudinal data. In other words, as intellectual abilities decline, belief in the power of others increases. However, elders can get caught in a negative cycle wherein they see some decline in their abilities, they believe they need more help from others, they then avoid intellectually demanding tasks, their abilities decline more, they believe more in powerful others, and so on. Therefore, a goal for those training older adults to perform new tasks or use new systems is to encourage older adults "to understand that they *can* do something to improve their memories by using greater effort or new strategies, because the belief that memory decline is inevitable can be detrimental to motivation" (Lachman, 1991, p. 172).

Whether you believe that you control your destiny, others control your destiny, or chance controls your destiny will influence your behaviors and your interactions with the world around you. Human factors specialists endeavor to improve the relationship between humans and systems. The evidence reviewed suggests that an understanding of an individual's control orientation will assist the human factors effort in a number of areas.

First, the choice of instructional format, feedback, and pacing of instruction will all benefit from knowledge of whether the learner is internal or believes in powerful others or chance. Moreover, expectations regarding the utilization of systems and technology might be influenced by an individual's locus of control classification.

Second is the issue of whether patients will take control of their health regimen, adhere to their medicines (see Park and Jones, Chapter 11, this volume), or adapt and utilize new medical technologies (see Gardner-Bonneau and Gosbee, Chapter 10, this volume). Locus of control assessments may provide information that is helpful in determining how to maximize healthy behavior. For example, the context in which information is presented could be varied for internals and externals. Bundek et al. (1993) suggest that a means of increasing breast self-examination (BSE) is to stress the "self-initiated nature of BSE and appointment setting to patients high in internal control . . . [and] for patients who measure high in control by powerful others, compliance with physician recommendations regarding BSE can be stressed as an important component of the physician-patient relationship" (p. 198). A similar approach could be adopted for other health-related behaviors.

GENERAL COGNITIVE ABILITIES

Adams (1989b) defined an *ability* as a "behavioral repertoire that is a determiner of performance in the various tasks that require the ability. A person has a number of abilities, and tasks require them in different combinations" (p. 367). The proposed number of abilities that individuals possess vary by theorist from a single general intelligence factor (Spearman, 1927) to a myriad of more than 100 different ability factors (Guilford, 1979).

Understanding individual differences in abilities is important for human factors specialists for a variety of reasons. First is selection. Different jobs require different abilities: the abilities required to be a pilot are very different from the abilities required to be a lathe operator, which in turn are very different from the abilities required to be a graphic artist. Recent task analytic approaches have emphasized the importance of understanding cognitive abilities for the successful understanding of the training needs within a task domain (e.g., Goldstein, 1993; Rogers, Maurer, Salas, & Fisk, 1996). The cognitive approach provides a link between determining the tasks and components that need to be trained and the best methods for training them. In addition, an understanding of the abilities required to perform a particular job will allow better selection of individuals for that job.

Training is another domain in which knowledge of individual differences in abilities can be informative. For example, Eberts and Brock (1987) suggest that the degree to which computer-aided instruction will be successful is dependent on the trainer's ability to accurately assess the individual student's level of ability. Then the difficulty level of the task can be tailored to the individual student to ensure that he or she is capable of doing the task yet sufficiently challenged to maintain motivated performance. More generally, Cronbach and Snow (1977) have shown that the degree to which an individual will benefit from a particular training program may be dependent on his or her ability level. Such "aptitude–treatment interactions" must be considered to maximize the benefits of training regimes.

The relationship between individual differences in abilities and learning has been investigated since the early 1900s (for a review, see Adams, 1989a). Ability–performance relationships change as a function of task practice. Initial performance on a novel task is dependent on broad cognitive abilities (Ackerman, 1988; Fleishman, 1972) whereas practiced performance may be dependent on a task-specific ability (Fleishman, 1972), psychomotor speed (Ackerman, 1988), working memory activation speed (Woltz, 1988), or some other ability that is dependent on the particular task. To select individuals who will successfully acquire the skill of interest, the appropriate abilities for skilled performance on that task must be measured. In addition, training development will benefit from an understanding of the abilities important for a particular phase of practice. For example, if working memory is critical for initial performance, memory aids may help individuals with lower working memory spans. This is the basis for some part-task training approaches such as augmentation (Wightman & Lintern, 1985).

Older adults have many new things to learn in their environments: home medical devices such as blood pressure monitors and glucose monitors; computers; home alarm systems; automatic teller machines; driving an automobile (e.g., widows); on-line card catalog system at the library; golf or other sports; bridge, chess, or other games; and job-related skills such as a new software system, new equipment, or automation of parts of the job component. Certainly it would be useful to understand if the abilities required to perform such tasks are the same for young and older adults. There is some suggestive research showing that ability–performance relationships may differ for young and older adults. For example, Rogers, Fisk, and Hertzog (1994) found that, although ability–performance relationships were similar for the task performance of young and old subjects during the acquisition of a visual search skill, independent assessment of learning revealed very different patterns. Similarly, Rogers, Gilbert, and Fisk (1993) have found that individual differences in performance on an associative learning task are predicted by semantic memory access speed for young adults but by associative memory ability for older adults.

The ability–performance data show that the underlying abilities that determine performance may differ for young and older adults. Such age differences may be the result of older individuals compensating for ability deficits through the reliance on intact abilities (Salthouse, 1984; Smith, 1986). The selection of individuals might differ across age groups, and the choice of a particular training program might also differ. For example, if older adults are relying on perceptual comparisons to perform a task, while younger adults are utilizing their working memory, the training aids for the two groups would differ.

Finally, it is important for human factors specialists to be aware of the cognitive abilities that do and do not change as we grow older. A distinction is often made between fluid intelligence and crystallized intelligence (e.g., Horn & Cattell, 1966). *Fluid intelligence* represents on-line reasoning and the ability to solve novel problems. *Crystallized intelligence* refers to the acquired knowledge that an individual possesses. Typical patterns of age-related differences are that fluid intelligence abilities such as inductive reasoning and problem solving begin to decline as early as age 25 or 30; on the contrary, older adults maintain their crystallized abilities such as vocabulary and general knowledge, well into their 60s and 70s (Horn, 1982; Schaie, 1983). Similarly, measures of wisdom dependent on one's knowledge base suggest that older adults' have an advantage (e.g., Baltes & Staudinger, 1993). Understanding these general patterns of age-related changes in cognitive ability can help training developers maximize the performance of older adults by relying more on their acquired knowledge base and less on their ability to perform fluid operations. Of course, it also important to remember that there are individual differences in the rate and magnitude of age-related changes in abilities (Hertzog, 1985; Schaie, 1989) and in an individual's acquired knowledge base (Ackerman, 1996). Hence, even within a group of older adults there may be a need for individualized training.

FIELD DEPENDENCE OR INDEPENDENCE

Field dependence or independence (FD/I) is an individual difference variable that represents how an individual interacts with his or her environment. More specifically, FD/I describes how individuals' perceptions are influenced by surrounding contexts. The construct was first defined by Witkin (for a review, see Witkin & Goodenough, 1981), who developed the most widely used measure of the construct: the Embedded Figures Test (EFT; Witkin, Oltman, Raskin, & Karp, 1971). The EFT requires subjects to disembed simple and complex figures from complex visual fields. Field independents are less influenced by the visual background than are field dependents.

The relationship of FD/I to learning has been widely investigated. From their extensive review of the literature, Jonassen and Grabowski (1993) reach the following conclusions: (1) field dependent learners will perform better in group-oriented and collaborative situations, will benefit from advanced organizers, will learn better with highly structured materials, and will benefit from specific feedback about their errors and the explicit provision of strategies; (2) field independent learners prefer less guidance and more opportunity for discovery, and learn better in individualized, self-paced, and loosely structured learning environments.

Older adults are more likely to be classified as field dependent rather than independent (e.g., Lambert & Fleury, 1994; Panek, 1985; Panek, Barrett, Sterns, & Alexander, 1977; Witkin et al., 1971). This trend toward field dependence has important implications for the ability of older adults to extract critical information from the environment. Cole and Gaeth (1990) studied the degree to which adults of all ages were able to extract nutritional information from cereal labels. FD/I, as measured by the EFT, was related to trials to criterion and the amount of time needed to make a decision about the most nutritious cereal. Cole and Gaeth reported two encouraging findings. First, a perceptual aid (highlighting the critically important information) improved performance for everyone, but especially for high field dependents. Second, older individuals who received the perceptual aid performed as well as younger adults who did not. Therefore, an external aid designed to improve the extraction of information from the perceptual environment improved performance. The success of perceptual aids to overcome limitations of field dependence should be investigated in other contexts.

COGNITIVE AND LEARNING STYLES

Cognitive styles represent the "characteristic approaches of individuals in acquiring and organizing information" (Jonassen & Grabowski, 1993, p. 173). Cognitive styles are represented by different dimensions: (1) visual–haptic represents a preference for gathering information through visual means or tactile means; (2) visualizer–verbalizer describes a preference for visual versus verbal information; (3) leveling–sharpening refers to whether individuals represent information more generally or attend to minutiae; and (4) serialist–holist is a dimension contrasting a procedural, detailed approach to a more global approach of selecting information.

Cognitive styles are typically measured through assessments of performance differences under the contrasting contexts (e.g., visual versus haptic).

Learning styles, on the other hand, are individuals' perceptions of their cognitive styles and are measured through self-report.* Thus learning styles are representative of learner preferences but may or may not correspond to actual performance differences.

Both cognitive and learning styles are presumed to be important variables for learning, processing new information, retaining old information, and so on. For example, when discussing the potential benefits of spatial versus verbal displays, Wickens (1984) concluded that "the experimental data do not clearly point to one mode as superior to the other. Some of the ambivalence may result because different modes are preferred by different categories of users" (p. 214).

Sein and Boström (1989) used Kolb's Learning Style Inventory to classify a group of young adults as either abstract or concrete learners and then compared their ability to learn using an abstract system model or a concrete analogical model. They discovered that the abstract learners scored almost three times better with the abstract model relative to the concrete model; conversely, the concrete learners performed better with the concrete model. Thus Sein and Boström provide evidence that one's preferred learning mode can influence the degree to which one will benefit from a particular type of training method.

Learning styles can be defined by different modalities: perceptual (how information is extracted from the environment), cognitive (mental processing of that information), and emotional (personal feelings and attitudes that may influence both the perceptual and cognitive modalities). With respect to perceptual learning styles, Galbraith and James (1984) compared the preferences of young and older adults. They discovered that the order of preference for young adults was visual, haptic, interactive, aural, print, kinesthetic, and olfactory. For older adults the order of preference was visual, interactive, aural, haptic, print, kinesthetic and olfactory. Thus older adults showed a preference for learning situations in which the information was presented visually and in an interactive mode. Galbraith and James suggest that, because learning styles can affect the degree to which information is processed initially and remembered later, an awareness of older adults' effective learning styles is necessary to maximize learning.

Kuznar, Falciglia, Wood, and Frankel (1991) used the Price, Dunn, and Dunn (1982) Productivity Environmental Preference Survey to analyze the personal preferences of younger and older women. "Both groups preferred a formal classroom situation . . . older adults preferred learning in the morn-

*This distinction between cognitive and learning styles is based on Jonassen and Grabowski's (1993) conceptualization of the two constructs.

ing, cooler temperatures, and indirect lighting . . . the young adults preferred learning in the afternoon, bright lighting, and food or drink during a learning situation" (p. 26). Kuznar et al. argued that the identification of learning styles via a screening device prior to the presentation of educational programs could allow the instructor to present the information in the most appropriate manner for particular individuals (i.e., tailored to their cognitive styles).

Thus, whether couched in terms of cognitive styles or learning styles, it is clear that people have learning preferences. The way information is presented, the type of information that is being learned, and the context in which the information is presented can all affect the success of the learning. Trainers should be cognizant of the importance of these factors and that young and older adults have different preferences. Consequently, to maximize the benefits of instruction, learning, and training, style variables should be considered and there should be a match between the preferences of the individuals and the mode of information transmission.

MOTIVATION

Motivation is an important variable to success of learning (e.g., Ackerman, 1989; Kanfer, 1987, 1990; Kanfer & Ackerman, 1989). Many years ago, Gilliland and Clark (1939) suggested that "One of the greatest problems in education and industry is that of motivation, or the arousal of interest" (p. 478). With respect to age differences, some researchers have argued that older adults perform more poorly on novel tasks simply because they are poorly motivated (for a review, see Kausler, 1990). Therefore, one might predict that older adults would not perform well on tasks involving a new system, for example, because they are not motivated to learn. However, at least in the case of computer use, attitude surveys suggest otherwise; older adults are often very willing to learn to use computer technology (see Morrell & Echt in press for a review).

Others have suggested that older adults may be overly motivated to perform well, which leads to overarousal and hence poor performance (Minton & Schneider, 1985). In research with young adults, Kanfer and her colleagues (e.g., Kanfer & Ackerman, 1989; Kanfer, Ackerman, Murtha, Dugdale, & Nelson, 1994) have demonstrated that external motivation in the form of goal setting can be detrimental for lower ability subjects. The same may hold true for older individuals. The idea is that having to keep a goal active in working memory requires resources and thus interferes with performance on the task.

There is a paucity of research on the effects of motivation manipulations on older adults. If, in fact, older adults are not motivated enough to perform well, external motivators may improve their performance. However, care will have to be taken not to overload them with motivational information that may itself interfere with task performance.

UNDERSTANDING DRIVING BEHAVIOR

The contribution of individual differences variables is an important human factors problem in determining the safety and ability of older drivers. The magnitude of the problem is exemplified by that fact that two special issues of *Human Factors* were devoted to the safety and mobility of elderly drivers (1991, edited by Barr & Eberhard; 1992, edited by Eberhard & Barr). A critical question involves the determination of which older drivers should continue to drive and which should not. One approach would be to disallow anyone over age 65 from driving. Obviously this is not a reasonable solution given individual differences. Instead, researchers have attempted to try to understand the individual difference variables that are predictive of driving success.

One such variable is the visual field that can be processed during a brief glance known as the *useful field of view* (UFOV). The UFOV varies as a function of the duration, salience, and eccentricity of the target as well as the degree of competing attentional demands (Ball & Owsley, 1991). The UFOV also varies between individuals, with older adults tending to have a smaller UFOV (Owsley, Ball, Sloane, Roenker, & Bruni, 1991). Ball and Owsley (1991) reported that a measure of UFOV alone can account for 13% of the variance of all accident in a sample of older drivers and 21% of the variance of intersection accidents in the same sample. Thus individual differences in UFOV appear to be related to individual differences in driving accidents. However, restricted UFOV's can be improved through training by as much as 133% after only five days of training (Ball, Beard, Roenker, Miller, & Griggs, 1988).

Perceptual style (i.e., field dependence or independence) also plays a role in driving behavior (e.g., Gilmore, Wenk, Naylor, & Stove, 1992; Panek et al., 1977). For example, Shinar, McDowell, Rackoff, and Rockwell (1978) showed that field dependence or independence is an important factor in the ability of drivers to adjust their searching pattern. They reported that "field dependent subjects are less able to adapt themselves to the changing environments encountered when moving from a straight road to a curved road segment" (p. 556). Additional evidence of the importance of perceptual styles for driving comes from Lambert and Fleury (1994). They demonstrated that performance on the Embedded Figures Test accounted for more than 53% of the variance in a task where subjects were required to recognize road signs in contexts of varying perceptual complexity. That is, field-dependent individuals were much slower to recognize and respond to familiar traffic signs (e.g., stop sign, yield sign) presented against complex backgrounds. This pattern of results was observed for young and older adults but the effect of perceptual style was greater for the older adults (i.e., there was a larger difference in response time between field dependent and independent individuals). An encouraging fact is that in a second study Lambert and Fleury improved the performance of the older, field-dependent individuals by increasing the readability of the traffic signs. They reduced the spatial frequency of the information on the signs, increased the color contrast, and consequently decreased response times. Thus, awareness of the potential difficulties of older adults' reading of sings might lead to improvement in the visibility of the signs, which would benefit all drivers.

Driving also requires rapid attention switching between sources of information. There are individual differences in the ability to shift attention, especially for older drivers with various types of dementia (Parasuraman & Nestor, 1991). Proctor and Van Zandt (1994) suggest that "because of these individual differences in attention-shifting ability, driving competence should be determined in part by tests of attention" (p. 194).

Another important variable to consider for driving is locus of control. Older individuals who are more internal have been shown to be less likely to believe that they will have an accident, in comparison to other individuals of the same age (Holland, 1993). However, as discussed earlier, in general, older individuals are more likely to believe in external control. Consequently, Holland (1993) suggested that "giving older people specific information of the risk factors [of driving] along with suggestions as to what to do to improve their safety, may not only make them safer but also put them 'back in control' increasing the internality of their locus of control" (p. 440).

The domain of driving provides one example of how knowledge of individual differences can aid in a practical problem; namely, how to select individuals who should be driving from those who should not. Although the definitive discriminative tests have not yet been determined, individual difference variables will almost certainly be part of the equation. In addition, as we develop a better understanding of driving behavior and the limitations of the driver (i.e., the human factor), we can improve the roadways, the signage, and through training, the capabilities of the individual to improve the overall driving situation for all drivers.

SUMMARY

There were three primary goals of this chapter. By way of summary, I will restate each goal and then provide the major points relevant to that goal.

1. *To review the importance of personality and other individual differences to the field of human factors.* The research reviewed suggests that individual differences variables are indeed relevant to human factors issues. For example, trainers and educators can tailor their programs to individual learners based on their awareness of the individual's locus of control, level of field dependence, cognitive ability, cognitive style, and learning style.
2. *To determine whether these variables change as a function of age.* Many of the individual difference variables do show age-related trends. Older adults tend to be more field dependent, more external in their locus of control (both in terms of chance and powerful others), and prefer visual and interactive learning situations. Moreover, certain cognitive abilities such as reasoning do decline with age. However, variables such as cognitive style and motivation have not received much attention and age-related differences therein are a yet unknown. Future research should focus on understanding the source and permanence of the age-related differences.
3. *To determine whether the relationships between the individual difference variables and performance are the same for young and older adults.* This remains the area about which we know the least. There is some evidence that older adults are more influenced by perceptual styles than are young adults (e.g., Lambert & Fleury, 1994). There is also evidence that cognitive ability–performance relationships may differ across age groups (e.g., Rogers et al., 1994; Rogers et al., 1993). However, the relationships between performance and cognitive styles, learning styles, motivation, and locus of control have not been investigated as a function of age. We need to learn more about the degree to which age mediates the relationships between individual differences and performance.

In summary, human factors practitioners should be aware of the importance of assessing individual difference variables for adults of all ages. In addition, human factors researchers should continue to uncover the degree to which such individual differences can be modified to improve human–system interactions (improved cognitive abilities, decreased field dependence, setting ideal motivation levels, etc.).

Conclusion

"The challenge to human factors researchers is to make it easier for elderly people to stay in touch with others and the world and to find ways to put their knowledge and talents to use" (Nickerson, 1992, p. 355).

The study of individual difference variables and whether they change as we grow older will aid human factors researchers in meeting the challenge. Clearly we must search for general laws of behavior. However, we must be aware of the likelihood that the generality of such laws may be limited to certain groups of individuals: young or old, field dependent or independent, motivated or apathetic, visual or verbal, and so on.

Acknowledgments

The author was supported in part by a grant from National Institutes of Health (National Institute on Aging) Grant No. P50 AG11715 under the auspices of the Center for Applied Cognitive Research on Aging (one of the Edward R. Roybal Centers for Research on Applied Gerontology). She would like to thank the students in her Human Factors seminar for their comments on an earlier draft of the chapter: Ragin Hause, Brian Jamieson, Gabe Rousseau, and Ken Watkins. She would also like to thank Dan Fisk for constructive criticisms of the chapter.

References

Ackerman, P. L. (1988). Determinants of individual differences during skill acquisition: A theory of cognitive abilities and information processing. *Journal of Experimental Psychology: General, 117,* 299–329.

Ackerman, P. L. (1989). Abilities, elementary information processes, and other sights to see at the zoo. In R. Kanfer, P. L. Ackerman, & R. Cudeck (Eds.), *Abilities, motivation, and methodology: The Minnesota Symposium on Learning and Individual Differences* (pp. 281–293). Hillsdale, NJ: Erlbaum.

Ackerman, P. L. (1996). Intelligence as process and knowledge: An integration for adult development and application. In W. A. Rogers, A. D. Fisk, and N. Walker (Eds.), *Aging and skilled performance: Advances in theory and application* (pp. 139–156). Hillsdale, NJ: Erlbaum.

Adams, J. A. (1989a). Historical background and appraisal of research on individual differences in learning. In R. Kanfer, P. L. Ackerman, & R. Cudeck (Eds.), *Abilities, motivation, and methodology: The Minnesota Symposium on Learning and Individual Differences* (pp. 3–22). Hillsdale, NJ: Erlbaum.

Adams, J. A. (1989b). *Human factors engineering.* New York: Macmillan.

Ball, K., Beard, B., Roenker, D., Miller, R., & Griggs, D. (1988). Age and visual search: Expanding the useful field of view. *Journal of the Optical Society of America, 5,* 2210–2219.

Ball, K., & Owsley, C. (1991). Identifying correlates of accident involvement for the older driver. *Human Factors, 33,* 583–595.

Baltes, P. B., & Staudinger, U. M. (1993). The search for a psychology of wisdom. *Current Directions in Psychological Science, 2,* 75–80.

Barr, R. A., & Eberhard, J. W. (1991). Special Issue: Safety and Mobility of Elderly Drivers, Part I, *Human Factors, 33(5),* 497–600.

Bazargan, M., Barbre, A. R., & Hamm, V. (1993). Failure to have prescriptions filled among black elderly. *Journal of Aging and Health, 5,* 264–282.

Bundek, N. I., Marks, G., & Richardson, J. L. (1993). Role of health locus of control beliefs in cancer screening of elderly Hispanic women. *Health Psychology, 12,* 193–199.

Cole, C. A., & Gaeth, G. J. (1990). Cognitive and age-related differences in the ability to use nutritional information in a complex environment. *Journal of Marketing Research, 27,* 175–184.

Cronbach, L. J., & Snow, R. E. (1977). *Aptitudes and instructional methods: A handbook for research on interactions.* New York: Irvington.

Devolder, P. A. (1991). Comparison of within-group variabilities across older and younger adults: A meta-analysis. *Experimental Aging Research, 17,* 113–117.

Eberhard, J. W., & Barr, R. A. (1992). Special Issue: Safety and Mobility of Elderly Drivers, Part II, *Human Factors, 34(1),* 1–120.

Eberts, R. E., & Brock, J. F. (1987). Computer-assisted and computer-managed instruction. In G. Salvendy (Ed.), *Handbook of human factors* (pp. 976–1011). New York: Wiley.

Fleishman, E. A. (1972). On the relation between abilities, learning, and individual differences. *American Psychologist, 27,* 1017–1032.

Galbraith, M. W., & James, W. B. (1984). Assessment of dominant perceptual learning styles of older adults. *Educational Gerontology, 10,* 449–457.

Gilliland, A. R., & Clark, E. L. (1939). *Psychology of individual differences.* New York: Prentice-Hall.

Gilmore, G. C., Wenk, H. E., Naylor, L. A., & Stove, T. A. (1992). Motion perception and age. *Psychological Aging, 4,* 654–660.

Goldstein, I. L. (1993). *Training in organizations: Needs assessment, development, and evaluation* (3rd ed.). Pacific Grove, CA: Brooks/Cole.

Grover, D. R., & Hertzog, C. (1991). Relationships between intellectual control beliefs and psychometric intelligence in adulthood. *Journal of Gerontology: Psychological Sciences, 46,* P109–P115.

Guilford, J. P. (1979). *Cognitive psychology with a frame of reference.* San Diego, CA: EdITS.

Hertzog, C. (1985). An individual differences perspective: Implications for cognitive research in gerontology. *Research on Aging, 7,* 7–45.

Holland, C. A. (1993). Self-bias in older drivers' judgments of accident likelihood. *Accident Analysis and Prevention, 25,* 431–441.

Horn, J. L. (1982). The theory of fluid and crystallized intelligence in relation to concepts of cognitive psychology and aging in adulthood. In F. I. M. Craik & S. Trehub (Eds.), *Aging and cognitive processes* (pp. 237–278). New York: Plenum.

Horn, J. L., & Cattell, R. B. (1968). Refinement of the theory of fluid and crystallized general intelligences. *Journal of Educational Psychology, 57,* 253–270.

Human Factors and Ergonomics Society. (1996). *Human Factors and Ergonomics Society Directory.* Santa Monica, CA: Author.

Jonassen, D. H., & Grabowski, B. L. (1993). *Handbook of individual differences, learning, and instruction.* Hillsdale, NJ: Erlbaum.

Kanfer, R. (1987). Task-specific motivation: An integrative approach to issues of measurement, mechanisms, processes, and determinants. *Journal of Social and Clinical Psychology, 5,* 237–264.

Kanfer, R. (1990). Motivation and individual differences in learning: An integration of developmental, differential, and cognitive perspectives. *Learning and Individual Differences, 2,* 221–239.

Kanfer, R., & Ackerman, P. L. (1989). Motivation and cognitive abilities: An integrative/aptitude-treatment interaction approach to skill acquisition. *Journal of Applied Psychology Monograph, 74,* 657–690.

Kanfer, R., Ackerman, P. L., Murtha, T. C., Dugdale, B., & Nelson, L. (1994). Goal setting, conditions of practice, and task performance: A resource allocation perspective. *Journal of Applied Psychology, 79,* 826–835.

Kausler, D. H. (1990). Motivation, human aging and cognitive performance. In J. E. Birren & K. W. Schaie (Eds.), *handbook of the psychology of aging* (pp. 171–182). San Diego, CA: Academic Press.

Kuznar, E., Falciglia, G. A., Wood, L., & Frankel, J. (1991). Learning style preferences: A comparison of younger and older adult females. *Journal of Nutrition for the Elderly, 10,* 1991.

Lachman, M. E. (1983). Perception of intellectual aging: Antecedent or consequent of intellectual functioning? *Developmental Psychology, 19,* 482–498.

Lachman, M. E. (1986). Locus of control in aging research: A case for multidimensional and domain-specific assessment. *Psychology and Aging, 1,* 34–40.

Lachman, M. E. (1991). Perceived control over memory aging: Developmental and intervention perspectives. *Journal of Social Issues, 47,* 159–175.

Lachman, M. E., & Leff, R. (1989). Perceived control and intellectual functioning in the elderly: A 5-year longitudinal study. *Developmental Psychology, 25,* 722–728.

Lambert, L. D., & Fleury, M. (1994). Age, cognitive style, and traffic signs. *Perceptual and Motor Skills, 78,* 611–624.

Levenson, H. (1974). Activism and powerful others: Distinctions within the concept of internal-external control. *Journal of Personality Assessment, 38,* 377–383.

Minton, H. L., & Schneider, F. W. (1985). *Differential psychology.* Monterey, CA: Brooks/Cole.

Morrell, R. W., & Echt, K. V. (in press). Instructional design for older computer users: The influence of cognitive factors. In W. A. Rogers, A. D. Fisk, and N. Walker (Eds.), *Aging and skilled performance: Advances in theory and application.* Hillsdale, NJ: Erlbaum.

Nickerson, R. S. (1992). *Looking ahead: Human factors challenges in a changing world.* Hillsdale, NJ: Erlbaum.

Owsley, C., Ball, K., Sloane, M. E., Roenker, D. L., & Bruni, J. R. (1991). Visual perceptual/cognitive correlates of vehicle accidents in older drivers. *Psychology and Aging, 6,* 403–415.

Panek, P. E. (1985). Age differences in field-dependence/independence. *Experimental Aging Research, 11,* 97–99.

Panek, P. E., Barrett, G. V., Sterns, H. L., & Alexander, R. A. (1977). A review of age changes in perceptual information processing ability with regard to driving. *Experimental Aging Research, 3,* 387–449.

Parasuraman, R., & Nestor, P. G. (1991). Attention and driving skills in aging and Alzheimer's disease. *Human Factors, 33,* 539–557.

Price, G. E., Dunn, R., & Dunn, K. (1982). *Productivity environment preference survey manual* (3rd ed.). Lawrence, KS: Price Systems.

Proctor, R. W., & Van Zandt, T. (1994). *Human factors in simple and complex systems.* Boston: Allyn & Bacon.

Rabbitt, P. (1990). Applied cognitive gerontology: Some problems, methodologies, and data. *Applied Cognitive Psychology, 4,* 225–246.

Robinson-Whelan, S., & Storandt, M. (1992). Factorial structure of two health belief measures among older adults. *Psychology and Aging, 7,* 209–213.

Rogers, W. A., Fisk, A. D., & Hertzog, C. (1994). Do ability-performance relationships differentiate age and practice effects in visual search? *Journal of Experimental Psychology: Learning, Memory, and Cognition, 20,* 710–738.

Rogers, W. A., Gilbert, D. K., & Fisk, A. D. (1993, October). Ability-performance relationships in memory skill tasks for young and old adults. In *Proceedings of Human Factors and Ergonomics Society 37th annual meeting.* (pp. 167–171). Santa Monica, CA: Human Factors and Ergonomics Society.

Rogers, W. A., Maurer, T. J., Salas, E., & Fisk, A. D. (1996). Training design and cognitive theory: Principles and a methodology (CAPTAM). In K. Ford (Ed.), *Improving training effectiveness in work organizations* (pp. 19–45). Hillsdale, NJ: Erlbaum.

Roome, P., & Humphrey, M. (1992). Personality factors in analgesic usage. *Psychology of Stress, 8,* 237–240.

Rotter, J. B. (1966). Generalized expectancies for internal versus external control of reinforcement. *Psychological Monographs, 81* (Whole No. 609).

Salthouse, T. A. (1984). Effects of age and skill in typing. *Journal of Experimental Psychology: General, 13,* 345–371.

Schaie, K. W. (1983). The Seattle longitudinal study: A twenty-one year exploration of psychometric intelligence in adulthood. In K. W. Schaie (ed.), *Longitudinal studies of adult psychological development* (pp. 64–135). New York: Guilford.

Schaie, K. W. (1989). Individual differences in rate of cognitive change in adulthood. In V. L. Bengston & K. W. Schaie (Eds.), *The course of later life: Research and reflections* (pp. 68–83). New York: Springer.

Sein, M. K., & Boström, R. P. (1989). Individual differences and conceptual models in training novice users. *Human Computer Interaction, 4,* 197–229.

Shinar, D., McDowell, E. D., Rackoff, N. J., & Rockwell, T. H. (1978). Field dependence and driver visual search behavior. *Human Factors, 20,* 553–559.

Smith, D. B. D. (1986). Human aging: Areas of challenge for human factors in the micro and macro design of organizational systems. In O. Brown & H. W. Hendrick (Eds.), *Human factors in organizational design and management* (pp. 3–12). Amsterdam: North-Holland.

Spearman, C. (1927). *The abilities of man: Their nature and measurement.* New York: Macmillan.

Wallston, K. A., Wallston, B. S., & DeVellis, R. (1978). Development of the multidimensional health locus of control (MHLOC) scales. *Health Education Monographs, 6,* 160–170.

Wickens, C. D. (1984). *Engineering psychology and human performance.* Columbus, OH: Bell and Howell.

Wightman, D. C., & Lintern, G. (1985). Part-task training for tracking and manual control. *Human Factors, 27,* 267–283.

Witkin, H. A., & Goodenough, D. R. (1981). *Cognitive styles: Essence and origins: Field dependence and independence.* New York: International Universities Press.

Witkin, H. A., Oltman, P., Raskin, E., & Karp, S. (1971). *A manual for the embedded figures test.* Palo Alto, CA: Consulting Psychologists Press.

Woltz, D. J. (1988). An investigation of the role of working memory in procedural skill acquisition. *Journal of Experimental Psychology: General, 117,* 319–331.

Chapter 8

Behavioral Pharmacology and Aging

M. Jackson Marr

RATIONALE

As every reader of this text will already know, the proportion of people over 65 is the most rapidly growing segment of our population, predicted to constitute some 20% by 2025. Among the more profound implications of this growth is the role of drug consumption in the aged population. Already, those aged 65 and older while representing 12% of the population account for more than 30% of drugs consumed, including both prescription and over-the-counter (OTC) agents (see Lamy, Salzman, & Nevis-Olesen, 1992, for a detailed review of drug-taking statistics). A substantial proportion of these drugs are taken explicitly to affect behavior. For example, sedative and hypnotic agents are third after cardiovascular and analgesic drugs in the proportion of drugs taken by the aged. And, of course, cardiovascular and analgesic drugs may also have significant behavioral effects.

Three major issues contribute to human factors concerns: (1) the large numbers of drugs taken by the aged with the attendant possibilities of separate and interactive toxicity; (2) the classes of agents consumed, which include major behaviorally active agents that are known to produce such side effects as sedation, confusion, movement disorders, orthostatic hypo-

Handbook of Human Factors and the Older Adult

tension and dizziness, memory loss, and cardiac dysfunction; and (3) the biological changes with age that not only contribute to the level and variety of drug consumption, but can modify significantly the toxicity of those drugs. These age-related modifications result from changes in how a drug is handled by the body, changes in the sensitivity to the drug at the various sites of action in the central nervous system and elsewhere, and behavioral variables that control differential sensitivities to drug effects.

Why are these problems of human factors interest? The increase in the proportion of the aged in the population means an increase in the proportion in the work force. Behaviorally active drugs may interfere with work performance, increasing the chances of errors, absenteeism, and accidents. These kinds of concerns by employers may already plague the older worker, independent of considerations of drug taking. How can we reduce possible performance deficits resulting from necessary drug usage?

For the nonworking aged population who may be actively retired, drug-related performance deficits present possible difficulties and dangers in the home and on the road. For those elderly confined either at home or in hospitals or nursing facilities, the problems may be compounded by the growing deficits contributed by age alone. How can we design safer and more comfortable environments for the aged, taking into consideration possible deleterious effects of extensive drug consumption? This question is in addition to considerations of compliance with drug regimens. Of course, noncompliance can potentiate drug-related problems, and effective compliance system design is another human factors challenge.

There is an additional issue of human factors interest. I have been emphasizing possible performance deficits resulting from therapeutic drug taking. But much research now is devoted to discovering agents that may enhance performance in the aged. Most of this work focuses on pathological conditions like Alzheimer's disease, but there is the possibility that agents might be developed to enhance performance in the healthy aged or retard the neural processes contributing to deficits characteristic of normal aging.

Whether one is focused on positive or negative effects of drugs, human factors research and methodology combined with the long-established field of behavioral pharmacology offers immense possibilities for basic understanding of and extensive application to drug-performance interactions. For example, O'Hanlon (1991) has called for a human factors role in human behavioral pharmacology:

> If human factors specialists are to survive professionally in anything like their present number, many must find new applications of their knowledge and skills. After acquiring experience and a reasonable working knowledge of the principles of pharmacology, psychiatry, and related medical disciplines, he or

she can become capable of conceiving, organizing, and managing projects related to drug development and regulation. (p. 1)

This chapter can be but a precis of a massive research and practice area in pharmacology and aging. Excellent books and reviews are available for the reader interested in more detail (e.g., Albert & Kneofel, 1994; Bloom & Shlom, 1993; Bressler & Katz, 1993; Iversen, Iversen, & Snyder, 1988; McKim & Mishara, 1987; Salzman, 1992; Vestal & Cusack, 1990). My task will be to provide an overview that may allow the reader to probe more deeply into other sources and approach some of the primary literature. The principal goal, however, is to sensitize the human factors community to the possible role of drug-behavior interactions in research and application. My emphasis will be on three principal topics: (1) the basic pharmacology of aging, (2) pharmacological implications of age-related neurobiological changes, and (3) pharmacology and performance.

SOME BASIC PHARMACOLOGY

Pharmacology is a diverse field comprising a variety of subfields and related specialties. Fields like toxicology, pharmacogenetics, pharmacognosy, pharmacy, molecular pharmacology, neuropharmacology, and behavioral pharmacology illustrate the range of interests in basic and applied research as well as clinical practice (e.g., Cooper, Bloom, & Roth, 1991; Gilman, Rall, Nies, & Taylor, 1990; Pratt & Taylor, 1990). Two topics, however, essentially define the basic science of pharmacology: pharmacokinetics and pharmacodynamics. Pharmacokinetics can be capsuled in the question, What does the body do to a drug? This includes processes of absorption, distribution, storage, metabolism, and excretion. Quantitative approaches to these processes measure and model the time course of concentration of a drug in various compartments of the body, which, in turn, determines the time course of action of the drug.

Absorption is the process by which a drug enters the circulation by crossing through various cell membranes, primarily via passive diffusion. Only in the case of intravenous administration is absorption bypassed because then the drug enters the circulation directly. Otherwise, some barrier(s) will stand between the site of administration and the bloodstream. The nature of those barriers depends on the route of administration. Most drugs of interest here are taken by mouth and subject to a number of complex processes before entering the circulation. The drug enters the stomach, where it may be destroyed by the acidic digestive environment or otherwise compromised by food present there. Following gastric emptying, most agents will be passed onto the small intestine for absorption.

Absorption in regions like the small intestine is relatively efficient because of the large surface area and extensive blood circulation. Additional factors controlling absorption include molecular size, concentration, degree of ionization, and lipid solubility. Cell membranes, including those in the central nervous system, are composed largely of lipids, thus for most drugs under most conditions, lipid solubility is a major parameter of absorption. Ionized or polar compounds are poorly lipid soluble. Most drugs are weak acids or bases, therefore, depending upon the pH of their environment, they may be relatively more or less ionized. It is well to keep in mind, however, that absorption at a given site may involve jointly all the factors previously mentioned, as well as others.

Once the drug enters the circulation, it is carried to all the tissues of the body, a process called *distribution*. The same factors that control absorption determine how a drug might be taken up into the tissues, including those containing the sites of action. Drugs of behavioral interest, that is, those entering the central nervous system, face the blood–brain barrier. This is not some sort of mysterious anatomical Great Wall of China, but rather largely the result of the tight junctions between the endothelial cells of the capillaries supplying blood to most of the brain. In other tissues, these capillary cells are not so tightly bound. Spaces are present between cells allowing substances to go back and forth between the capillary interior and the surrounding tissue, depending on their concentration gradients. As for the brain, the lack of such easy access means that a premium is placed on lipid solubility. Virtually all drugs of behavioral interest are lipid soluble.

An important factor contributing to distribution is the availability of the unbound fraction of the drug in the circulation, for only that fraction can enter the tissues. Within the blood many drugs bind to proteins (mostly albumin), thus taking them out of circulation as far as distribution is concerned. This binding is reversible; and as the unbound fraction is distributed to the tissues, more is released from the bound state. Blood proteins therefore act as storage depots and thus may slow the availability of a drug to its sites of action. Drugs may also be stored in other tissues. For example, poisons like DDT and lead are stored in fat and bone, respectively, and can continue to produce toxic actions long after initial exposure by "leaching" back into the circulation.

Prior to their excretion, drugs typically undergo biotransformation; that is, metabolic conversion to other compounds. This occurs mostly in different cell fractions of the liver and is the result of actions of various enzyme systems. This is commonly a two-step process. The first step, Phase I or nonsynthetic reaction, typically involves oxidation, reduction, or hydrolysis. The products of these reactions may be active or inactive. The second class of biotransformation, Phase II or synthetic reactions, nearly always results in an inactive compound. Synthetic reactions involve the production of new compounds by combining with endogenous substances such as glucuronide. The result is an increase in excretability by the kidney because the compound is more polar or ionized and hence less lipid soluble. As blood is filtered through the kidney, these products tend not to be reabsorbed and enter the urine to be excreted.

Drugs absorbed from the gastrointestinal (GI) tract enter the hepatic portal system carrying them directly to the liver before they enter the general circulation. They are then exposed to metabolic enzymatic action, possibly deactivating them. This is called a *first-pass effect.* Alternatively, enzymatic action of a Phase I type may initially produce active products, in some cases much more active than the original drug, to be then passed on to the rest of the body.

All the pharmacokinetic processes I have so far discussed—absorption, distribution, biotransformation, and elimination—account for the time course of concentration and thus the time course of actions of a drug. A key concept here is bioavailability; that is, the proportion of administered drug (including its active metabolites) that actually reaches sites of action. Any changes in parameters affecting pharmacokinetic processes may alter the intensity and duration of action of a drug by either increasing or decreasing its bioavailability. Our primary concern is how aging might alter pharmacokinetic parameters.

AGING AND PHARMACOKINETICS

Age-related changes in body processes can, at least in principle, contribute to virtually every facet of pharmacokinetics. I emphasize *at least in principle* because such changes do not always have functional effects. Reviewing the now extensive but still very incomplete literature on pharmacokinetics and aging yields no simple conclusions. There is considerable variability in findings (a common outcome with the aged), a lack of substantial evidence relating drug effects to age per se, especially in the nonhospitalized population, a strong drug class dependence, counterbalancing effects so that one age-related change can be attenuated by another, and questionable experimental designs. All these factors and more make consistent interpretations difficult, if not impossible. Two excellent reviews are provided by Abernethy (1992) and Vestal and Cusak (1990) that consider these problems in some detail.

Absorption

If we confine ourselves to absorption via the GI tract, then a number of age-related changes could be relevant. These include increases in gastric pH, delayed gastric emptying, reduced absorptive surface and blood flow, and reduced gastric motility (Abernethy, 1992). While these factors would seem to retard the uptake to the circulation of most drugs, functionally, they seem to be of little effect. Possible exceptions are anticholinergic drugs, including such agents as atropine and tricyclic antidepressants. These can reduce intestinal motility to a point where absorption and thus clinical effects of these and other drugs may be delayed. Anticholinergics are potential troublemakers on a number of fronts as I shall subsequently detail.

Distribution

Two principal factors potentially affect drug distribution to sites of action: changes in the ratio of fat to body water and changes in protein binding in the blood. Age brings increases in the proportion of body fat, in males virtually a doubling from the 30s to the 60s, in females an increase of about a third (Vestal & Cusack, 1990). For highly lipid-soluble drugs this increases the volume of distribution, meaning that it takes longer for the drug to clear the body. On the other hand, the peak levels at sites of action may be reduced or delayed. For drugs like ethanol and lithium, which are water soluble, the volume of distribution will be decreased so that peak concentrations will be higher with attendant increased effects.

As discussed already, binding sites play both storage and release roles in the blood and other tissues. Lipid storage prolongs the time a lipid-soluble drug remains in the body, as mentioned earlier. Binding blood proteins such as albumin are reduced with age, but others may increase; for example, alpha 1-acid glycoprotein. The outcome will depend minimally on the class of drugs because different drugs have different affinities for the binding proteins. Although some adverse effects are said to result from reduction in protein binding (e.g., with some benzodiazepines), at least in normal aging, this process does not seem to be a significant factor in toxicity (Abernethy, 1992).

Biotransformation, Clearance, and Excretion

The half-life of a drug in the body is directly proportional to the volume of distribution and inversely proportional to the clearance. Clearance is measured in units of flow rate (ml/min) and specifies the amount of blood cleared of the drug per minute. This is the index of the person's ability to eliminate a drug. Actually, clearance can be specified with respect to a given organ, for example, the liver. The index then represents the efficiency of the organ in removing the drug from the blood. This, in turn, will be a joint function of the blood flow to that organ and the metabolic activity within the organ. Both these factors may change with age.

An estimate of 30% reduction in blood flow to the liver from ages 30–75 has been given (Vestal & Cusack, 1990). This figure may contribute to significant increases in the half-life of several behaviorally active drugs, including some benzodiazepines and tricyclic antidepressants (Abernethy, 1992). The half-life periods of these agents may be tripled in the aged. The interactions between blood flow and alterations in biotransformation in the liver are complex. As mentioned previously, a drug absorbed from the GI tract is carried via the hepatic portal system to the liver before reaching the general circulation. In the liver, metabolic processes begin producing new compounds from the drug. This first-pass effect may remove as much as 80% of the drug before it is passed on the rest of the body. For those drugs whose primary metabolites are inactive, reduced blood flow will mean prolonged action because a larger amount will appear in the general circulation. But with Phase I biotransformations, some, or even all, the products will be active. For example, the tricyclic antidepressant amitriptyline is converted to nortryptyline, an active antidepressant. Prolongation of biotransformation may occur not only from reduced blood flow but also from reduced enzymatic action, especially of Phase I reactions. The evidence on age-related deficits on Phase I biotransformations is inconsistent in both species and gender. However, some data indicate an age-related deficit in hepatic oxidative metabolism in men but not women (Vestal & Cusack, 1990). There is no evidence of age-related changes in Phase II hepatic biotransformations.

Renal clearance is another possible source of toxicity and prolongation of action. Both renal blood flow and filtration rate decrease with age, and these factors may be further compromised by cardiovascular diseases so common in the elderly.

All of the pharmacokinetic mechanisms just discussed, of course, will apply to multiple dosing, the most common practice with psychoactive drugs. Antidepressants and neuroleptics typically take two or more weeks to reach effective levels. Repeated dosing at intervals less than the half-life of the drug will result in accumulation in the body. Eventually equilibration is reached when absorption equals clearance. With the aged, this steady state may take longer for a given dose schedule than for younger individuals. What is more, the steady-state plasma levels will be higher. This should call for a more carefully considered and monitored dose regimen for the older patient.

AGING AND PHARMACODYNAMICS

Pharmacodynamics is the study of the mechanisms of drug actions—what they do the body and to behavior. Behaviorally active drugs act at sites in the central nervous system, primarily to modify mechanisms of neural transmission. The relationships of these actions to changes in behavior is a primary research agendum in neuro–behavioral pharmacology. For the most part, we have only a vague understanding of drug–brain–behavior interactions. One source of information on this problem has been the study of psychotherapeutic agents, their sites of action, and relations to behavioral modification. Yet we remain woefully ignorant of transmitter mechanisms in behavior. One of the problems is that behaviorally active drugs often act at many sites, so that attempting to isolate neural mechanisms in behavior via pharmacological intervention is a significant challenge. Conversely, unless an appropriate in-depth behavior analysis is consistently coupled with neural events, neither the behaviors nor the neural events can be interpreted in terms of each other (see, e.g., Marr, 1990). Four essential and interlocking research efforts have contributed to advances in this area. First, identifying anatomical localization of transmitter systems that can yield functional properties of neural circuitry. Second, elucidating synaptic mechanisms, including synthesis, degradation, and interactions of transmitters and related substances, receptor identification, chemistry, and synthesis, and intra-, extra-, and multicellular mechanisms—all of which are essential to understand how pharmacological agents can exert their effects at the cellular and tissue level. Third, synthesizing compounds with increasing specificity, which is necessary if we are to understand mechanisms of action, molecular and cellular, and associated neural processes. Fourth, designing sophisticated and selective behavioral procedures, including a range of animal and human models, to assess the interrelations of findings from the other three research areas to provide an integrative perspective on brain–behavior dynamics.

The primary research focus of particular interest to behavioral pharmacologists is the assessment of changes in synaptic transmitter mechanisms as a function of age. This work has consisted largely of measuring levels and activities of various neural transmitters and their associated enzymes and receptors. Human data have been gathered mostly from postmortem analyses. These data are subject to a variety of problems in interpretation (see, for example, DeKosky & Palmer, 1994). More stringent controls and sophisticated procedures are possible with nonhuman subjects, but the data obtained with different species, including nonhuman primates, can differ significantly from each other and from the available human data. The sheer number of studies is staggering (see, for example the long table of studies and results through 1988 in Morgan & May, 1990). The present chapter cannot do justice to this mass of information, including the variations and difficulties of interpretation. However, it is possible to discern some trends useful in understanding both pharmacological problems and promises for therapeutic intervention.

Receptors

The concept of receptor in pharmacology is one of those very rare examples of a hypothetical construct that made good. Since the 19th century the possibility was entertained that a drug reacted with an endogenous "receptor substance" to produce its effects. In this century developments in the physiology and biochemistry of the nervous system, first in the periphery with the motor and the autonomic nervous systems, and much later in the central nervous system, resulted in the discovery of a very large number of neural transmitter substances, their anatomical and metabolic pathways, and a host of receptors for each. This work continues at an ever accelerating pace, accounting for the enormous literature on the relatively narrow topic of neural transmitters and aging (see, e.g., Cooper et al., 1991; Hall, 1992).

Each neural transmitter bonds with a group of more-or-less specific receptors found in both pre- and post-synaptic neural membranes. Transmitter–receptor binding functions in excitatory and inhibitory postsynaptic actions and in the regulation of neural transmitter synthesis and, indeed, in the synthesis of the receptors themselves. Presynaptic receptors, for example, may be sensitive to the availability of transmitter released; too little, and more transmitter is synthesized; too much, and less is synthesized.

Receptors are protein molecules imbedded in the neural membrane or sequestered within the cell. In some cases, the molecular structure has been determined well enough to understand how a given transmitter (and associated drug class) bonds with the receptor and leads to the events characteristic of the particular transmitter system. This work offers the promise of designing and synthesizing drugs specific to a given receptor and thus producing a very specific effect.

Receptors, like neural transmitters, are subject to regulation. A chronic low level of transmitter substance released can lead to "upregulation"; that is, increased synthesis of receptors. This has the effect of increasing the sensitivity of the post–synaptic neuron to the released transmitter. Alternatively, too much transmitter may lead to "downregulation," a reduction in available receptors with a concomitant reduction in sensitivity.

In addition to sensitivity change brought about by up- or downregulation, at least two other general mechanisms could contribute to modification of receptor action. Affinity, that is, the ability of a transmitter or associated drug to bind with the receptor, may be changed. This has generally not been found to be a significant factor associated with aging. Also possible, but more difficult to assess, are alterations in receptor mechanisms that involve steps beyond the initial transmitter–receptor binding. For example, activated receptors often set in motion a series of "second messenger" processes dependent on G-proteins within the neuron, which in turn drive other mechanisms involving cyclic AMP (Adenosine 3′, 5′ - monophosphate) or GMP, (Guanosine monophasphate) that lead ultimately to changes in neural excitability.

A major caveat is that transmitter systems should not be viewed as operating in isolation from each other or from other, numerous, neurochemical processes (e.g., Siegal, Agranoff, Albers, & Molinoff, 1989). This means that changes in the functions of one transmitter may have major influences on others. This is an enduring concern in attempting to interpret changes in sensitivity to drug classes as a result of age-related alterations in transmitter functions.

Transmitter Function and Aging

Two interconnected topics are of interest here. First are the neural transmitter alterations associated with behavioral deficits characteristic of either normal or pathological aging. This issue is of primary concern when pharmacological melioration of deficits is sought. The second topic follows from my earlier consideration of pharmacokinetic variables and how they might be associated with changes in sensitivity to drugs in the elderly. From the perspective of pharmacodynamics, the important issue is how changes in transmitter function with age may affect the mechanisms of action or sensitivity of the nervous system to drugs.

Of the many possible transmitters, neuromodulators, neurotropics and the like that one might discuss, space permits only a few examples. I have chosen acetycholine, dopamine, and GABA. These transmitters are particularly important in the neuropharmacology of behaviorally active drugs, and in addition, they may play significant roles in age-related dysfunction (DeKosky & Palmer, 1994).

Acetycholine

This transmitter is widely distributed in both the central and peripheral nervous systems. In the periphery, acetycholine is the transmitter at the neuromuscular junction and also acts at the autonomic ganglia and at the postganglionic terminals in the parasympathetic nervous system. In the central nervous system, its functions are much less well understood, but extensive research has indicated a possible major role in working memory processes as well as sensory and motor function. Two general classes of receptors, nicotinic and muscarinic, with subclasses of each, bind acetycholine at postsynaptic sites. Muscarinic (M2) presynaptic autoregulatory sites have also been identified. Acetycholine is synthesized from choline, largely dietary, and acetyl-CoA via the enzyme choline acetyltransferase (CAT). Once released by nerve terminals, acetycholine is rapidly destroyed by acetycholinesterase. Acetycholine is apparently unique among transmitters in having its synaptic actions terminated directly by enzymatic action. Other transmitters have their actions terminated by active transport (reuptake) mostly into the presynaptic nerve terminal.

Cholinergic function has received an intensive research focus in the aged for several reasons. A major role in Alzheimer's disease has been suggested since the 1970s; it is implicated as well in Parkinson's disease, especially in associated dementia. In addition, aged individuals may show an increased sensitivity to anticholinergic agents, displaying symptoms of memory loss and other cognitive dysfunctions, confusion, and disorientation, all of which could result in a misdiagnosis of dementia, including Alzheimer's disease. It remains to be demonstrated, however, if the hypersensitivity to anticholinergics in the normal aged are related to similar alterations of cholinergic function seen in dementia. This kind of issue lies at the heart of controversies over the relations between normal and pathological aging; indeed, what aging actually is as far as brain–behavior relations are concerned. A careful assessment of drug effects as a function of age in both normal subjects and those with neuropathology should contribute to enlightenment on this vexing question.

What changes in cholinergic function contribute to age-related drug effects? Despite much research, a clear answer is not yet available. The principal experimental markers of cholinergic function have been CAT activity and anatomical alterations in cholinergic neurons and fiber tracts. Reductions in both these classes of markers have been seen, particularly in the basal forebrain, where fibers arise to connect with the neocortex, hippocampus, and amygdala. Reductions in synthesis of acetycholine and muscarinic binding have been reported with aged-animal studies (Morgan & May, 1990). The significance of reductions in CAT activity is difficult to interpret because CAT is not the rate-limiting step in acetycholine synthesis; there is plenty to go around, so changes one way or another should not matter directly. The same is true of acetycholinesterase. Choline uptake is the rate-limiting step; perhaps there are age-related changes with this variable, but I could find no study devoted to this problem.

The role of acetycholine in memory function (or dysfunction) remains controversial. While memory loss does occur with anticholinergics such as atropine, scopolamine, and some tricyclic antidepressants with anticholinergic activity (e.g., amitriptyline), this effect is not always overcome by agents that increase the available acetycholine (e.g., Tariot, 1992). I shall discuss this problem further in a later section of the chapter.

As for symptoms of confusion and disorientation, in the laboratory, anticholinergics may interfere with stimulus control, especially under conditions of distractability and "attentional challenge" (Heise & Milar, 1984). Perhaps these findings are related to the those common age-related side effects.

Dopamine

Dopamine serves as a neurotransmitter in several distinct systems in the brain, including the olfactory bulb and retina, connections between the hypothalamus and the anterior pituitary, the nigrostriatal system, and other connections between the ventral tegmentum and the cortex and limbic system. Each of these dopamine subsystems has its own peculiarities with regard to receptor function and pharmacological profile. As one might expect from anatomical considerations alone, dopamine has been implicated in a variety of normal and dysfunctional behaviors including reinforcement mechanisms and mood, memory functions, schizophrenia, and most convincing, motor disorders such as Parkinson's disease.

The biochemistry of dopamine, and that of other monoamines, is more complex than acetycholine. Dopamine, along with norepinephrine and epinephrine is synthesized from the amino acid tyrosine, actively transported from the circulation across the blood–brain barrier into the central nervous system. The first synthetic step is the rate-limiting one, tyrosine hydroxylase converts tyrosine to L-dopa. The next step is carried out by the relatively nonspecific enzyme aromatic-amino-acid decarboxylase, which converts L-dopa to dopamine. Norepinephrine and epinephrine are further steps along the synthetic chain. The three monoamines have multiple functions as neural transmitters, neuromodulators, and hormones. As a central transmitter and neuromodulator, dopamine appears to have primarily inhibitory neural effects.

The postsynaptic actions are terminated by active reuptake into the presynaptic ending. Monoamine oxidase (actually MAO-B, one of two forms of monoamine oxidase), found mostly within the neuron, degrades dopamine into dihydorxyphenylacetic acid (DOPAC). Outside the neuron, dopamine is converted to homovanillic acid (HVA) by the sequential action of catechol-O-methyltransferase (COMT) and MAO. HVA in the brain or spinal cord has been a principal marker of dopamine activity.

Although several more are known, two types of receptors, designated D1 and D2, are of particular interest here. D1 receptors are postsynaptic and found in several dopaminergic systems, including those associated with motor function and reinforcement mechanisms. D2 receptors are also found postsynaptically, but they play a major role as presynaptic autoreceptors regulating dopamine synthesis, release, and impulse flow. Both these receptor types are subject to up- and downregulation through actions of agonist and antagonist drugs as well as availability of dopamine itself.

Several age-related changes in dopamine systems have been noted. The most well documented are the reductions in dopamine neurons and dopamine in the nigro–striatal pathway characteristic of Parkinson's disease. The loss of dopaminergic cells in the substantia nigra exceeds 80% in the earliest manifestations of this disease. However, in normal aging, tyrosine hydroxlyase, aromatic amino acid decarboxlyase, and dopamine neurons decrease in the striatum, accompanied by increases in MAO (Sunderland, 1992). The effects of these changes, in the absence of any significant motor deficits, are made manifest by the sensitivity of the aged to dopaminergic antagonists. The major culprits are the neuroleptics. Some 50%–75% of elderly patients show movement-disorder side effects as a result of treatment with these drugs (Comella & Klawans, 1994). These agents are prescribed not only for such severe conditions as late-onset schizophrenia but for the more common symptoms of restlessness, agitation, anxiety, irritability, aggressiveness, delusions, confusion, and disorientation. Virtually all classes of these agents can produce at least moderate motor dysfunctions. These classes include the phenothiazines (e.g., chlopromazine), butyrophenones (e.g., haloperidol), thiozanthenes (e.g., thiothixene), and dibenzoxazepines (e.g., loxzapine).

In addition to parkinsonlike symptoms of tremor, rigidity, postural disorders, and poverty of movement, other extrapyramidal side effects can occur, including akathisia (a motor restlessness that can be misdiagnosed as agitation), resulting in increases in neuroleptic doses with, of course, increases in side effects. Extrapyramidal symptoms may not directly involve dopamine; the origins are not always known, but may involve anticholinergic effects. As mentioned previously, anticholinergic side effects of neuroleptics can be severe.

An extremely serious motor deficit called *tardive dyskinesia* can occur as a side effect of neuroleptic treatment. Clinical features include choreatic movements of the mouth and face such as chewing, lip smacking, and tongue protrusion, along with spasms and writhing movements of the arms, legs, and trunk. This often incurable disorder is thought to result from dopamine receptor hypersensitivity brought about by their chronic blockade by the neuroleptic agents. The incidence of tardive dyskinesia can be as high as 60% of neuroleptic treated patients over 70, more than three times that seen in patients younger than 50 (Comella & Klawans, 1994). The older the patient, the more severe are the symptoms. The disease may arise from a course of chronic neuroleptic treatment as short as 3 months.

Dopamine receptors D1 and D2 undergo changes in binding with age, but the consequences are difficult to assess. Present data indicate an increase in D1 receptors in some regions of the brain (e.g., striatum) accompanied by a decrease in D2 receptors. Dopaminergic mechanisms appear to depend in a close interdependence of D1 and D2 activities (Cooper et al., 1991) so that the dynamics of neural function may not easily be interpreted from changes in binding of one or the other class of receptor.

GABA

Gamma-aminobutyric acid of GABA is a major inhibitory transmitter in the CNS and found throughout the brain. The principal source for GABA is glucose via the Krebs cycle. Alpha-ketoglutarate, a Krebs cycle intermediate, feeds a metabolic pathway, called the *GABA shunt,* with the remarkable property of conserving the supply of GABA. Alpha-ketoglutarate is converted to glutamate by the enzyme GABA-T. (Glutamate is the most prevalent neural transmitter in the CNS.) Glutamate can then be converted to GABA by glutamic acid decarboxylase (GAD). The same enzyme that began the process, GABA-T, can destroy GABA by converting it to succinic semialdehyde, but only if alpha-ketoglutarate is converted to glutamate at the same time. Thus, in this metabolic pathway a molecule of GABA can only be degraded if a molecule of precursor is synthesized (McGeer & McGeer, 1989).

The inhibitory action of GABA comes about at postsynaptic ionotropic receptors (GABA-A) by increasing the cellular permeability to the influx of chlorine (C1-), thus resisting depolarization. These GABA-A receptors have a complex structure whose subunit proteins act as separate binding sites for the benzodiazepines, the barbiturates, and ethanol, in addition to GABA itself. The general effect of these drugs, even though they bind at different sites, is to enhance the effect of GABA in increasing the influx of C1-. This common action helps explain their long-known shared behavioral and pharmacological actions. For example, all these drug classes can restore behavior suppressed by punishment. This effect is one laboratory screening procedure for indicating if a new agent may have anxiolytic properties. These agents also show somewhat similar withdrawal symptoms after chronic dosing (e.g., Julien, 1995).

There are differences between them, however, indicating their attachment to different binding sites, as well as the possibility of other, non-GABA-related actions. There are also differences within each of the classes. For example, various benzodiazepines (more than a dozen are available) differ in their sedative, muscle relaxation, or anticonvulsant actions. Discounting the pharmacokinetic differences, mostly in biotransformation, distinctions in the spectra of action are probably due to binding at as yet unidentified subclasses of GABA-A receptors. An additional possibility is the relative binding to the other major GABA receptor, GABA-B.

GABA-B receptors are presynaptic neuromodulators located not only on GABA neurons but also can be found on terminals releasing other transmitters such as dopamine, 5-HT, glutamate, and others. Their function appears to be to inhibit the release of neurotransmitters, possibly by altering calcium (Ca^{++}) influx into the terminals.

Virtually all markers of GABA activity, in all of its major pathways in the CNS—cortex, hippocampus, striatum—show age-related declines. This decrement may play a role in the expression of some pathological conditions such as Huntington's disease, parkinsonism, tardive dyskinesia, and epilepsy. The functional consequences for normal aging, however, are less clear. As mentioned previously, the benzodiazepines show increased toxicity in the aged. At least some of these effects are accountable by pharmacokinetics, primarily in metabolic alterations increasing half-life. However, these processes cannot account for observed increased sensitivity to benzodiazepines in the aged (Sunderland, 1992). Presumably this effect arises from changes in binding in the benzodiazepine–GABA receptor complex. The mechanism underlying this is, to my knowledge, unknown, although changes in binding are known to occur in other ligand–receptor interactions. The possible lesson here is in the interactive nature of neural transmitter processes. Because in aging so many transmitters and their associated processes could be altered, bewildering complexities may arise, particularly if one focuses only on each transmitter system in isolation. The reader may have already been puzzled by how responsiveness to benzodiazepines is enhanced in the aged though increased sensitivity of GABA receptors, yet these same receptors have decreased in number! I am puzzled, too. If any of these mechanisms are relevant, then perhaps the increased sensitivity of receptors overwhelms their decreased number. To make the situation more confusing, decreased GABA (also noted in the aged) would be expected to lead to increased numbers of receptors (upregulation), but such is apparently not the case. We have much to learn about neurochemistry and behavior at any age.

What is without dispute is that the elderly may manifest what Julien describes as a "drug-induced brain syndrome" (Julien, 1995, p. 57) when inappropriately treated with benzodiazepines or, especially, barbiturates. The latter are generally not recommended for the elderly except under special circumstances. The syndrome Julien refers to includes those features associated with senile dementia such as confusion, disorientation, memory dysfunction, poor judgment, inappropriate affect, delusions, hallucinations, and confabulations. These symptoms may be misinterpreted so as to lead to increase dosages or the addition of antipsychotic or antidepressant agents to the regimen, making an already bad situation worse. These toxic effects could also occur with excess consumption of alcohol. Interestingly, alcohol consumption tends to decrease with age, perhaps because of increased sensitivity to its effects.

Though drug-induced dementia calls for vigilance by physicians and other caregivers, the principal side effect of the GABA-associated agents is sedation. This can have profound, indeed dangerous, consequences in the workplace, the home, or on the highway.

The previous discussion of neural transmitter functions related to drug effects in the aged terminates in a general principle: attempting to predict classes of drug effects from knowing that the amounts of endogenous transmitter components have changed or, indeed, any other particular function has changed is, at best, risky. As I have tried to point out, these neurochemical systems are not static entities, but exhibit complex dynamic and interactive adjustments to variations in availability of components, level of activity, agonist or antagonist exposure, and possibly a host of behavioral variables. Until we have a better understanding of neural transmitter, neuromodular, neurotropic, and behavioral mechanisms in all their dynamic interactive glory, we cannot hope to be very specific in predicting drug effects in the aged, or any other population for that matter, by looking at only the brain. Our prime source of data and theory will continue to be experimental, clinical, and applied analyses of drug–behavior interactions.

DRUG EFFECTS AND PERFORMANCE

As readers of this volume will have become aware, intensive research over many years in both basic and applied settings have attempted to characterize significant behavioral changes related to aging. This is an immensely difficult task both methodologically and conceptually. The success of this enterprise depends not only on the careful empirical and theoretical analyses of behavioral variables in the young, which are then applied to the elderly, but results from the study of the aged also throw light backward on our understanding of behavior in the young. That is, there can be no such thing as an isolated field dealing with behavior of the aged, but rather a more comprehensive field of behavior analysis in which age plays an interactive role and from which we may derive general principles of behavior.

The same kind of interactive dynamics applies to behavioral pharmacology. I have discussed the possible effects of drugs in the elderly from the perspective of pharmacokinetics and pharmacodynamics. A strictly reductionist perspective would have me describe and account for the behavioral actions of drugs only the basis of how they are handled by the body and their mechanisms of actions within the central nervous system. But this is an exceedingly parochial view. A major limitation to any strictly physiological approach is that we simply do not understand (except in the grossest terms) either the physiology or the pharmacology of behavior. What is more, advances in the physiology and pharmacology of behavior will come not only from advances in those fields themselves, but just as important, advances in behavior analysis. No proper interpretation of central physiological or pharmacological events is possible in a behavioral vacuum. Drug effects on behavior are often not clearly related to known molecular or physiological mechanisms or even identifiable in terms of drug classification. If all this seems strange, simply consider the different effects of the same "dose" of alcohol, one consumed at a loud boisterous party with old friends, the other when alone in a drab hotel room in a strange city. No known physiological or pharmacological measurement could have accounted for, let alone predicted, the likely profound differences in ensuing behaviors. In a different example, agents as seemingly different as d-amphetamine, scopolamine, and diazepam may all produce deficits in remembering. Thus, to the traditional pharmacological mechanisms, pharmacokinetic and pharmacodynamic, we must add behavioral mechanisms of action.

Perhaps the major contribution of behavioral pharmacology is the demonstration that a given drug not only has multiple behavioral effects, but these effects depend in turn on many behavioral variables—history, context, prevailing contingencies, ongoing behavior, and so on—all of which may interact with each other (Barrett & Witkin, 1986; Branch, 1991; Carlton, 1983). Complexities are further amplified when one considers that the potential variables can also interact with age. There is a clear need for a conceptual framework, particularly in the service of a pragmatic, human factors perspective, for predicting and interpreting the behavioral effects of drugs in the aged based on those variables shown to be significant in behavioral pharmacology investigations. What is proposed is both a reflection of the behavior-analytic origins of behavioral pharmacology and the generally cognitive orientation of modern human factors psychology. Because the two fields have emerged from different sources, with different conceptual frames, it is necessary to reformulate or reorganize at least some of the issues. Fortunately, this is not really very difficult, because fundamentally, whether you are a cognitive psychologist or a behavior analyst, the primary subject matter of interest is behavior, overt or covert. The pragmatic stance of human factors is also advantageous because it pays particular interest to conditions controlling and modifying behavior, as embodied in task analysis. The same goals lie at the heart of behavior analysis.

What age-related behaviors are of special interest in the joint context of drug effects and human factors? Two relatively uncontroversial effects, sedation and motor dysfunction have obvious human factors implications. More subtle, but perhaps just as significant, are behaviors (or "processes") labeled as "cognitive." These include a range of activities such as remembering, learning new skills, maintaining old skills, problem solving, planning and the like. Much of the cognitive aging literature is devoted to an experimental and conceptual analysis of age-related changes in these kinds of cognitive functioning. How might we organize cognitive functions into a behavior-analytic framework more easily to draw on the available literature to predict or interpret drug effects?

Two key interlocking concepts in behavioral analysis helpful in this endeavor are *contingency* and *stimulus control*. Contingency refers to discriminative stimulus–behavior–consequence relations. Loosely speaking, what properties of behavior (rate, pattern, topography, quantity, quality, etc.), under what context, leads to what consequences. The consequences in turn, feed back to affect the ongoing behavior and discriminative control in a dynamical-system interplay essential for the shaping, maintenance, and modification of behavior.

Stimulus control refers to the extent to which variations in stimulus conditions control variations in behavior. Such control is ubiquitous and manifested in discriminative stimuli, conditional discrimination, generalization, psychophysical functions, relational frames, conceptual behavior, rule-governed behavior, and control via previously encountered stimuli, better known as remembering. For behavior analysts, much of the subject matter of interest to cognitive psychologists is more comfortably cast into a functional analysis of contingencies of stimulus control; that is, the conditions necessary to bring about, maintain, or alter behavior through stimulus arrangements.

Application to Memory and Learning

Of all the potential deficits encountered in normal aging, those collectively characterized as memory losses are perhaps the most common and the most disturbing. In addition to sedation, memory dysfunction is also the most commonly reported side effect of behaviorally active drug treatment in the elderly. Memory loss may occur with antidepressants, antianxiety agents, stimulants, and a variety of centrally acting anticholinergic agents. The latter, in particular, have been singled out as being especially troublesome in producing this side effect. Scopolamine-induced memory dysfunction has served as a model for age-associated memory loss (e.g., Dean & Bartus, 1988; Sahakian, 1988). This status has been earned by demonstrating that young subjects, when appropriately dosed with scopolamine, show memory deficits similar to those displayed by nondrugged old subjects.

A fundamental question arises when there are indications of memory problems after exposure to a drug. Just what is the drug doing? In addition to eliminating alterations in sensory–motor functioning, or motivational factors, our principal task should be characterize in a functional sense what age-related memory changes are. This requires, of course, some theory or conceptual framework about memory. Memory is probably the most active research area in cognitive aging (e.g., Smith 1996), and present results provide the beginning of a behavioral analysis of drug effects on remembering. Smith (1996) has written a very useful review from the cognitive perspective of this complex area that can serve as a starting point.

Much memory-related theory and experimentation has described and made use of distinctions between various kinds of memory (episodic, semantic, procedural, prospective, retrospective, implicit, explicit, sensory, short term, working, long term, etc.) and associated processes (attention, encoding, storage, retrieval) and contingencies of measurement (recall, recognition, savings, etc.)—all presumably reflective of distinct "processes." Aging, and presumably a host of other conditions including drug exposure, could show differential effects with respect to any of these kinds of processes. The problem is that the experimental aging literature contains a bewildering variety of findings, which render many of the standard taxonomic categories basically nonfunctional. Fortunately, if the data are looked at along the proper dimensions, some order emerges. As Smith describes it, the primary factor determining the probability of successful remembering is degree of "effortful processing"; that is, the more difficult is the memory task, the less one can remember. This would be a useless truism if there were no independent means of controlling or assessing difficulty, by characterizing what is remembered under what conditions. Craik (1986) had earlier suggested the importance of environmental support in controlling successful memory in the aged. This is a direct application of the contingencies defining stimulus control in behavior analysis. To take perhaps the simplest possible example, if a person's name is clearly written before you, there is little or nothing to remember (assuming you can read). If we gradually fade the name away (perhaps the name tag is written in disappearing ink), then we have withdrawn important sources of control. Other sources may remain, such as the person's face, or even an image of that face, but these are different stimulus conditions, operating under different contingencies, and perhaps controlling different classes of behaviors. It is certainly more difficult to generate an image of a person's face than simply to look at that face when the person is present. Thus, difficulty in the context of remembering is related to strength of stimulus control, in turn a function of the contingencies necessary to develop and maintain that control and the history of exposure to those contingencies.

With age, an additional variable comes to interact with stimulus control contingencies; namely, speed. If a single dependent variable is most characteristic of aging, it is slowing (see, e.g., Salthouse, 1993). This applies to virtually all major classes of performance—motor, sensory, and cognitive. When slowing is added to a gradient of complexity in contingencies for acquisition and maintenance of stimulus control, differences in remembering performance between the young and the old are likely to emerge. I should add that even simple reaction time in the nonaged is increased by many drugs (McKim, 1991).

A third factor may come into play in determining performance differences in the face of stimulus control complexity. This is the degree to which a performance may be described as "automatic" versus "controlled." Here *controlled* refers loosely to conscious, deliberate effort in executing a performance, usually under conditions of low levels of practice or insurmountable complexity. Very well-practiced performance, on the other hand, tends to be executed with fluency and relatively little effort, demonstrated, for example, by concurrently engaging in another task. Carrying on a conversation while driving is a common example. Automaticity may occur with very complex tasks, given extended practice and some degree of consistency in task characteristics (Fisk, Ackerman, & Schneider, 1987). Thus, it is not simply the nominal complexity of a task that determines how an intervention may affect it, but the ongoing performance level on the task as well as the need to carry out other tasks concurrently.

With this long prelude I am ready to deal more directly with drug effects on cognitive performances such as acquisition and remembering. Interventions, drugs included, may have differential effects depending on the strength of stimulus control maintaining the behavior. That control, in turn, will depend on current and historical contingencies that shape differential attentional control, as well as the particular task-related sensory–motor and cognitive skills. Because multiple and interactive variable control any performance moment to moment, the experimental analysis of the effects of drugs on complex performance is a challenging task. Although much of this analysis originates in nonhuman animal studies, where contingencies may be more easily specified and controlled, human studies have both extended and corroborated the animal work. Several very useful references on drugs and stimulus control are available; for example, Eckerman and Bushnell (1992), Heise and Milar (1984), and Katz (1990). The kinds of contingencies include analysis of basic sensory functions via psychophysical methods, single trial learning (largely with passive avoidance), vigilance procedures, simple and complex discrimination, repeated acquisition versus maintained performance, delayed matching or oddity, spatial control under immediate and delayed conditions, temporal control, habituation, Pavlovian conditioning, and others. This is not the place to review all this vast literature but rather to select and interpret it in the context of possible age-related drug effects. It should be emphasized that relatively few (though a large absolute number) of these studies have manipulated age as a variable. However, results so far obtained indicate that if a significant drug effect on behavior is seen in nonaged subjects, then it will not only be seen in aged subjects but the effects are likely to be greater.

A huge number of drugs have been shown to affect in some way behavior under various stimulus control procedures. To list but a few, pentobarbital, d-amphetamine, imipramine, chlorpromazine, morphine, scopolamine, chlordiazepoxide, and alcohol; in other words, representatives of all the major classes of agents most likely to be part of the routine intake of an aged person. Curiously perhaps, while distinctions both within and among the classes represented by these agents can be made as to their relative potencies or efficacies, as well as particular spectra of effects, these are generally less important than the characteristic behaviors controlled by the various contingencies or procedures studied. That is, there are primary behavioral determinants of drug action.

An example of a well-studied procedure having relevance to a number of cognitive processing variables is repeated acquisition of behavior sequences, first studied by Boren (1963), and extensively used in behavior pharmacology experiments by Thompson and Moeschbaecker (see, e.g., Moeschbaecker & Thompson, 1980). The subject (pigeons, rats, monkeys, and humans have served as subjects) must learn a particular sequence of responses (ranging from 3 to 10, depending on details of procedure and subject species). This sequence changes from session to session and constitutes the acquisition component of the procedure. In addition, there is usually a performance component where the sequence remains constant under explicit discriminative control, or is varied, but again with explicit discriminative control. This procedure allows for comparisons between acquisition, that is, "learning," and a steady-state, well-controlled performance. Over a number of such studies, involving many different classes of drugs, the acquisition component is typically more sensitive to drugs than the performance component. This is congruent with the previous discussion asserting that the magnitude of drug effects should be correlated with the more effortful, less automatic performance.

An instructive example using human subjects is a study by Bickel, Higgins, and Griffiths (1989) of the effects of multiple administrations of the benzodiazepine anxiolytic diazepam. Each session the subjects were required to learn a 10-response sequence. Along with this acquisition component was a performance component with an invariant sequence. After some training, essentially no errors occurred in the latter, while an average of 20 errors per session were made in the acquisition component. On first administration diazepam (80 mg) impaired both acquisition and performance, but by the second administration on the next day, acquisition was very much more affected than the performance component. An average of more than 60 errors occurred during acquisition, while the performance had returned to near control levels, demonstrating the characteristic result of greater sensitivity of the acquisition component. By the third day, complete tolerance was demonstrated by both the acquisition and performance components having returned to their control levels. This third-day effect was probably a manifestation of "contingent tolerance"; that is, a behavioral tolerance engendered by compensatory adjustments to changes in behavior–consequent relations. This effect is shown by a number of agents under appropriate conditions, including ethanol and d-amphetamine (see, e.g., Branch, 1994). I shall return to this effect shortly.

Various delay procedures, most notably delayed matching to sample (DMTS), have been commonly employed to evaluate drug effects on working memory or control by a previously encountered stimulus. As with the repeated acquisition contingencies, the persistent issue with delay conditions centers on just what aspects of the procedures control what aspects of behavior and, in turn, on which of these contingency–behavior functions do drugs act. As mentioned previously, anticholinergic agents like scopolamine are said to interfere with remembering, but just what does this mean? Delay procedures coupled with analysis of aspects of attention have contributed to separating, at least to some degree, various task components. For example, in a delay task an age-related effect on retention would be measured by an interaction of delay with age (older subjects showing a greater slope in errors as a function of delay than young subjects). Likewise, a specific action of a drug on retention would be revealed by larger effects at longer delays.

In the classic experiments of Bartus and his colleagues (Bartus, 1980; Bartus, Dean, Pontecorvo, & Flicker, 1985) with scopolamine among other drugs, rhesus or cebus monkeys were required to demonstrate recall of which one of nine panels in a 3 × 3 matrix had been illuminated after a delay by pressing the appropriate panel. This is a recall task, unlike most memory procedures in the nonhuman experimental literature, which are basically recognition tasks. In general, recall contingencies show greater age-deficits in humans than recognition contingencies (Smith, 1996). Under nondrug conditions, aged monkeys show greater deficits at longer delays than young monkeys, thus indicating an age-specific retention effect. Scopolamine in young monkeys shows significant dose by delay interactions of the kind seen with old monkeys under control conditions. In older monkeys, scopolamine, as expected, renders an already poor performance worse.

In summary, a stimulus control analysis predicts that drug effects on performance will depend on the degree of control exerted by contingencies controlling that performance. This control, in turn, may involve a history of extensive practice or, alternatively, a novel or inconsistent task. The imposition of additional concurrent tasks will tend to weaken control even with some well-practices performances. Also, differential control may be reflected in variations in stimulus support, as exemplified by recognition as opposed to recall contingencies of remembering.

Demonstration of the strength of control in any situation is a functional task, not a nominal one; that is, in the absence of any prior experimental analysis with at least similar situations, it may be difficult to predict how a drug may modify behavior. To complicate matters further, drugs, as well as other interventions, do not always continue to have the same effects on a given performance. I have already mentioned contingent tolerance. Initially, drug exposure may have a major effect in modifying performance. After continued exposure, the performance may return to control levels. I am not talking here about pharmacological tolerance, but behavioral tolerance. Essentially, the consequences of altered performance under the drug feedback to control restoration of the predrug performance. This effect may be of considerable significance in the aged individual under chronic dosing with a performance-altering drug, especially with long-practiced (i.e., "automatic") tasks such as driving. Unfortunately, there are little data on the role of drugs in driving performance in the aged (Ray, Gurwitz, Decker, & Kennedy, 1992).

Performance Maintenance and Enhancement

While I have focused almost entirely on the possible deleterious effects of drugs in the aged, a very active area of research is devoted to the development and testing of agents for the alleviation of performance deficits inherent in aging. The primary thrust of this work is toward effective pharmacological treatment for severe dementias, particularly Alzheimer's disease. However, there would be an obvious benefit simply to performance maintenance in the normal aged; that is, maintaining relatively youthful levels of behavioral functioning via pharmacological or other means.

Unfortunately, to date no "wonder drug" is on the horizon to treat, for example, memory deficits in the aged. However, there are some promising developments (see, e.g., Dean & Bartus, 1988; Porsolt, Roux, & Lenegre, 1994). Among several possible candidates, two general classes have received the most experimental attention in the animal laboratory and the clinic. As expected, one class is comprised of cholinergic agonists, either direct acting such as the muscarinic drug oxytremorine or indirect agonists (e.g., acetylcholinesterase inhibitors) such as physostigmine. The second group includes the racetam compounds, commonly known as *nootropics,* although this term actually refers a variety of different compounds. Piracetam and aniracetam are exemplars. The mechanism of action of these drugs remains a matter of debate but may involve transport, metabolic, or specific transmitter-related functions (Gouliaev & Senning, 1994).

Tests of so-called cognitive enhancers have included a variety of animal models of cognition as well as tests of cognitive functioning in healthy and clinical human subjects (e.g., Gouliaev & Senning, 1994; Albernoni, Bressi, & Cattaneo, 1993; Woodruff-Pak & Li, 1994). While many positive results have been obtained, they have tended to be small (i.e., statistically but not necessarily functionally significant). By no means have all studies reported positive effects, and considerable variability with respect to subject, species, test, and the like has been a common finding. Thus considerable caution is warranted about expecting any "breakthroughs" in this area. Most researchers are sensitive both to the complexity of cognitive functions and our ignorance of the interrelations between behavioral and neurochemical evens. There will be no "magic bullet" to slay the dragon of dementia or the ogre of aging.

CODA

As initially indicated, this has been a quick primer of the potential role of behavioral pharmacology to human factors issues. Because of space limitations, some important topics were not discussed, such as the effects of drugs on sensory functions and motor skills. However, I hope that what was presented not only will be of some aid in approaching the vast and complex literature in the field, but perhaps more important, provided a convincing argument that the combination of functional cognitive psychology, behavior analysis, and neuropharmacology yields an empirical and theoretical framework with which to approach human factors research and practice. Moreover, armed with this foundation, human factors stands to make substantial contributions to our understanding of how drugs may affect human behavior—positively or negatively, young or old.

References

Albert, M. L., & Knoefel, J. E. (Eds.). (1994). *Clinical neurology of aging.* New York: Oxford University Press.

Abernethy, D. R. (1992). Psychotrophic drugs and the aging process: Pharmacokinetics and pharmacodynamics. In C. Salzman (Ed.), *Clinical geriatric psychopharmacology* (2nd ed., pp. 61–76). Baltimore: Williams & Wilkins.

Barrett, J. E., & Witkin, J. M. (1986). The role of behavioral and pharmacological history in determining the effects of abused drugs. In S. R. Goldberg & I. P. Stolerman (Eds.), *Behavioral analysis of drug dependence* (pp. 195–223). Orlando, FL: Academic Press.

Bartus, R. T. (1980). Cholinergic drug effects on memory and cognition in animals. In L. W. Poon (Ed.), *Aging in the 80's: Psychological issues* (pp. 163–180). Washington, DC: American Psychological Association.

Bartus, R. T., Dean, R. L., Pontecorvo, M. J., & Flicker, C. (1985). The cholinergic hypothesis: A historical overview, current perspective, and future directions. *Annals of the New York Academy of Sciences, 444,* 332–358.

Bickel, W. K., Higgins, S. T., & Griffiths, R. R. (1989). Repeated diazepam administration: Effects on the acquisition and performance of response chains in humans. *Journal of the Experimental Analysis of Behavior, 52,* 47–56.

Bloom, H. G., & Shlom, E. A. (1993). *Drug prescribing for the elderly.* New York: Raven Press.

Boren, J. J. (1963). Repeated acquisition of new behavioral chains. *American Psychologist, 18,* 421.

Branch, M. N. (1991). Behavioral pharmacology. In L. H. Iversen & K. A. Lattal (Eds.), *Experimental analysis of behavior* (Part 2, pp. 21–77). Amsterdam: Elsevier.

Branch, M. N. (1994). Behavioral factors in drug tolerance. In F. van Haaren (Ed.), *Methods in behavioral pharmacology.* (pp. 329–347). Amsterdam: Elsevier.

Bressler, R., & Katz, M. D. (1993). *Geriatric pharmacology.* New York: McGraw-Hill.

Carlton, P. L. (1983). *A primer of behavioral pharmacology.* New York: Freeman.

Comella, C. L. & Klawans, H. L. (1994). NonParkinsonian movement disorders in the elderly. In M. L. Albert & J. E. Knoefel (Eds.), *Clinical neurology of aging* (2nd Ed., pp. 502–520). NY: Oxford University Press.

Cooper, J. R., Bloom, F. E., & Roth, R. H. (1991). *The biochemical basis of neuropharmacology* (7th ed.). New York: Oxford University Press.

Craik, F. I. M. (1986). A functional account of age differences in memory. In F. Klix & H. Hagendorf (Eds.), *Human memory and cognitive capabilities, mechanisms, and performance* (pp. 409–422). North-Holland: Elsevier.

Dean, R. L., & Bartus, R. T. (1988). Behavioral models of aging in non-human primates. In L. L. Iversen, S. D. Iversen, & S. H. Snyder (Eds.), *Handbook of psychopharmacology: Vol. 20. Psychopharmacology of the aging nervous system* (pp. 325–392). New York: Plenum.

DeKosky, S. T., & Palmer, A. M. (1994). Neurochemistry of aging. In M. L. Albert & J. E. Knoefel (Eds.), *Clinical neurology of aging* (pp. 79–101). New York: Oxford University Press.

Eckerman, D. A., & Bushnell, P. J. (1992). The neurotoxicology of cognition: Attention, learning, and memory. In H. A. Tilson & C. L. Mitchell (Eds.), *Neurotoxicology* (pp. 213–270). New York: Raven Press.

Fisk, A. D., Ackerman, P. L., & Schneider, W. (1987). Automatic and controlled processing

theory and its application to human factors. In P. Hancock (Ed.), *Human factors psychology*. New York: North-Holland.
Gilman, A. G., Rall, T. W., Nies, A. S., & Taylor, P. (Eds.). (1990). *Goodman and Gilman's The Pharmacological Basis of Therapeutics* (8th ed.). New York: McGraw-Hill.
Gouliaev, A. H., & Senning, A. (1994). Piracitam and other structurally related nootropics. *Brain Research Reviews, 19,* 180–222.
Hall, Z. W. (1992). *An introduction to molecular neurobiology.* Sunderland, MA: Sinauer.
Heise, G., & Milar, K. (1984). Drugs and stimulus control. In L. L. Iversen, S. D. Iversen, & S. H. Snyder (Eds.), *Handbook of psychopharmacology: Vol. 18. Drugs, neurotransmitters, and behavior* (pp. 129–190). New York: Plenum.
Iversen, L. L., Iversen, S. D., & Snyder, S. H. (Eds.). (1988). *Handbook of psychopharmacology: Vol. 20. Psychopharmacology of the aging nervous system.* New York: Plenum.
Julien, R. M. (1995). *A primer of drug action* (7th ed.). New York: Freeman.
Katz, J. (1990). Effects of drugs on stimulus control of behavior under schedules of reinforcement. In J. E. Barrett, T. Thompson, & P. Dews (Eds.), *Advances in behavioral pharmacology* (Vol. 7, pp. 13–38). Hillsdale, NJ: Erlbaum.
Lamy, P. P., Salzman, C., & Nevis-Olesen, J. (1992). Drug prescribing patterns, risks, and compliance guidelines. In C. Salzman (Ed.), *Clinical geriatric psychopharmacology* (2nd ed., pp. 15–37). Baltimore: Williams & Wilkins.
Marr, M. J. (1990). Behavioral pharmacology: Issues of reductionism and causality. In J. E. Barrett, T. Thompson, & P. Dews (Eds.), *Advances in behavioral pharmacology* (Vol. 7, pp. 1–12). Hillsdale, NJ: Erlbaum.
McGeer, P. L., & McGeer, E. G. (1989). Amino acid neurotransmitters. In G. J. Siegal, B. W. Agranoff, R. W. Albers, & P. B. Molinoff (Eds.), *Basic neurochemistry* (pp. 311–332). New York: Raven Press.
McKim, W. A. (1991). *Drugs and behavior* (2nd ed.). Englewood Cliffs, NJ: Prentice-Hall.
McKim, W. A., & Mishara, B. (1987). *Drugs and aging.* Toronto: Butterworth.
Moeschbaecker, J., & Thompson, D. (1980). Effects of d-amphetamine, cocaine, and phencyclidine on the acquisition of response sequences with and without stimulus fading. *Journal of the Experimental Analysis of Behavior, 33,* 369–381.
Morgan, D. G., & May, P. C. (1990). Age-related changes in synaptic neurochemistry. In E. L. Schneider & J. W. Rowe (Eds.), *Handbook of the biology of aging* (3rd ed., pp. 219–254). San Diego, CA: Academic Press.
O'Hanlon, J. F. (1991). Human factors in psychoactive drug development: A new challenge and opportunity. *Human Factors Society Bulletin, 34* (4), 1–3.
Porsolt, R., Roux, S., & Lenegre, A. (1994). Critical issues in cognition enhancement research. In T. Palomo, T. Archer, & R. Beninger (Eds.), *Strategies for studying brain disorders: Vol. 2. Schizophrenia, movement disorders and related cognitive disorders* (pp. 285–297). London: Farrand Press.
Pratt, W. B., & Taylor, P. (Eds.). (1990). *Principles of drug action* (3rd ed.). New York: Churchill-Livingstone.
Preda, L., Alberoni, M., Bressi, S., & Cattaneo, C. (1993). Effects of acute doses of oxiracetam in the scopolomine model of human amnesia. *Psychopharmacology, 110,* 421–426.
Ray, W. A., Gurwitz, J., Decker, M. D., & Kennedy, D. L. (1992). Medications and the safety of the older driver: Is there a basis for concern? *Human Factors, 34,* 33–47.
Sahakian, B. J. (1988). Cholinergic drugs and human cognitive performance. In L. L. Iversen, S. D. Iversen, & S. H. Snyder (Eds.), *Handbook of psychopharmacology: Vol. 20. Psychopharmacology of the aging nervous system* (pp. 393–424). New York: Plenum.
Salthouse, T. (1993). Speed mediation of adult age differences in cognition. *Developmental Psychology, 29,* 722–738.

Salzman, C. (Ed.). (1992). *Clinical geriatric psychopharmacology* (2nd ed.). Baltimore: Williams & Wilkins.
Siegal, G. J., Agranoff, B. W., Albers, R. W., & Molinoff, P. B. (Eds.). (1989). *Basic neurochemistry.* New York: Raven Press.
Smith, A. D. (1996). Memory. In J. E. Birren & K. W. Schaie (Eds.), *Handbook of the psychology of aging* (4th ed. pp. 236–250). New York: Academic Press.
Sunderland, T. (1992). Neurotransmission in the aging central nervous system. In C. Salzman (Ed.), *Clinical geriatric psychopharmacology* (2nd ed., pp. 41–59). Baltimore: Williams & Wilkins.
Tariot, P. N. (1992). Neurobiology and treatment of dementia. In C. Salzman (Ed.), *Clinical geriatric psychopharmacology* (2nd ed., pp. 277–299). Baltimore: Williams & Wilkins.
Vestal, R. E., & Cusack, B. J. (1990). Pharmacology and aging. In E. L. Schneider & J. W. Rowe (Eds.), *Handbook of the biology of aging* (3rd ed., pp. 349–383). San Diego, CA: Academic Press.
Woodruff-Pak, D. S., & Li, -Yong-Tong (1994). Nefiracetam (DM-9384): Effect on eyeblink classical conditioning in older rabbits. *Psychopharmacology, 114,* 200–208.

Part 2

APPLICATIONS

Chapter 9

Aging, Pilot Performance, and Expertise

Daniel Morrow
Von Leirer

INTRODUCTION

There is a long history of psychologists working with engineers to improve the fit between pilot and aircraft (e.g., Fitts & Jones, 1947; McFarland, 1953). While the pilot has often been generically described in this research, the present volume attests to the growing awareness that human factors should encompass individual differences in abilities, experience, and interests. Pilot age relates to all of these factors. The influence of age on pilot performance is especially important to consider at the present time for the following reasons.

First, the pilot's job is rapidly changing. Commercial operations are becoming more complex, in part because of increased congestion in the airspace around airports. This complexity may translate into higher pilot workload because of more frequent communication, decision making, and other components of pilot performance. Piloting is also changing because of increasing flight deck and Air Traffic Control automation, which is shifting pilot workload from manual control to more cognitive tasks such as system monitoring and decision making (Billings, 1991). Therefore, it is important

Handbook of Human Factors and the Older Adult

to consider how pilot factors such as age and experience influence performance in this increasingly complex cognitive domain.

Second, the work force in the United States is aging. For example, 12% of the U.S. population was age 65 or older in 1988, whereas this proportion is expected to increase to 17% by the year 2020 (Transportation Research Board, 1988). If the same trend holds for pilots, it is important to identify when and how aging limits pilot performance and if age declines can be mitigated by experience and by training and design interventions.

Third, aviation policy issues also relate to pilot age. The age 60 retirement rule for pilots flying large commercial aircraft assumes that age represents an unacceptable risk to public safety after age 60 because of increasing risk of sudden incapacitation due to medical problems or physiological and cognitive deficits associated with normal aging (U.S. General Account Office, 1989). This policy has prompted much discussion about issues such as the appropriate chronological age cutoff for retirement or whether this criterion can be replaced by a proficiency-based criterion that reflects functional age (e.g., Braune & Wickens, 1984; Mohler, 1981).

Finally, recent developments in cognitive aging and expertise theory have generated interest in when and how experience mitigates age declines in complex task performance. The present chapter focuses on the relevance of these theories to pilot performance. For example, cognitive aging and expertise theory can guide design and training interventions that may minimize age effects in pilot performance (see the Conclusions section). At the same time, aviation research points to the need for these theories to address the nature of the environment within which experts perform (Kirlik, 1995). In sum, both practical and theoretical developments focus attention on two important issues: under what conditions is age likely to limit pilot performance, and how can deficits be minimized? The present chapter addresses these issues.

Overview

Age is clearly only one of many factors that influence complex task performance. Therefore, the influence of age on pilot performance is likely to depend on a variety of pilot, task, and environmental factors. For example, age-related declines in cognitive resources may be offset by experience, health status, or other pilot factors. In addition, task factors such as complexity and familiarity and environmental factors related to stress (e.g., temperature, noise) may amplify effects of aging or minimize the benefits of experience. We examine the influence of age on pilot performance in the context of a range of factors, focusing on theory and research that relates age, experience, and pilot performance. We first summarize several theories of how cognition changes with age in the general population. Next, we discuss research related to expertise, task factors, and aging in complex task domains. The rest of the chapter concentrates on pilot performance research, beginning with a brief overview of cognitive components of piloting and methodological issues related to aging and pilot performance research. Studies of age and expertise effects on overall or global pilot performance are followed by research about the effects of these factors on components of piloting, from perceptual and attentional processes to complex tasks such as communication and decision making. Because relatively few aging studies have involved pilots, we also review research in other complex task domains such as driving. The chapter concludes with implications for minimizing age effects in pilot performance and with suggestions for future research that will provide more precise answers to when (and how) age influences pilot performance.

AGING AND COGNITION IN THE GENERAL POPULATION

Theories of Cognitive Aging

Laboratory studies reveal age-related declines on a range of sensory and cognitive abilities, including visual and auditory perception (Corso, 1987), divided and focused attention (McDowd & Birren, 1990), the efficiency of processing information in working memory (Stine, 1995), encoding and retrieval (Poon, 1985), and language understanding and production (Stine, Soederberg, & Morrow, 1996). These declines are gradual, beginning in the middle to late 20s and progressing to the middle 70s, after which they become more precipitous (Salthouse, 1991b). Performance is more likely to reflect age-related declines under complex task conditions (e.g., Cerella, Poon, & Williams, 1980). Several general theories have been proposed to explain these age-related declines.

Cognitive Slowing

Perhaps the most widely accepted theory argues that age declines reflect a gradual reduction in the rate of processing (e.g., Salthouse, 1991b; Welford, 1958). Slowing occurs for both sensorimotor or response processes and central or cognitive processes (Earles & Salthouse, 1995). There is, however, disagreement about how much slowing reflects an irreversible biological process and the extent to which it reflects experiential factors that can be reversed by training (Willis & Schaie, 1986).

Reduced Working Memory Capacity

Age may also bring a decline in the cognitive resources available for the storage and processing of information in working memory (Craik & Byrd, 1982), although declining working memory capacity may partly reflect age-related slowing (Salthouse, 1991a). Therefore, older adults should have particular difficulty when tasks impose heavy demands on storage or processing. For example, age differences tend to increase for free recall rather than cued recall tasks (Craik & McDowd, 1987). Working memory capacity has been measured by tasks such as sentence span (Daneman & Carpenter, 1980), and age differences in span scores partly account for differences in recall (e.g., Stine & Wingfield, 1990). There may also be separate verbal and spatial working memories (Baddeley, 1986), which is consistent with multiple resources theories that posit separate resources for input and output processes in verbal and spatial domains (Wickens, 1992).

Failure to Inhibit

Age differences in performance may also reflect a decreased ability to inhibit task-irrelevant information (Hasher & Zacks, 1988). This information competes with more relevant information for working memory capacity. Hence, older adults are likely to be more susceptible to interference; they are more vulnerable to interference effects in the Stroop task (Cohn, Dustman, & Bradford, 1984) and less able to ignore irrelevant information in visual search (Plude & Hoyer, 1985).

Whether viewed as speed or capacity, declining processing resources are likely to impair pilot performance, which involves a range of cognitive abilities in a multitask environment (see Components of Flying section). Moreover, inhibition failure may make older pilots more vulnerable to distraction, a recognized problem in piloting.

Aging and Expertise

While laboratory studies tend to present a dismal view of aging and cognition, everyday observation suggests that as we age we often maintain high levels of competence at home and in the workplace. To resolve this discrepancy, many researchers point out that aging is associated with stable or increasing knowledge and experience, which may offset declining cognitive resources (e.g., Rybash, Hoyer, & Roodin, 1986; Salthouse, 1990). This prediction is supported by the expertise literature, which shows that experts outperform novices even though the two groups do not differ in general cognitive abilities. Supported by domain knowledge, expert performance on domain-relevant tasks appears to be less constrained by resource limits than novice performance (e.g., Chi, Glaser, & Farr, 1988; Ericsson & Smith, 1991). It follows that experts may also be less constrained than novices by age-related declines in cognitive resources. Several mechanisms relevant to pilot performance may account for how expertise can offset such age declines in resources.

Maintenance

According to skill acquisition theory, some skill components become automatized with practice (Anderson, 1983). Thus, high levels of training may circumvent age-related resource declines, with highly practiced skills maintained in later adulthood. However, evidence for this position is mixed—practice reduces age differences for some tasks but not others (for a review, see Salthouse, 1990). Job-related experience may also reduce age differences on skills. Some studies examined if older graphic designers (Lindenberger, Kleigl, & Baltes, 1992) or architects (Salthouse, Babcock, Skovronek, Mitchell, & Palmon, 1990) are as proficient as younger professionals on spatial tasks, which may tap skills maintained by work-related practice. However, expertise did not reduce age differences in either study. Declining resources may hamper skill acquisition by older adults (Bosman & Charness, 1996; Fisk & Rogers, 1991). This is an important aviation issue because evolving technology requires pilots to continually update skills.

Compensation

Compensation involves developing new ways to perform tasks in order to offset age declines in cognitive resources. Therefore, older adults should perform tasks differently than younger adults in response to a perceived deficit (Backman & Dixon, 1992). For example, older transcription typists tend to have larger preview spans than younger typists, allowing more time for motor response (Salthouse, 1984). Thus, a "top-down" strategy compensates for age-related slowing on some task components (also see Charness, 1991). Compensation may involve external as well as internal strategies. Older adults may rely on external memory aids such as diaries or calendars to remember appointments or other tasks (Charness & Bosman, 1995). Other strategies take advantage of the social environment. People may adopt collaborative strategies that pool individual cognitive resources to accomplish a joint task. Shared resources may compensate for declining resources at the individual level. For example, typical age differences in narrative recall occur for individuals and pairs of unrelated individuals, but not for married couples (Dixon, 1996). We will review evidence for compensatory strategies in pilot time-sharing ability and communication tasks.

Accommodation

Instead of developing new means to accomplish the same task, older adults may cope with declining resources by selectively avoiding demanding conditions, thereby redefining the task. For example, older adults may increasingly avoid nighttime or rush hour driving. Older workers may make a transition to more administrative positions, relying on others to accomplish more manual jobs (Abraham & Hansson, 1995). In aviation, older commercial pilots tend to have more seniority and may select less taxing routes with fewer takeoffs and landings. While this seems likely, there is virtually no research on accommodative strategies among pilots.

Expertise and Environmental Support

Expertise is most likely to mitigate age declines when the task supports knowledge use. Experts tend to outperform novices when materials (displays, instructions) are organized in terms of domain principles, and expertise benefits increase with organization (Abernathy, Neal, & Koning, 1994; Chase & Simon, 1973; Gilhooly, Wood, Kinnear, & Green, 1988; Vicente, 1992). Thus, experts excell on highly domain-relevant tasks, which are compatible with their domain knowledge and goals. These findings are consistent with theories emphasizing that expertise is embedded in specific task environments (Kirlik, 1995). Thus, pilots are experts in particular cockpit and system environments (Hutchins, 1991).

Domain-relevant tasks should provide environmental support for older adults. According to Craik and Jennings (1992), environmental support minimizes age differences by reducing demands on encoding and retrieval processes. Domain-relevant tasks may provide environmental support by enabling knowledge-based strategies that circumvent age declines in cognitive resources. However, very complex or unfamiliar tasks are unlikely to support such strategies. Indeed, studies that test experts on highly domain-relevant tasks such as typing provide evidence for mitigation (e.g., Salthouse, 1984), while studies with more domain-general tests do not (e.g., Lindenberger, et al., 1992; Salthouse et al., 1990). Similarly, Clancy and Hoyer (1994) found that expertise reduces age differences in visual search only for domain-relevant contexts. Similar findings for piloting are described in the Pilot Communication section.

Opportunities for knowledge-based mitigation of age declines in cognitive resources depend on factors in addition to the task. According to Murphy (1989), relationships between task demands, experience, and cognitive resources often change during the course of a career (Park, 1992, extends this view to cognitive aging). Careers such as commercial piloting have typical trajectories with transition and maintenance phases. Transitional phases are characterized by learning new tasks, with heavy demands on cognitive resources. Pilots make transitions to new crew positions (e.g., from flight engineer to first officer) and to new types of aircraft. Transitions are followed by maintenance phases, characterized by stable task demands. Knowledge-based mitigation of declining resources may be more likely during maintenance periods, when older workers use highly practiced skills to accomplish familiar tasks. These skills may be maintained in the face of declining cognitive resources. Transitional phases, on the other hand, pose greater challenges for older workers because of declining cognitive resources. In fact, older adults may need more time than younger adults to acquire new skills (Fisk & Rogers, 1991). Therefore, designing the environment to promote knowledge-based strategies may be particularly important during transitions (Park, 1992). Transitions bring opportunities as well as new challenges. For example, older commercial pilots who become captains have more leverage to redefine tasks to accommodate declining resources, perhaps by choosing less taxing routes. Other aspects of the job may increase workload, such as managing crew coordination. Pilot aging research has not yet addressed experience/age tradeoffs over the course of pilot careers.

Predictions about Aging and Pilot Performance

This brief review of aging and expertise research in the general population suggests several predictions about aging and pilot performance, which help refine the question about when age is likely to influence pilot performance. (1) More experienced pilots are less likely to show age-related decrements, although the type of flying experience may be more important than amount of experience—older pilots may be at greatest risk when they have little recent experience, or few hours in a new aircraft. (2) Age has less impact on more knowledge-based piloting abilities and tasks, reflecting compensatory or maintenance strategies. (3) Age has more impact on difficult or novel tasks, which are more likely to tax limited resources. (4) Assessing performance with domain-independent tasks may underestimate the influence of expertise on age differences in pilot performance. Research relevant to these predictions is presented in the next section.

AGING AND PILOT PERFORMANCE RESEARCH

We present a general description of piloting to identify the cognitive processes likely to be influenced by pilot age and experience.

Cognitive Processes in Piloting

Flying an aircraft is a good example of a multitask environment (Roscoe, 1980). Pilots must accomplish several functions more or less simultaneously: maintain control (of aircraft attitude and state, the three-dimensional flight path); remain informed of aircraft state, destination, and conditions; and communicate (with Air Traffic Control, other aircraft, the airline company [Billings, 1991]). Piloting is also very dynamic, with variable demands on pilot cognitive resources. For example, resource demands may vary with (1) flight phase (takeoffs and landings are generally more demanding than cruise phases); (2) operations (nonroutine operations such as equipment failure are more demanding than routine operations; long haul flights impose different demands than short haul flights); and (3) flight conditions (e.g., bad weather).

Several cognitive processes and structures are required to accomplish these functions. Psychomotor, or "stick and rudder," skills are required to control the aircraft (e.g., using the yoke to maintain heading and altitude). This function also involves visual perception (e.g., scanning instruments or searching for other air traffic) and auditory perception (e.g., listening to the engine or to the radio for Air Traffic Control [ATC] messages). Because pilots continually perform multiple tasks, they must time share and schedule these tasks (e.g., talking to Air Traffic Control while scanning instruments). Therefore, piloting requires the ability to divide or switch attention among multiple tasks, and the ability to focus attention on a single task while ignoring irrelevant information.

Working memory is also essential. Pilots often need to temporarily store verbal (e.g., ATC clearance) and spatial (traffic location) information. Working memory involves processing as well as storage, with information encoded into long-term memory (Baddeley, 1986; Daneman & Carpenter, 1980). It is also involved in integrating information from instruments, ATC communication and other sources to update a mental model of current and anticipated flight conditions (Wickens & Flach, 1988). The mental model supports monitoring and planning (Sarter & Woods, 1991). Thus, working memory capacity is essential to pilot communication and decision making. Several studies have examined how age-related declines in working memory capacity constrain this component of flying (see the Pilot Communication section). Prospective memory, remembering to perform actions at the appropriate time, is also important; pilots must remember to set flaps or contact ATC at the appropriate time. Pilots manage memory demands in part by relying on checklists, manuals, and displays. Thus, pilot expertise involves knowing what information is available in the cockpit (Kirlik, 1995).

Finally, piloting involves social or collaborative processes. Commercial pilots are usually members of a crew, and flying requires effective crew coordination and communication (e.g., Kanki, Lozito, & Foushee, 1989; Linde, 1988).

The relative importance of these components is changing as flying becomes more automated. Pilots increasingly interact with computerized flight management systems that automate many of the aircraft control functions and assist in monitoring aircraft conditions. Thus, automation shifts pilot workload from the psychomotor processes involved in aircraft control to more cognitively demanding components such as decision making and information management. Collaboration has also become more important because crew members must often coordinate their efforts to use automated systems (Billings, 1991).

This description of piloting provides a framework for reviewing the aging and pilot performance literature. We first examine how age and experience influence overall pilot performance and then focus on the impact of these factors on components of piloting, from more domain-general perceptual, attentional, and memory abilities involved in pilot performance to tasks such as communication and decision making, which involve knowledge-based as well as domain-independent cognitive processes. To better understand this research, we take a brief detour to consider several methodological issues.

Methodological Issues

Measuring Pilot Performance

Pilot performance can be measured in a variety of ways. Accident rates are most directly related to flight safety. While it is fortunate that accidents are rare events, this also limits their value as a measure of performance. Such low base-rate events are unlikely to be a sensitive index of age differences in performance because subtle aging effects may not be manifested in accidents. Flight incidents (e.g., deviation from assigned altitude) are more frequent than accidents and thus may be more informative (e.g., Billings & Cheaney, 1981), but pilot age is often not included in incident databases. Observer ratings of performance during actual or simulated flight is another common measure. Indeed, the FAA typically assesses pilot proficiency in this way. However, observer ratings may be influenced by unconscious biases related to age or other factors. Studies of age in the workplace sometimes find that age is negatively related to supervisor ratings but is not related to more objective measures such as production records (see Sparrow & Davies, 1988, for a review). Another limitation of both accident rate and observer rating measures is that they provide little information about which cognitive processes are influenced by age and under what conditions.

Laboratory tasks that tap cognitive processes related to piloting enable precise measurement under controlled conditions. While age differences on such tasks are assumed to reflect age differences in piloting (e.g., Glanzer & Glaser, 1959; Szafran, 1969), these tasks may underestimate expertise effects on performance, perhaps by precluding knowledge-based strategies that compensate for age declines on components of piloting (e.g., Morrow, Leirer, Altieri, & Fitzsimmons, 1994).

High-fidelity aircraft simulators allow researchers to quantify pilot performance under both realistic and controlled conditions. Simulators are used by many airlines for line-oriented flight training (LOFT), which involves realistic, complex scenarios (Kanki et al., 1989). While simulator studies have traditionally relied on expert ratings of crew performance, researchers are beginning to take advantage of computerized recording and analysis of simulator performance output to provide more precise, quantitative measures (e.g., Hyland, 1993; Leirer, Yesavage, & Morrow, 1989; Ross & Mundt, 1988).

Pilot expertise is also measured in different ways. The most common measure is hours of flying, either total accumulated hours, recent hours (e.g., in the last year), or hours in particular aircraft types. This is a fairly coarse measure because amount of experience is only loosely related to expertise (Charness, 1991). Some aspects of expertise have also been measured more directly, for example by exploring domain-relevant knowledge structures (e.g., Schvaneveldt et al., 1985). However, these measures have not been related to pilot performance.

Assessing Age Differences in Pilot Performance

Cross-sectional designs are most commonly used to assess age differences in pilot performance. This design, which involves comparing two or more age groups at the same point in time, requires matching the groups on relevant factors such as cognitive ability and pilot experience (e.g., hours of flying). Equating older and younger pilot groups on experience is difficult because older pilots tend to be more experienced. In addition, the expertise literature suggests that the type as well as amount of experience is important to consider. It is especially difficult to match age groups on type of flying experience because the aviation industry changes over time, so that older pilots may have had different educational, training, and flying experience when they were younger. Such cohort effects may be minimized if both older and younger pilots have high levels of similar recent flying experience. However, this strategy is impossible when comparing commercial pilots over age 60 to younger pilots. Because these older pilots are retired from commercial operations, they are unlikely to have similar recent experience. Yet, restricting the older pilot group to those under age 60 may attenuate age effects.

Pilot age can also be assessed by longitudinal studies, where the same pilots are repeatedly tested over time. While this design has its own difficulties, longitudinal comparisons with different cohorts allow assessment of performance changes related to age, uncontaminated by cohort effects

(Schaie, 1988). Longitudinal designs have rarely been used in pilot aging research (but see Kay et al., 1993).

A final point relates to integrating findings in these studies. We will see that different studies focus on different types of pilots, such as military, commercial, and general aviation pilots. Variation in pilot experience across studies complicate direct comparisons of age effects in these studies.

The Influence of Age and Experience on Global Measures of Pilot Performance

Despite problems with global measures of pilot performance such as accident rates, these measures provide an initial picture of the influence of pilot age and experience on overall performance. Kay et al. (1993) analyzed records from the Federal Aviation Administration and the National Transportation Safety Board databases to compare accident rates for pilots of different ages, experience levels, and medical certificates. Cross-sectional and longitudinal comparisons revealed a modest decrease in accident rates with age (from 30–34) that leveled off for pilots in their 50s (the pattern was similar across medical certificate classes). There was a trend for accident rates to increase after age 63 for Class II and Class III pilots (most Class I pilots are eliminated after age 60 because of the retirement rule). The trend for accidents to decrease through the 40s and 50s may reflect the effects of increased flying experience because older pilots tend to accumulate more flying hours. However, this trend may also reflect the effects of selection over time—older groups may have a greater proportion of high-ability pilots.

Greater recent flying experience was also associated with lower accident rates and was more predictive than pilot age. Level of recent experience was also more important than total flying hours, suggesting the importance of the type as well as amount of flying experience.

Pilot age may also be associated with different kinds of errors, reflecting different types of limitations. Eyraud and Borowsky (1985) compared incident rates for naval fighter and helicopter pilots from age 22 to 40+. The youngest fighter pilots were involved in more incidents than the older groups, and the mishaps often related to controlling the aircraft. Incidents for older pilots more frequently related to poor judgment and violation of regulations. Younger pilot errors may reflect lack of skill in controlling aircraft, while older pilot errors may reflect forgetting or failure to maintain awareness of flight conditions. However, any conclusions are limited by a restricted age range (only 8% of pilots were over age 40) and the fact that older pilots had more experience. More generally, analyses of accident rates provide scant information about the specific pilot and operational conditions related to performance. For example, we do not know if the older and younger pilots flew different kinds of missions.

Other global measures include ratings by expert observers. Cobb (1968) examined supervisor and peer ratings of air traffic controllers, who, like pilots, perform in a multitask environment involving a range of cognitive skills. Analysis of ratings for 568 center controllers found small but significant negative correlations between age and observer ratings, with no significant correlations between ratings and experience. Like the previous studies, this study had a restricted age range (max age = 50). In a study of commercial pilots flying a 727 simulator, Hyland (1993) found that age was associated with lower expert ratings of global performance, but was not related to a more objective system of scoring deviation from ideal performance. Like the research on aging and work performance (e.g., Sparrow & Davies, 1988), this finding suggests the possibility of age-related bias in observer ratings in pilot and aging studies. We will see that objective scoring of simulator performance tends to find few age differences except under demanding task conditions (see the Pilot Communication section).

Summary

Studies that investigate overall pilot performances suggest that age is associated with safer flying through midadulthood, with decreasing margins of safety for pilots in their later 60s and 70s. This pattern suggests either that increasing experience mitigates age declines in component processes, or that pilot selection (e.g., through FAA proficiency checks) has changed the composition of older groups. The studies also hint at the possibility that age effects depend on level of pilot experience, particularly recent flying experience. However, these studies use global measures of performance and provide little direct information about which aspects of piloting are influenced by age and experience and under what conditions. For a more fine-grained picture, we turn to laboratory and simulator studies of pilot performance and aging.

The Influence of Aging and Experience on Components of Piloting

Pilot Domain Knowledge

Aging and expertise research suggests that experience is more likely to mitigate age declines for more knowledge-based tasks. This prediction assumes that older pilots have roughly the same knowledge as younger pilots, which offsets declining cognitive resources. This assumption seems reasonable, considering the finding of minimal age differences in general knowledge structures such as scripts (e.g., Arbuckle, Vanderleck, Harsany, &

Lapidus, 1990). However, few studies have examined age differences in aviation knowledge. Obviously, domain knowledge is necessary for flying at any age. In fact, knowledge-based measures, such as the ability to match a sequence of ATC messages to the correct flight situation, is a better predictor of simulator performance than domain-independent tasks (Stokes, Belger, & Zhang, 1990; but see Hyland, 1993). Hyland (1993) found age differences in the ATC message task mentioned previously, perhaps because the task required active processing of domain knowledge that taxed older pilots' cognitive resources (cf. Arbuckle et al., 1990). Similarly, Glanzer and Glaser (1959) found older pilots were less able to identify aircraft position from a compass and artificial horizon, which requires ability to integrate domain-relevant information in working memory. On the other hand, Morrow, Leirer et al. (1994) found some evidence that expertise reduced age differences among commercial pilots for ATC tasks that are similar to actual piloting (see the Pilot Communication section). These age differences also contrast with more substantial and qualitative effects of pilot expertise on knowledge structures (e.g., Schvaneveldt et al., 1985). Hence, there is little evidence that older and younger pilots differ on direct measures of expertise, although this conclusion is qualified by limited research. The following sections examine if and when this expertise reduces age differences in pilot performance.

Perceptual and Psychomotor Processing

Pilots continually process visual and auditory information to monitor flight conditions, control the aircraft, and communicate. While relationships between age declines in pilot perceptual abilities and flying accidents have not been documented, such relationships have been found for driving (Institute of Medicine, 1981). Age-related changes in peripheral sensory systems occur for pilots as well as nonpilots. For example, age-related declines in lens accommodation reduce acuity in the general population (Corso, 1987). Szafran (1969) also found small but significant correlations between age and ability to accommodate and adapt to dark among pilots, but argued that these modest relationships are operationally negligible. However, this study had a restricted age range and involved domain-general tasks.

Age also influences the ability to process visual information in complex tasks such as driving (Ball & Owsley, 1991). Glanzer and Glaser (1959) tested Air National Guard pilots and commercial pilots between the ages of 20 and 50 on a range of laboratory tasks. Pilot age correlated .29 with accuracy of identifying masked objects, and .10 with performance on mental rotation tasks. Braune and Wickens (1984), using instrument-rated pilots (20–60 years), found older pilots were slower to perform the hidden figures task.

Because piloting often demands rapid responses, researchers have focused on how pilot age influences perceptual speed tasks. Studies with nonpilots find age differences increase for more complex reaction time (RT) tasks such as choice vs. simple RT (Welford, 1958). A similar pattern occurs for pilots. In a study of 560 civil air pilots, Spieth (1964) found age correlated with choice RT despite a restricted age range. Szafran (1969) varied the number of alternatives in a choice reaction time task and whether the task was performed alone or concurrently with a short-term memory task. Age declines occurred only in the more difficult concurrent condition.

Tracking tasks, a common measure of age differences in psychomotor skills, presumably tap control abilities necessary for flying or driving. In fact, psychomotor skill correlates with driving performance (Barrett, Mihal, Panek, Sterns, & Alexander, 1977). Hours of flying experience may be more important than age for predicting tracking performance (Braune & Wickens, 1984), while age effects occur for nonpilots on the same task (Braune & Wickens, 1985). However, Mertens, Higgins, and McKenzie (1983) found that age decrements in tracking increased with workload level.

Variable relations between age and experience across studies may reflect task factors. As predicted by resource deficit models of cognitive aging, age differences in these perceptual studies were more likely to occur as task difficulty increased. The domain relevance of the task may also be important. Most of the studies reviewed in the present section used domain-independent laboratory tasks. However, moderating effects of pilot experience on age effects are more likely to occur for domain-relevant tasks, which may trigger highly practiced skills that circumvent age declines in cognitive resources (Bosman & Charness, 1996). Support for this explanation comes from several studies that find few effects of pilot age on perceptual tasks such as time to detect equipment failures or aircraft targets, which were embedded in realistic simulator scenarios (Morrow, Yesavage, Leirer, & Tinklenberg, 1993; Taylor, Dohlert, Morrow, Friedman, & Yesavage, 1994). Age also had little effect on the ability to control the aircraft in these studies, except under high workload conditions such as an approach with turbulence and crosswind (Leirer et al., 1989; Morrow, Leirer, & Yesavage, 1990). These studies involved primarily general aviation pilots and may underestimate expertise effects on performance.

Attentional Processing

Piloting is also highly dependent on the ability to allocate attention across multiple tasks such as monitoring, communicating, and decision making (Roscoe, 1980; Wickens & Flach, 1988). Indeed, the ability to divide attention may be an important predictor of pilot training success (Gopher, Well, & Bareket, 1994). According to resource deficit theories of aging, older pilots should have particular trouble dividing attention as task complexity increases. Research on aging and divided attention in the general population presents a complex picture, but suggests that older adults are less able to perform multiple tasks when the component tasks are complex (e.g., Ponds, Brouwer, & van Wolffelaar, 1988; Salthouse, Rogan, & Prill, 1984). Older adults may have particular difficulty switching attention between visual and auditory tasks, a frequent requirement of piloting (Stine, Wingfield, & Meyers, 1990). However, Braune and Wickens (1985) found no evidence for age differences in time-sharing ability. While little research has examined the impact of age on pilots' ability to divide attention, one study compared pilots and nonpilots and found age declines in time-sharing efficiency (measured by dual task decrement) and resource allocation (shifting priority when instructed) for both groups (Tsang & Shaner, 1994). Notably, pilot expertise reduced, but did not eliminate, age differences.

Aging also appears to reduce the ability to focus attention and ignore irrelevant information. For example, older adults are more susceptible to irrelevant information in visual research (Plude & Hoyer, 1985). Older (nonpilot) adults are less able to focus attention in dichotic listening tasks (Braune & Wickens, 1985). However, research on expertise in nonaviation domains suggests that expertise facilitates focal as well as divided attention. For example, expertise (experience interpreting gram stains) reduces age differences in visual search accuracy among medical technologists, primarily when the context is familiar (Clancy & Hoyer, 1994). In the aviation domain, Glanzer and Glaser (1959) found that age reduced the ability to ignore irrelevant information in visual tasks, suggesting that age reduces the ability to focus attention among pilots as well as nonpilots.

In summary, age differences tend to occur for difficult divided attention tasks among pilots as well as nonpilots, as predicted by resource deficit models. Age-related difficulty with ignoring irrelevant information among pilots is consistent with inhibition failure accounts of aging (McDowd & Birren, 1990). More positively, the few studies of expertise and attention suggest that experience may help maintain attentional skills among pilots, at least for familiar tasks. Thus, expertise may help mitigate age declines even for "lower level" components of piloting that primarily involve perception and attention. This finding is consistent with expertise models that emphasize perceptual cues (e.g., Kirlik, 1995). The impact of pilot age and experience level on divided and focused attention should be investigated during simulated flight while varying opportunity for knowledge-based strategies (e.g., task familiarity).

Working Memory

Working memory is a fundamental constraint on information processing—it serves as a temporary store (remembering a frequency until it is dialed on the radio) and as a workspace where information is encoded for long-term memory (Baddeley, 1986). Working memory capacity should also constrain pilot performance (Wickens & Flach, 1988). In the present section, we review studies of pilot age and expertise effects on temporary storage of information in working memory and on long-term memory for domain-relevant information.

Research on aging and memory in the general population finds few age differences in short-term storage, although differences tend to arise when information must be simultaneously processed and stored (Poon, 1985). One measure of the ability to simultaneously store and process information in working memory is the sentence span task (Daneman & Carpenter, 1980). Older adults typically have smaller sentence spans than younger adults, indicating age declines in working memory capacity (Stine & Wingfield, 1990). Such declines are true of pilots as well as nonpilots, even for aviation-related span materials (Morrow, Leirer, & Altieri, 1992). This suggests that expertise does not reduce age differences in working memory capacity, at least as it is measured by laboratory tasks that assess short-term storage.

According to models of text processing, working memory is a critical constraint on the ability to encode and retrieve information from long-term memory. Age differences in working memory capacity (measured by sentence span) help explain age differences in text recall (see Stine et al., 1996, for a review). In the aviation domain, age also appears to limit pilots' ability to recall aviation information, perhaps because of declining working memory capacity. Glanzer and Glaser (1959) found small but significant correlations between pilot age and recall for a briefing about new aviation-related equipment and procedures. Morrow et al. (1992) found that pilots were better than nonpilots at understanding and remembering aviation-related narratives, but expertise did not reduce age differences. The finding that expertise did not reduce age differences may reflect the fact that the narrative recall task was not directly related to piloting and thus did not support knowledge use among older pilots (see the Pilot Communication section).

Piloting also depends on the ability to integrate information from multiple sources into a mental model of the flight conditions (Sarter & Woods, 1991). Because integration is limited by working memory capacity (Wickens & Flach, 1988), age-related differences in working memory might impair the ability to update a mental model from ATC messages (producing pilot communication problems) or the ability to use the mental model to support situation awareness and decision making. On the other hand, domain expertise may facilitate the process of updating mental models—experts are adept at creating mental models from text, and expertise sometimes reduces age differences in comprehension (see Morrow, Leirer et al., 1994, for a review). We next consider the influence of pilot age and expertise on pilot communication and decision making.

Pilot Communication

Commercial pilots communicate with air traffic controllers before, during, and after the flight. In the current ATC environment, pilots and controllers communicate by radio, which requires the perceptual, attentional, and memory processes described previously. It is an often demanding task—words must be recognized and grammatical structure parsed and this linguistic information must be integrated with contextual information (e.g., from flight instruments). Moreover, pilots often perform other tasks while communicating. Therefore, it is not surprising that pilots and controllers occasionally miscommunicate. Communication problems are a factor in the majority of safety incidents (Billings & Cheaney, 1981) as well as many accidents (Cushing, 1994). Pilots and controllers use several collaborative strategies to guard against miscommunication. For example, pilots repeat, or "read back," ATC clearances to controllers, giving them the opportunity to check that the pilot correctly understood the message (Morrow & Rodvold, in press).

Problems tend to arise when ATC communication overloads pilot memory, suggesting that age-related declines in working memory contribute to miscommunication. First, longer ATC messages (i.e., more commands per message) increase the frequency of incorrect or partial readbacks. Analysis of these readback errors suggest that multiple commands in the same message increase interference in working memory (Cardosi, 1993; Morrow & Rodvold, in press; Taylor, Yesavage, Morrow, Dolhert, & Poon, 1994). Second, rapidly presented ATC messages appear to increase memory demands. High speech rates by controllers, or "speedfeed," is cited as a factor in incident reports (Billings & Cheaney, 1981), and it increased readback errors in one study in which pilots responded to ATC messages while flying a simulator (Taylor, Yesavage, et al., 1994).

A third piece of evidence that communication problems reflect working memory demands relates to the modality by which ATC messages are delivered. Communication problems in the current radio environment (among other reasons) have prompted plans to introduce a computer data link between air and ground (Kerns, 1994). Data link provides a more permanent print medium for ATC messages because pilots will read messages on a computer screen, thereby reducing memory load. Studies of prototype data link systems suggest that longer ATC messages do not increase communication problems when presented visually rather than auditorially. However, new problems may arise. Short intervals between two successive ATC messages slow pilot response to the messages in both data link and radio environments, in part because pilots do not have time to respond to one message before the next is presented. Moreover, this message interval effect is magnified when a voice message follows a data link message (such "mixed," voice and data link, environments are likely to occur when the data link is introduced into the ATC system), perhaps because pilots have difficulty rapidly switching attention between auditory and visual modalities (Morrow, Rodvold, McGann, & Mackintosh, 1994).

Older pilots may be especially vulnerable to complex ATC communication because of declining cognitive resources. Age differences in pilot communication have been examined by several studies involving noncommercial pilots flying a light aircraft simulator. Pilots in these studies flew scenarios involving ATC messages to change heading, altitude, and radio frequencies. Older pilots made more message readback and execution errors than younger pilots, but there were few age differences in performing routine maneuvers such as takeoff and landing (Morrow et al., 1990; Morrow, Yesavage, Leirer, & Tinklenberg, 1993). Both older and younger pilot performance on the communication and routine flying tasks improved with practice, although practice did not reduce age differences in performance (Morrow, Yesavage, Leirer, & Tinklenberg, 1993). Similarly, laboratory research finds little evidence that practice reduces age differences among nonpilots (see Salthouse, 1990, for a review). Finally, Morrow et al. (1990) found age declines for pilots in their 30s and 40s (also see Leirer et al., 1989).

The finding that age influenced communication tasks more than routine maneuvers, like the laboratory studies of perception and attention described earlier, suggests that age differences increase for more difficult tasks. To directly test this prediction, Taylor, Yesavage et al. (1994) examined if longer and more rapidly presented messages increase age differences in communication errors. Readback and execution errors increased in response to longer and faster messages, but age differences did not increase. The absence of an age by message complexity interaction may reflect methodological difficulties (e.g., floor effects for older pilots). It is also possible that the older pilots drew on knowledge of ATC message organization to offset the increased demands of the longer, more rapidly presented messages. This possibility is supported by more general studies of aging and memory for spoken discourse, which find that rapid speech only differentially penalizes older adults for discourse without normal prosodic and semantic structure. Thus, older adults take advantage of prosodic and semantic context to circumvent demands on their limited cognitive resources (Wingfield & Stine, 1991).

These pilot communication studies provide little direct evidence that expertise mitigates age declines. However, they may underestimate expertise effects because they involved noncommercial pilots. Commercial airline pilots, on the other hand, routinely talk with controllers and are more likely to develop schemas that represent regularities in how ATC messages are organized and presented. Morrow, Leirer et al. (1994) compared older and younger commercial pilots to older and younger nonpilots on several tasks varying in similarity to actual piloting. Expertise was expected to reduce age differences for tasks directly related to piloting because these tasks should support older pilots' use of domain knowledge (see the Aging and Expertise section). Participants listened to a set of ATC messages that described a route through the airspace around an airport. They read back the commands after each message and then recalled the route after the entire set of messages. The readback task is domain-relevant because it is a routine ATC procedure, but the recall procedure is not typically part of piloting. Expertise reduced age differences on some components of the readback task. While expertise also improved recall of the route, it did not reduce age differences. A similar pattern occurred for recall of aviation-related narratives (Morrow et al., 1992).

These findings suggest that domain-relevant tasks, with materials and procedures that are compatible with expert schemas, support knowledge-based strategies that compensate for age declines in cognitive resources. These strategies might reduce processing demands by streamlining recognition, parsing, inferencing, or other components of ATC message comprehension. However, the Morrow, Leier et al. (1994) study did not rule out the possibility that older pilots maintain communication skills because of years of practice, so that age differences are reduced by maintenance rather than compensatory mechanisms. This study may also have underestimated expertise effects. Because the older pilots were retired from commercial flying, they differed from the younger pilots in recent commercial flying experience. The study also used a single-pilot scenario and was unable to examine collaboration among crew members, which may be an important source of compensation. We next turn to this aspect of pilot performance.

Crew Communication

Crew communication and coordination is essential to flying many commercial aircraft. Effective crews appear to have distinctive communication patterns such as explicit responses to questions and commands (Kanki et al., 1989), and miscommunication among crew members has been implicated in several accidents (Linde, 1988). Communication may become even more important in the future because automation requires joint information management and decision making (Billings, 1991). While there are no studies of aging and crew communication, other research points to collaborative strategies as a source of compensation for age-related declines in cognitive resources. For example, typical age differences in narrative recall occur for pairs of unrelated adults but not for married couples (Dixon, 1996). This finding suggests that the common ground provided by prior interaction supports collaborative strategies that mitigate age declines in the cognitive resources necessary for recall. Even though changing crew composition may limit opportunity for such common ground among airline crews, collaborative strategies such as explicit acknowledgments may still support compensation.

Decision Making

Pilots continually make decisions that involve assessing dynamic or uncertain situations and choosing a course of action (Wickens & Flach, 1988). Poor decision making may be a factor in many accidents and incidents (Jensen & Benel, 1977). There are several reasons why pilot age may have little influence on decision making. First, decision making in familiar situations may not be highly resource consuming for experts because they rely on schemas to quickly recognize situations and evaluate alternatives (e.g., Klein, Orasanu, Calderwood, & Zsambok, 1993). Second, experts often rely more on environmental cues than on memory to make decisions, which can minimize highly resource-consuming strategies (Kirlik, 1995). Finally, collaborative strategies may support crew decision making. For example, captains of more effective crews tend to be more proactive, "keeping ahead of the aircraft" and allowing more time for planning and decision making (Klein et al., 1993). Proactive planning may help compensate for age declines in the cognitive resources needed for assessing and selecting a course of action by providing more time. To sum up, decision making in familiar circumstances may not be impaired by pilot age.

On the other hand, pilots also make decisions about uncertain, unfamiliar, and highly dynamic situations, requiring them to maintain an accurate mental model of the flight situation (Sarter & Woods, 1991). Age declines in cognitive resources are more likely to influence decision making in such situations, although expertise may still mitigate age declines under these circumstances—Stokes et al. (1990) found that stress influenced decision-making strategies for low- but not high-experience pilots. Therefore, as we have seen in several areas of pilot research, age and expertise effects depend on task and situational factors. Unfortunately, there are few studies of pilot age and decision making. Mohler (1981) describes several incidents where older pilots avoided accidents or minimized their consequences by rapid decision making. Szafran (1969) found no evidence that age influenced performance on a laboratory decision-making task. However, research has not systematically investigated the influence of pilot age on individual and crew decision making in situations varying in familiarity and complexity.

Summary of Aging and Pilot Performance Research

Studies of age and experience effects on components of pilot performance suggest that age is more likely to impair perception, attention, and working memory processes as task complexity increases. Age effects also influence pilot communication when the task loads working memory. On the other hand, expertise may reduce age differences for familiar, domain-relevant tasks. Such tasks may either support knowledge-based strategies that compensate for older pilots' declining resources or trigger highly practiced skills that are maintained into later adulthood.

Other Factors That Mediate Age Effects in Pilot Performance

Age effects in pilot performance may depend on several factors in addition to expertise. This final section briefly mentions several factors related to pilots and environmental conditions.

Health and Fitness

Health status predicts improved performance on memory and other cognitive tasks among older adults in the general population (Hultsch, Hammer, & Small, 1993), although age remains a factor when health status is controlled (Earles & Salthouse, 1995). Health status also influences pilot performance. For example, Szafran (1966) found that cardiopulmonary status was more important than pilot age for predicting performance on laboratory tasks (also see Spieth, 1964). However, health is less likely to be a limiting factor among pilots than in the general population because pilots are continually screened for medical problems and are generally in better health (Gerathewohl, 1977). For example, rates of sudden incapacitation during flight are very low for pilots in their 50s and 60s, and do not increase with age (Booze, 1989). Health status also does not explain all age-related declines in pilot performance. For example, several studies find age differences on difficult piloting tasks even when age groups do not differ in self-reported health (Morrow, Leire et al., 1994; Morrow, Yesavage, Leirer, & Tinklenberg, 1993).

Level of aerobic fitness and amount of exercise also improves performance on a range of laboratory tasks among older adults in the general population (Clarkson-Smith & Hartley, 1990). Thus, good health and regular exercise may be important for maintaining skills among older pilots, although it is unclear to what extent these factors attenuate age differences in complex task performance.

More generally, a range of factors tend to predict relatively high levels of cognitive function in late adulthood, including education level, active engagement in daily tasks, and social support (e.g., Baltes & Baltes, 1990). These "successful aging" factors may particularly characterize older commercial pilots and help mitigate age declines (Mohler, 1981; Tsang, 1989).

Fatigue

While health, fitness, and other pilot factors may reduce the chance of age-related impairment in pilot performance, some flying conditions may increase this possibility. Older pilots may be more susceptible to flight conditions that produce fatigue (Gerathewohl, 1977). For example, older pilots tend to lose more sleep during long flights, which may interfere with circadian rhythms (Gander, De Nguyen, Rosekind, & Connell, 1993). However, conditions that produce fatigue do not always increase age differences in performance. Mertens and Collins (1986) found that sleep deprivation equally impaired older and younger subject performance on a battery of laboratory tasks. Fatigue may increase susceptibility to distraction (Broadbent, 1953), which might differentially impair older pilots because of an age-related inhibition failure. It may particularly disrupt newly learned tasks.

Stress

Environmental sources of acute stress such as noise and temperature reduce working memory capacity necessary for pilot decision making (Wickens, 1992) and thus may differentially penalize older pilots with reduced working memory capacity. On the other hand, pilot experience may minimize effects of stress on decision making (Stokes et al., 1990). Acute stress may differentially tax older pilots because they have trouble inhibiting task-irrelevant events. Indeed, this might be one cause of age by task complexity interactions found in pilot as well as nonpilot studies. However, we have found no studies that examine how pilots of different ages and experience levels respond to sources of stress.

Drugs

Intoxication from alcohol or other drugs influences flying as well as other types of complex task performance. While age appears to selectively impair pilot performance, acute alcohol intoxication has pervasive effects on piloting components, which may last as long as 8–14 hours after drinking (Morrow et al., 1990; Morrow, Yesavage, Leirer, Dolhert et al., 1993; Ross & Mundt, 1988; Taylor, Dolhert et al., 1994). However, evidence for interactive effects of age and alcohol are mixed (e.g., Taylor, Dolhert et al., 1994). Older and younger pilot performance is similarly impaired by marijuana intoxication (Leirer et al., 1989).

CONCLUSIONS

We began this chapter by asking when age is likely to influence pilot performance and how age decrements can be minimized. It is difficult to draw specific conclusions from aging and pilot performance research because task complexity is defined differently across studies. Similarly, pilot experience varies across studies, with some studies involving general aviation pilots, others focusing on commercial airline pilots. Despite such limitations, the pattern of findings provides partial answers to our questions and supports several general predictions from cognitive aging and expertise theories. We summarize these findings and then mention several implications for design and training interventions. Finally, we outline topics and methods for future research.

When Is Aging Likely to Influence Piloting?

Both slowing and reduced working memory capacity theories of aging (Salthouse, 1991b) suggest that age decrements are more likely to occur for more complex piloting tasks. For the most part, this general prediction is supported by pilot aging research. Both laboratory and simulator studies show that age differences tend to occur when pilots must consider more alternatives in choice RT tasks and under concurrent memory load (Szafran, 1969), when attention is shared across several tasks (Mertens & Collins, 1986; Tsang & Shaner, 1994) and when they respond to complex ATC messages (e.g., Taylor, Yesavage et al., 1994). Inhibition failure theory (e.g., Hasher & Zacks, 1988) suggests that age differences also occur when pilots must ignore irrelevant information. While aviation research has not focused on this prediction, it receives some support (Glanzer & Glaser, 1959). Cognitive aging theories also predict that age is more likely to influence pilot performance when fatigue or stress diminishes the cognitive resources necessary for piloting, but little research has examined this issue.

Pilot expertise, on the other hand, can reduce age differences for familiar and relevant tasks, either by enabling compensatory strategies or by maintaining skilled performance (e.g., Morrow, Leirer et al., 1994). Pilot experience may also mitigate the effects of flight conditions such as stress (Stokes et al., 1990).

Minimizing Age Effects in Pilot Performance

Cognitive aging theories and existing research on aging and pilot performance have several implications for reducing pilot age decrements, either by modifying the environment through design or by influencing pilots through training.

Design

Resource deficit theories emphasize the importance of reducing task difficulty, for example, by providing environmental support. Careful design of cockpit displays and crew procedures should benefit all pilots, particularly older pilots.

Displays

Several principles of aircraft display design may help support older pilot performance. First, flight displays are often more effective when task-related information is perceptually integrated (Wickens & Andre, 1990). For example, compared to voice presentation, graphic weather displays may reduce inferencing required to integrate weather and aircraft route information (Kerns, 1994). Such displays may particularly benefit older pilots by reducing storage and computing demands on working memory.

Second, displays should take advantage of pilot expertise (see the Expertise and Environmental Support section). Roske-Hofstrand and Paap (1985) found that pilots more quickly programmed the control display unit (CDU) of a prototype flight management system when the CDU menu matched pilot preferences for organizing the system (also see Vicente, 1992). Such displays may reduce age-related performance decrements by supporting knowledge-based compensatory strategies.

Third, displays should be concise. The inhibition failure theory suggests that older pilots will be penalized if displays are cluttered with information not directly relevant to the task. Thus, concern about flight deck distraction is particularly relevant to older pilots. The same concerns holds for auditory stimuli. For example, new warning systems with voice messages may compete with ongoing ATC and crew communication for attention.

ATC Communication Procedures

Problems in controller–pilot communication suggest a breakdown in collaboration—controllers may minimize their own workload by rapidly delivering long messages, which load pilot working memory (Morrow, Rodvold et al., 1994). Collaboration may be improved if controllers present shorter messages with enough time between successive messages to avoid time pressure on pilots. Routine, explicit acknowledgments also support collaboration between controllers and pilots (Morrow & Rodvold, in press). These communication procedures may benefit particularly older pilots by minimizing working memory demands. For the same reason, visual data link communication between air and ground may differentially benefit older pilots. However, benefits will depend on appropriate implementation of this new technology. For example, a keystroke-based interface might penalize older pilots—older adults learn word processing applications more slowly when the interface is keystroke based rather than menu based, presumably because the keystroke system imposes greater memory demands (Kelly, Charness, Mottram, & Bosman, 1994). Data link systems might also complicate communication procedures. In one study, communication problems associated with voice ATC messages were more frequent when these messages followed data link messages compared to a condition with only voice messages, perhaps reflecting difficulty switching attention between auditory and visual modalities (Morrow, Rodvold et al., 1994). Mixing data link and voice messages might actually penalize older pilots because of age-related difficulty in switching attention between visual and auditory modalities (Stine et al., 1990). Well-designed procedures and displays are particularly important when older pilots make a transition to new cockpits. For example, it may be helpful to design new interfaces and procedures to be compatible with pilots' knowledge of aircraft systems (Roske-Hofstrand and Paap, 1985).

Training

Age differences in pilot performance may also be reduced by pilot training. Cognitive slowing suggests that older pilots may need more training time than younger pilots to acquire new skills. Research on training older workers shows that older as well as younger adults benefit from training, and sometimes such training reduces age effects (Sparrow & Davies, 1988). Studies of aging and pilot communication also show that older as well as younger pilots benefit from training, although the practice did not reduce age differences (Morrow, Yesavage, Leirer, & Tinklenberg, 1993; Taylor, Yesavage et al., 1994). Training effects for older pilots may be enhanced by well-defined training goals (Park, 1992).

Training, like design-based support, may be particularly important during transitions to new crew positions or new aircraft. If older adults have trouble inhibiting irrelevant information, they may be penalized by training that conflicts with past experience. Declining cognitive resources may also hamper skill acquisition among older adults. For example, Fisk and Rogers (1991) found that older adults have more trouble automatizing newly acquired skills. Therefore, skill acquisition by older pilots may be facilitated if the new skill builds on existing expertise. For example, prior computer experience reduces age differences in learning new computer applications (Kelly et al., 1994).

Future Research

Several important questions about the impact of aging on pilot performance should be addressed by future research. First, when does age begin to influence pilot performance? The accident studies suggest that performance generally improves over time for pilots in their 30s and 40s, while some simulator studies find decrements on demanding tasks for noncommercial pilots in this age group (e.g., Leirer et al., 1989; Morrow et al., 1990).

Second, when does expertise mitigate age differences? For example, flying experience may differentially benefit older commercial pilots during maintenance rather than transition phases of their career (Murphy, 1989). Most important, more focused studies are needed to examine how age and experience tradeoffs depend on task and flight condition factors—benefits of experience are more likely for more relevant, familiar tasks but may be less likely for more complex tasks. Novel tasks may penalize older pilots, particularly when pilots are fatigued.

Third, how does expertise mitigate age-related declines in cognitive resources? Older pilots might use compensatory, maintenance, or accommodative strategies to maintain performance for different tasks or under different conditions (Abraham & Hansson, 1995). It is important to identify when different strategies are used because they might be supported by different design and training interventions.

A research program that addresses these issues requires appropriate performance measures, pilot samples, and experimental designs. It should involve high fidelity simulators with realistic scenarios that systematically manipulate task conditions. Crew as well as individual pilot performance should be assessed by combining simulator performance data with more qualitative analysis of crew procedures and communication. Pilot age and experience level should be varied within the same study, focusing on commercial pilots from 50 to 70 years of age. Airline pilots over age 60 will differ from younger pilots in recent experience because they no longer fly commercially. This problem might be addressed by including older pilots who actively fly commuter or corporate operations (which are not subject to the age 60 rule). Longitudinal as well as cross-sectional comparisons for different age cohorts would provide a more definitive picture of how pilot performance changes over time (for similar proposals, see Hyland, Kay, Deimler, & Gurman, 1994; Institute of Medicine, 1981). A longitudinal design could also provide information about the differential impact of age and experience during transition and maintenance phases of pilot careers. Finally, it is also important to examine tradeoffs between flying experience and age in general aviation (GA), which is a large part of the aviation system. GA operations and conditions also tend to be less predictable than commercial operations and GA pilots are often less highly selected than airline pilots, so that age may have a greater impact on performance.

This research program should produce several general benefits. First, it will help identify conditions that disadvantage older pilots. Second, it will evaluate design and training interventions that may minimize age differences in pilot performance. Third, it will provide a broader empirical foundation for age-related aviation policies. For example, identifying conditions that place older pilots at greater risk for unsafe flight will help develop guidelines related to flight schedules, training requirements, and other pilot activities that encompass pilots of all ages. This information will also help decide if a chronological cutoff should remain the basis for commercial pilot retirement, or if assessment of functional age is feasible. Finally, this type of research will help forge closer links between theoretical accounts of aging and expertise, on the one hand, and training and design interventions, on the other.

Acknowledgment

Preparation of this chapter was supported by NIA grants R01 AGO9254 and R01 AG12163. Address correspondence to Daniel Morrow, Department of Psychology, Conant Hall, University of New Hampshire, Durham, NH 03824.

References

Abernathy, B., Neal, R. J., & Koning, P. (1994). Visual-perceptual and cognitive differences between expert, intermediate, and novice snooker players. *Applied Cognitive Psychology, 8,* 185–212.

Abraham, J. D., & Hansson, R. O. (1995). Successful aging at work: An applied study of selection, optimization, and compensation through impression management. *Journal of Gerontology: Psychological Sciences, 50B,* P94–P103.

Anderson, J. R. (1983). *The architecture of cognition.* Cambridge, MA: Harvard University Press.

Arbuckle, T., Vanderleck, V., Harsany, M., & Lapidus, S. (1990). Adult age differences in memory in relation to availability and accessibility of knowledge-based schemas. *Journal of Experimental Psychology: Learning, Memory, and Cognition, 16,* 305–315.

Backman, L., & Dixon, R. A. (1992). Psychological compensation: A theoretical framework. *Psychological Bulletin, 112,* 259–283.

Baddely A. (1986). *Working memory.* New York: Oxford University Press.

Ball, K., & Owsley, C. (1991). Identifying correlates of accident involvement for the older driver. *Human Factors, 33,* 583–595.

Baltes, P. B., & Baltes, M. M. (1990). *Successful aging: Perspectives from the behavioral sciences.* Cambridge, UK: Cambridge University Press.

Barrett, G. V., Mihal, W. L., Panek, P. E., Sterns, H. L., & Alexander, R. A. (1977). Information processing skills predictive of accident involvement for younger and older commercial drivers. *Industrial Gerontology, 4,* 173–182.

Billings, C. E. (1991). *Human-centered aircraft automation: A concept and guidelines* (NASA Tech. Memor. 103885). Moffett Field, CA: NASA Ames Research Center.

Billings, C. E., & Cheaney, E. (1981). *Information transfer problems in the aviation system* (NASA Tech. Paper 1875). Moffett Field, CA: NASA Ames Research Center.

Booze, C. F. (1989). Sudden inflight incapacitation in general aviation. *Aviation, Space, and Environmental Medicine, 60,* 332–335.

Bosman, E. A., & Charness, N. (1996). Age-related differences in skilled performance and skill acquisition. In F. Blanchard-Fields & T. Hess (Eds.), *Perspectives on cognition in adulthood and aging* (pp. 428–453). New York: McGraw-Hill.

Braune, R., & Wickens, C. D. (1984). *Individual differences and age-related performance assessment in aviators. Part 1: Battery development and assessment* (Final Tech. Rep. EPL-83-4/NAMRL-83-1). Urbana-Champaign: University of Illinois, Engineering-Psychology Laboratory.

Braune, R., & Wickens, C. D. (1985). The functional age profile: An objective decision criterion for the assessment of pilot performance capacities and capabilities. *Human Factors, 27,* 681–693.

Broadbent, D. E. (1953). Neglect of the surroundings in relation to fatigue decrements in output. In W. Floyd & A. Welford (Eds.), *Fatigue* (pp. 173–178). London: Lewis.

Cardosi, K. (1993). *An analysis of en route pilot-controller voice communications.* Washington, DC: U.S. Department of Transportation, Federal Aviation Administration.

Cerella, J., Poon, L. W., & Williams, D. (1980). Age and the complexity hypothesis. In L. W. Poon (Ed.), *Aging in the 1980's* (pp. 332–340). Washington, DC: American Psychological Association.

Charness, N. (1991). Expertise in chess: The balance between knowledge and search. In K. A. Ericsson & J. Smith (Eds.), *Toward a general theory of expertise: Prospects and limits* (pp. 39–63). Cambridge, UK: Cambridge University Press.

Charness, N., & Bosman, E. A. (1995). Compensation through environmental modification. In R. Dixon & L. Backman (Eds.), *Psychological compensation: Managing losses and promoting gains* (pp. 147–168). Mahway, NJ: Erlbaum.

Chase, W., & Simon, H. (1973). Perception in chess. *Cognitive Psychology, 4,* 55–81.

Chi, M., Glaser, R., & Farr, M. J. (1988). *The nature of expertise.* (pp. xv-xxvii). Hillsdale, NJ: Hove & London.

Clancy, S. N., & Hoyer, W. J. (1994). Age and skill in visual search. *Developmental Psychology, 30,* 545–552.

Clarkson-Smith, L., & Hartley, A. A. (1990). Structural equation models of relationships between exercise and cognitive abilities. *Psychology and Aging, 5,* 437–446.

Cobb, B. B. (1968). Relationships among chronological age, length of experience, and job performance ratings of air route traffic control specialists. *Aerospace Medicine, 39,* 119–124.

Cohn, N. B., Dustman, R. E., & Bradford, D. C. (1984). Age-related decrements in Stroop color test performance. *Journal of Clinical Psychology, 40,* 1244–1250.

Corso, J. (1987). Sensory-perceptual processes and aging. In W. Schaie (Ed.), *Annual review of gerontology and geriatrics* (pp. 29–56). New York: Springer.

Craik, F. I. M., & Byrd, M. (1982). Aging and cognitive deficits: The role of attentional resources. In F. I. M. Craik & S. Trehub (Eds.), *Aging and cognitive processes* (pp. 191–211). New York: Plenum.

Craik, F. I. M., & Jennings, J. M. (1992). Aging and memory. In F I. M. Craik & T. A. Salthouse (Eds.), *The handbook of aging and cognition* (pp. 51–110). Hillsdale, NJ: Erlbaum.

Craik, F. I. M., & McDowd, J. (1987). Age differences in recall and recognition. *Journal of Experimental Psychology: Learning, Memory, and Cognition, 13,* 474–479.

Cushing, S. (1994). *Fatal words.* Chicago: University of Chicago Press.

Daneman, M., & Carpenter, P. (1980). Individual differences in working memory and reading. *Journal of Verbal Learning and Verbal Behavior. 19,* 450–466.

Dixon, R. (1996). Collaborative memory and aging. In D. J. Hermann, M. K. Johnson, C. L. McEvoy, C. Hertzog, & P. Hertel (Eds.), *Basic and applied memory: Theory in context* (pp. 359–383). Hillsdale, NJ: Erlbaum.

Earles, J. L., & Salthouse, T. A. (1995). Interrelations of age, health, and speed. *Journal of Gerontology: Psychological Sciences, 50B,* P33–P41.

Ericsson, K. A., & Smith, J. (1991). *Toward a general theory of expertise: Prospects and limits.* Cambridge, UK: Cambridge University Press.

Eyraud, M. Y., & Borowsky, B. S. (1985). Age and pilot performance. *Aviation, Space, and Environmental Medicine, 56,* 553–558.

Fisk, A. D., & Rogers, W. A. (1991). Toward an understanding of age-related memory and visual search effects: Why older adults are deficient in automatic process development. *Journal of Experimental Psychology: General, 120,* 131–149.

Fitts, P. M., & Jones, R. E. (1947). *Analysis of 270 "pilot error" experiences in reading and interpreting aircraft instruments* (Report TSEAA-694-12A). Dayton, OH: Wright-Patterson Air Force Base, Aeromedical Laboratory.

Gander, P. H., De Nguyen, B. E., Rosekind, M. R., & Connell, L. J. (1993). Age, circadian rhythms, and sleep loss in flight crews. *Aviation, Space, and Environmental Medicine, 64,* 189–195.

Gerathewohl, S. J. (1977). *Psychophysiological effects of aging: Developing a functional age index for pilots: I. A survey of the pertinent literature* (Report No. FAA-AM-77-6). Washington, DC: Federal Aviation Administration; Office of Aviation Medicine.

Gilhooly, K. J., Wood, M., Kinnear, P. R., & Green, C. (1988). Skill in map reading and memory for maps. *Quarterly Journal of Experimental Psychology, 40A,* 87–107.

Glanzer, M., & Glaser, R. (1959). Cross-sectional and longitudinal results in a study of age-related changes. *Educational and Psychological Measurement, 19,* 89–101.

Gopher, D., Weil, M., & Bareket, T. (1994). Transfer of skill from a computer game trainer to flight. *Human Factors, 36,* 387–405.

Hasher, L., & Zacks, R. (1988). Working memory, comprehension, and aging: A review and a new view. *Psychology of Learning and Motivation, 22,* 193–225.

Hultsch, D. F., Hammer, M., & Small, B. J. (1993). Age differences in cognitive performance in later life: Relationships to self-reported health and activity life style. *Journal of Gerontology: Psychological Sciences. 48,* P1–P11.

Hutchins, E. (1991). *How a cockpit remembers its speed*(Technical Report). San Diego: University of California, Distributed Cognition Laboratory.

Hyland, D. T. (1993). *Experimental evaluation of aging and pilot performance.* Paper presented at the 7th Symposium on Aviation Psychology, Ohio State University, Columbus.

Hyland, D. T., Kay, E. J., Deimler, J. D., & Gurman, E. B. (1994). *Age 60 study: Part II. Airline pilot age and performance—A review of the scientific literature* (Report No. DOT/FAA/AM-94/21). Washington, DC: U.S. Department of Transportation, Federal Aviation Administration.

Institute of Medicine, National Academy of Sciences. (1981). *Airline pilot age, health, and performance.* Washington, DC: National Academy Press.

Jensen, R. S., & Benel, R. A. (1977). *Judgment evaluation and instruction in civil pilot training* (Final Report FAA-RD-78-24). Springfield, VA: National Technical Information.

Kanki, B. G., Lozito, S., & Foushee, H. C. (1989). Communication indices of crew coordination. *Aviation, Space, and Environmental Medicine. 60,* 56–60.

Kay, E. J., Harris, R. M., Voros, R. S., Hillman, D. J., Hyland, D. T., & Deimler, J. D. (1993). *Age 60 Project: Consolidated database experiments* (Hilton Systems Tech. Rep. 8025-3C (R2). Cherry Hill, NJ: Hilton Systems, Inc.

Kelly, C. L., Charness, N., Mottram, M., & Bosman, E. A. (1994, April). *The effects of cognitive aging and prior computer experience on learning to use a word processor.* Fifth Cognitive Aging Conference, Atlanta, GA.

Kerns, K. (1994). *Human factors in ATC/flight deck integration: Implications of data link simulation research* (Report MP94W0000098). McLean, VA: The Mitre Corporation.

Kirlik, A. (1995). Requirements for psychological models to support design: Towards ecological task analysis. In J. M. Flach, P. A. Hancock, J. K. Caird, & K. J. Vicente (Eds.), *Global perspectives on the ecology of human-machine system* (pp. 68–120). Hillsdale, NJ: Erlbaum.

Klein, G. A., Orasanu, J., Calderwood, R., & Zsambok, C. (1993). *Decision making in action: Models and methods.* Norwood, NJ: Ablex.

Leirer, V. O., Yesavage, J., & Morrow, D. G. (1989). Marijuana, aging, and task difficulty effects on pilot performance. *Aviation, Space, and Environmental Medicine. 60,* 1145–1152.

Linde, C. (1988). The quantitative study of communicative success: Politeness and accidents in aviation discourse. *Language in Society, 17,* 375–399.

Lindenberger, U., Kliegl, R., & Baltes, P. B. (1992). Professional expertise does not eliminate age differences in imagery-based memory performance during adulthood. *Psychology and Aging, 7,* 585–593.

McDowd, J. M., & Birren, J. E. (1990). Aging and attentional processes. In J. E. Birren & K. W. Schaie (Eds.), *Handbook of the psychology of aging* (pp. 222–230). San Diego, CA: Academic Press.

McFarland, R. A. (1953). *Human factors in air transportation.* New York: McGraw-Hill.

Mertens, H. W., & Collins, W. (1986). The effects of age, sleep deprivation, and altitude on complex performance. *Human Factors, 28,* 541–551.

Mertens, H. W., Higgins, E. A., & McKenzie, J. M. (1983). *Age, altitude, and workload effects on complex task performance* (NTIS No. FAA-AM-83-15). Oklahoma City, OK: Federal Aviation Administration, Civil Aeromedical Institute.

Mohler, S. R. (1981). Reasons for eliminating the "Age 60" regulation for airline pilots. *Aviation, Space, and Environmental Medicine. 52,* 455–454.

Morrow, D. G., Leirer, V. O., & Altieri, P. (1992). Aging, expertise, and narrative processing. *Psychology and Aging, 7,* 376–388.

Morrow, D. G., Leirer, V. O., Altieri, P., & Fitzsimmons, C. (1994). When expertise reduces age differences in performance. *Psychology and Aging, 9,* 134–148.

Morrow, D. G., Leirer, V. O., & Yesavage, J. (1990). The effect of alcohol and aging on communication during flight. *Aviation, Space, and Environmental Medicine, 61,* 12–20.

Morrow, D. G., & Rodvold, M. (in press). Issues in Air Traffic Control communication. In M. Smolensky & E. Stein (Eds.), *Human factors in air traffic control.* San Diego, CA: Academic press.

Morrow, D. G., Rodvold, M., McGann, A., & Mackintosh, M. A. (1994). Collaborative strategies in air-ground communication. *Proceedings of the Areotech '94 Conference.* Paper No. 942138.

Morrow, D. G., Yesavage, J., Leirer, V., Dohlert, N., Taylor, J., & Tinklenberg, J. (1993). The time-course of alcohol impairment of general aviation pilot performance in a Frasca 141 simulator. *Aviation, Space, and Environmental Medicine. 64,* 697–705.

Morrow, D. G., Yesavage, J., Leirer, V., & Tinklenberg, J. (1993). Aging and practice effects on piloting tasks. *Experimental Aging Research, 19,* 53–70.

Murphy, K. R. (1989). Is the relationship between cognitive ability and job performance stable over time? *Human Performance, 2,* 183–200.

Park, D. C. (1992). Applied cognitive aging research. In F. I. M. Craik & T. A. Salthouse (Eds.), *The handbook of aging and cognition* (pp. 449–493). Hillsdale, NJ: Erlbaum.

Plude, D. J., & Hoyer, W. J. (1985). Attention and performance: Identifying and localizing age defects. In N. Charness (Ed.), *Aging and human performance* (pp. 97–99). New York: Wiley.

Ponds, R. W., Brouwer, W. H., & van Wolffelaar, P. C. (1988). Age differences in divided attention in a simulated driving task. *Journal of Gerontology: Psychological Sciences, 43,* 151–156.

Poon, L. (1985). Differences in human memory with aging: Nature, causes, and clinical implications. In J. Birren & K. Schaie (Eds.), *Handbook of the psychology of aging (2nd ed., pp. 427–462).* New York: Van Nostrand.

Roscoe, S. (1980). *Aviation psychology.* Ames: Ohio State University Press.

Roske-Hofstrand, R., & Paap, K. (1985). *Cognitive network organization and cockpit automation, 3rd Symposium on Aviation Psychology.* Columbus: Ohio State University.

Ross, L. E., & Mundt, J. C. (1988). Multiattribute modeling analysis of the effects of a low blood alcohol level on pilot performance. *Human Factors, 30,* 293–304.

Rybash, J. M., Hoyer, W. J., & Roodin, P. A. (1986). *Adult cognition and aging.* New York: Pergamon.

Salthouse, T. A. (1984). Effects of age and skill in typing. *Journal of Experimental Psychology, 113,* 345–371.

Salthouse, T. A. (1990). Influence of experience on age differences in cognitive functioning. *Human Factors, 32,* 551–569.

Salthouse, T. A. (1991a). Mediation of adult age differences in cognition by reductions in working memory and speed of processing. *Psychological Science, 2,* 179–183.

Salthouse, T. A. (1991b). *Theoretical perspectives on cognitive aging.* Hillsdale, NJ: Erlbaum.

Salthouse, T. A., Babcock, R., Skovronek, E., Mitchell, D., & Palmon, R. (1990). Age and experience effects in spatial visualization. *Developmental Psychology, 26,* 128–36.

Salthouse, T. A., Rogan, J., & Prill, K. A. (1984). Division of attention: Age differences on a visually presented memory task. *Memory & Cognition, 12,* 613–620.

Sarter, N. R., & Woods, D. D. (1991). Situation awareness: A critical but ill-defined phenomenon. *International Journal of Aviation Psychology, 1,* 45–57.

Schaie, K. W. (1988). Internal validity threats in studies of adult cognitive development. In M. L. Howe & C. J. Brainerd (Eds.), *Cognitive development in adulthood: Progress in cognitive development research* (pp. 241–272). New York: Springer-Verlag.

Schvaneveldt, R. W., Durso, F. T., Goldsmith, T. E., Breen, T. J., Cooke, N. M., Tucker, R. G., & De Maio, J. C. (1985). Measuring the structure of expertise. *International Journal of Man-Machine Studies, 23,* 699–728.

Sparrow, P. R., & Davies, D. R. (1988). Effects of age, training, and job complexity on technical performance. *Psychology and Aging, 3,* 307–314.

Spieth, W. (1964). Cardiovascular health status, age, and psychological performance. *Journal of Gerontology, 19,* 277–284.

Stine, E. A. L. (1995). Aging and the distribution of resources in working memory. In P. Allen & T. Bashore (Eds.), *Age differences in word and language processing* (pp. 171–186). Amsterdam: North-Holland.

Stine, E. A. L., Soederberg, L. M., & Morrow, D. G. (1996). Language and discourse processing through adulthood. In F. Blanchard-Fields & T. Hess (Eds.), *Perspectives on cognition in adulthood and aging* (pp. 255–290). New York: McGraw-Hill.

Stine, E., & Wingfield, A. (1990). The assessment of qualitative age differences in discourse processing. In T. Hess (Ed.), *Aging and cognition: Knowledge organization and utilization* (pp. 33–92). Amsterdam: North-Holland.

Stine, E. A. L., Wingfield, A., & Myers, S. D. (1990). Age differences in processing information from television news: The effects of bisensory augmentation. *Journal of Gerontology: Psychological Sciences, 45,* P1–P8.

Stokes, A. F., Belger, A., & Zhang, K. (1990). *Investigation of factors comprising a model of pilot decision making: Part II. Anxiety and cognitive strategies in expert and novice avia-*

tors (Final Tech. Rep. ARL-90-8/SCEEE-90-2). Dayton, OH: AMRL, Wright-Patterson Air Force Base, Human Engineering Division.

Szafran, J. (1966). Age differences in the rate of gain of information, signal detection strategy, and cardiovascular status among pilots. *Gerontologia, 12,* 6–17.

Szafran, J. (1969). Psychological studies of aging in pilots. *Aerospace Medicine, 40,* 543–553.

Taylor, J., Dolhert, N., Morrow, D., Friedman, L., & Yesavage, J. (1994). Acute and 8-hour effects of alcohol on younger and older pilot's simulator performance. *Aviation, Space, and Environmental Medicine, 65,* 718–725.

Taylor, J., Yesavage, J., Morrow, D., Dolhert, N., & Poon, L. (1994). Effects of information load and speech rate on young and older aircraft pilots' ability to read back and execute Air Traffic Controller instructions. *Journal of Gerontology: Psychological Sciences, 49,* P191–P200.

Transportation Research Board. (1988). *Transportation in an aging society* (Vol. 1: Special Report 218). Washington, DC: National Research Council.

Tsang, P. S. (1989). *A reappraisal of aging and pilot performance.* Presented at the Fifth International Symposium of Aviation Psychology, Columbus, OH.

Tsang, P. S., & Shaner, T. L. (1994, April). *Aging and expertise in time-sharing performance.* Fifth Cognitive Aging Conference, Atlanta, GA.

U.S. General Accounting Office. (1989). *Aviation safety: Information on FAA's Age 60 Rule for pilots.* Washington, DC: GAO/RCED-90-45FS.

Vicente, K. J. (1992). Memory recall in a process recall system: A measure of expertise and display effectiveness. *Memory & Cognition, 20,* 356–373.

Welford, A. (1958). *Ageing and human skill.* Oxford: Oxford University Press.

Wickens, C. D. (1992). *Engineering psychology and human performance* (2nd ed.). New York: Harper Collins.

Wickens, C. D., & Andre, A. D. (1990). Proximity compatibility and information display: Effects of color, space, and objectness. *Human Factors, 32,* 61–77.

Wickens, C. D., & Flach, J. (1988). Information processing. In E. Wiener & D. Nagel (Eds.), *Human factors in aviation* (pp. 111–156). San Diego, CA: Academic Press.

Willis, S. L., & Schaie, K. W. (1986). Training the elderly on the ability factors of spatial orientation and inductive reasoning. *Psychology and Aging, 1,* 239–247.

Wingfield, A., & Stine, E. A. L. (1991). Expert systems in nature: Spoken language processing and adult aging. In J. Sinnott & J. Cavanaugh (Eds.), *Bridging paradigms. Positive development in adulthood and cognitive aging* (pp. 237–258). New York: Praeger.

Chapter 10

Health Care and Rehabilitation

Daryle Gardner-Bonneau
John Gosbee

INTRODUCTION

This chapter, perhaps more than many of the others, takes a process approach to its two title topics. A search of the literature quickly shows a paucity of research studies jointly addressing human factors, aging, and health care or rehabilitation, except in some specific topical areas (e.g., medication adherence, assistive technology), which receive treatment in other chapters within this book. Furthermore, to stress the point, health care, medical systems, and rehabilitation have not received much interest from the human factors profession generally, until recently, as evidenced by the fact that the Medical Systems and Rehabilitation Technical Group of the Human Factors and Ergonomics Society has existed since only 1993.

Much of this chapter, therefore, is devoted to laying out broad-based issues in health care and rehabilitation that require human factors attention, particularly as they apply to the older adult. In so doing, we hope to provide a sufficiently explicit picture of the health care and rehabilitation contexts such that more human factors professionals will feel comfortable exploring the many possibilities that exist for valuable contributions to the field, both in research and applications.

Handbook of Human Factors and the Older Adult

HEALTH CARE

The Nature of the Older Adult Health Care Population

The elderly health care "market" is an increasingly educated group and also an increasingly healthy group (Wiklund, 1992). Nevertheless, of the 30 million Americans 65 or older, 23% are disabled in one or more aspects of self-care. Of those 75 and over, 40% have multiple chronic illnesses or dementia (Lonergan & Krevans, 1991). It is also true that the 85 and over age group, which could be expected to have even higher levels of disabling conditions, is growing at a rate six times that of the general population (Lonergan & Krevans, 1991). However, Soldo and Longino (1988) have noted that even at the age of 84 and over, one-half of those individuals living at home had no substantial loss in carrying out the activities of daily living. Because the population of elderly therefore, is heterogeneous, older adults are often classified as well, moderately impaired, or frail (Regnier & Pynoos, 1987). Between 27% and 51% of the elderly fall into the well category at any given time (Stahl, 1984).

The health care problems in the elderly population are different than those in younger age groups (Wiklund, 1992). Even among the healthy elderly, sensory impairments are common. Over 30% of the population composed of individuals over the age of 75 has a hearing impairment or static visual acuity of 20/50 or worse (Small, 1987). Hearing impairments differ among men and women, with men having losses in the 3000–6000 Hz range, but women tending to have impairments in the 550–1000 Hz range. Reaction times of older adults will also be longer, on average. Simple reaction time increases by about 20% by age 60, and complex reaction time increases to an even greater extent by this age. Similarly, strength decreases by 10–20% by ages 60 to 70, and mobility may also be decreased in those with joint diseases. Kovar and La Croix (1987) found, also, that of those individuals in their study who retired for health reasons, 5 in 10 had decreases in lower and upper body strength, endurance, or mobility. (Please consult the Fundamentals part of this book for a thorough review of these issues).

In terms of health problems of the elderly, the Institute of Medicine of the National Academy of Sciences, in a special report published in 1991 (see Lonergan & Krevans, 1991), identified the following geriatric syndromes as frequently occurring and due additional research attention because of the potential for treatment advances: (1) failure to thrive; (2) impaired postural stability, strength, and mobility; (3) mismanagement of medications; (4) urinary incontinence; and (5) delirium or acute confusional states (which occur in one-third of hospitalized older patients). In addition, the Institute of Medicine identified the following as "the important diseases of old age" and indicated that more research is necessary to understand the interaction between age-related physiological changes and these diseases: (1) cardiovascular disease; (2) dementia and affective disorders; (3) musculoskeletal disorders; (4) infectious disease and diminished immunologie competence; (5) neoplasia; and (6) disorders of metabolism and homeostasis. The same report also called for more research on the delivery of health services to the elderly, including studies concerning transitioning between types of care (acute, nursing home, home, ambulatory, and residential care).

What the Future Is Bringing

The health care cost for older persons with disabilities or chronic illnesses is currently more than $160 billion per year and is expected to double in the 1990s (Lonergan & Krevans, 1991). Several transitions are occurring in health care that directly affect the design of systems and devices for elderly. Table 1 summarizes old and new emphases. There are many reasons for these changes, including cost control, improved understanding of optimal medical care, and cultural changes in thinking about "wellness."

Devoting resources to prevention and focusing on the continuum of care have been the cornerstones of public health and the specialty of preventive medicine for several years. However, many of the changes described in Table 1 are just beginning to have an impact on many areas of the country. Most health care organizations have been rewarded by fee-for-service for doing the "old." Managed care incentives have the potential to move organiza-

TABLE 1
Old and New Emphases in Health Care

	Old	New
Main place for care	Hospital	Clinic or home
Doctor–patient relation	Paternal	Cooperative
Emphasis for resources	Acute treatment	Prevention
Payer or provider focus	Episodic	Continuum
Gatekeeper or manager	None	Family physician
Expectations	Better at any cost	Living will
Following treatment plan	Compliance	Adherence
Caregivers	Physicians	Nurse practitioners Physician assistants

tions to the "new." Many medical device and medical computer companies have taken the strategy to build and market to the "new."

The fact that one in four older persons lives in a rural area (Coward & Cutler, 1989) poses special problems with respect to health care, particularly *access to* health care, for this group. According to Lassey and Lassey (1985), two bodies of literature concern health care and the rural elderly, and both are deficient. We need to (1) better understand the life circumstances, health status, and health care needs of the rural elderly and (2) develop and deliver effective, efficient health services in the rural context. Specialty care is especially scarce in rural areas, where 53% of the care is provided by general or family practitioners, as compared to metropolitan areas, where the figure is 12% (Norton & McManus, 1989).

Providing specialty care as well as access to care in general are among the goals of telemedicine. Telemedicine is the electronic transmission of patient information to a clinician at a remote site. It is not a new concept (see the historical review in Greenberger & Puffer, 1989) but is seeing a recent "rebirth" because of the advent of managed care, the need for better access to care in rural areas, improvements in the technology available for its delivery, and lower capital and transmission costs (Grigsby et al., 1994).

A Telemedicine Case Study

The promise of telemedicine in the health care of the elderly was aptly demonstrated in a recent study conducted at the University of Kansas Medical Center (UKMC: Hubble, Pahwa, Michalek, Thomas, & Koller, 1993). The goal of the study was to investigate the utility of interactive video conferencing (IVC) for the interim assessment and care of patients suffering from Parkinson's disease, a disease that occurs in 1% of individuals over 65 years of age. Figure 1 shows a typical setup for an IVC system used for telemedicine.

The treatment and management of Parkinson's disease requires a medical specialist, the neurologist, to assess and balance side effects from treatment medication with the progressively worsening effects of the disease. On a regular basis, daily living problems caused by the disease need to be evaluated and addressed, as well. Access to such specialists via telemedicine would be of significant benefit to elderly Parkinson's patients. In this case, for example, many elderly Kansans live several dozen miles away from the nearest neurologist.

In the UKMC study, nine Parkinson's patients were assessed by different physicians who performed their evaluations either through IVC or with the patient in the clinic. Both sets of physicians evaluated the subject on the Unified Parkinson's Disease Rating Scale, which has both subjective mea-

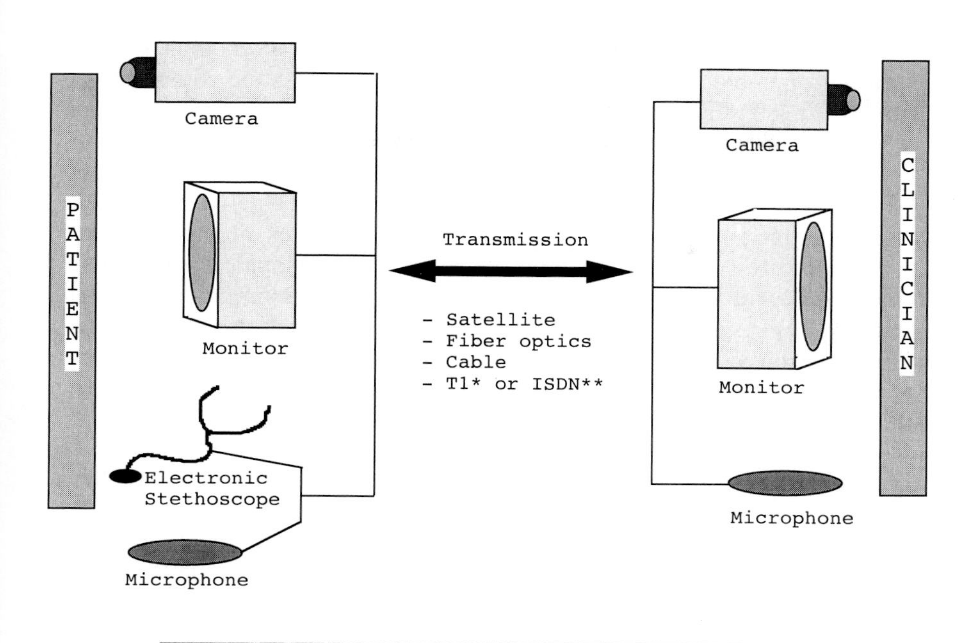

* T1 is a dedicated data transmission service (1.2 MB/sec)
** ISDN = Integrated Services Digital Network: A switched data transmission service (two 64 KB/sec lines)

FIGURE 1 Typical interactive video communication system used for telemedicine.

sures (mood, mentation) and objective measures of motor status. The use of this scale is crucial to the management of debilitation for this incurable, chronic disease. The results of the UKMC evaluation showed no differences in the Unified Parkinson's Disease Rating Scale results between the physicians using IVC and those seeing the patient directly in the clinic. Furthermore, patients liked the system and thought it improved their access to care.

Although telemedicine was successfully used for disease management and treatment under these circumstances, many human factors issues and other factors can affect both its usefulness and its acceptability to patients in a given instance. Research concerning video-mediated communication issues in telemedicine has only begun to take place (Bocker & Muhlbach, 1993), and it has not yet been targeted at age-related concerns. In addition, the cost–benefit tradeoffs of telemedicine, particularly for the elderly who might well be major users, have yet to be determined (Grigsby et al., 1994).

The potential applications of telemedicine, as well as its definition, extend well beyond the diagnostic and treatment management situation just described. Telemedicine also includes other methods of access to health care information, including the telephone, facsimile machine, and computer networks. While IVC may be technologically complex and costly, many forms of telemedicine are much less so.

Greenberger and Puffer (1989), for example, describe a telemedicine system they designed to promote self-care among the elderly. In doing so they note that, to be successful, telemedicine applications targeting self-care for the elderly must be (1) simple to access; (2) personal as opposed to impersonal, and (3) operable without the need for a communication intermediary. Their system, called HealthCom, is a health care information system accessible via a Touch-Tone phone. It allows patients to request and access health care information that is personally meaningful, without the need for a direct encounter with a physician. In addition to allowing patients access to information, they can record questions to a physician or nurse practitioner, request appointments, and record any needs they have for immediate attention. Recorded questions are reviewed and responses are made the same day, via direct phone calls to the patient or recorded responses.

Interestingly, many home visits by nurses are not for hands-on care but for observing the patient doing some task (Allen, 1995). Examples of these observations include watching to ensure that medications are taken on time and properly, double-checking a glucose level reported by a patient, and assessing the cognitive status of a patient. Some have proposed, or are attempting, the use of video and data communications for accomplishing these types of tasks. An analysis of cost efficiency for the state of Kansas showed a potential savings of $8.1 million per year with the use of these media (Allen, 1995). The answers to important questions about which observations and activities can be done remotely are less well-known, however. Certainly, operators on both ends of such systems would need systems that are easy to learn and use and that have a low potential for error. For example, most video systems require significant expertise to ensure accurate color representation; otherwise, a blue cyanotic person might look pink as a posey.

The health care-specific human-system interactions that occur with these telemedicine systems are crucial. Diseases can cause cognitive or physical limitations that make barely usable communication systems unusable. Unfortunately, these limitations usually are not considered in most evaluations. In general, industry and medical personnel in charge of development and implementation do not subscribe to the user-centered process. Many of those involved in the development process also equate clinical efficacy (e.g., am I able to diagnose pneumonia?) with viability and usability (Gosbee, in press).

Medical Device Design and Self-Care

In the future, more emphasis will be on self-care and an increasing number of medical devices in the home. The efficacy and safety of these devices will depend on their usability (Wiklund, 1992). However, as Smith (1990) has noted, most of the data collected with respect to aging has been to age differences and the aging process, not to guide design. Therefore, quantitative data relevant to device usability is lacking, particularly on subgroups within the population of older adults. Nevertheless, Wiklund (1992) and Koncelik (1982) have both formulated a number of design principles relevant to the design of medical devices used by the elderly. These design principles are summarized in Table 2.

TABLE 2
Design Principles for Medical Device Design

Impairment or limitation	Example	Relevant design principle
Cognitive rigidity	Memorization of many steps	Number of steps in procedure kept low
		Use of familiar features that are common to other products used by the elderly
Sensory deficits	See following	Redundant cues, like auditory, visual, and tactile feedback
		Videotaped product instructions and demonstrations
Hearing impairments	High-frequency loss in males	Auditory signals in the 1500–2500 Hz range
Visual impairments	Visual acuity	Labels should employ large fonts
	Visual acuity and diminished low-light vision	Supplemental illumination for devices used in low-light conditions
	Increased sensitivity to glare	Matte finishes should be used for control panels and antiglare coating should be used on displays
	Loss of color sensitivity	Displays will be read most easily by this population if they employ white characters on a black background
Mobility limitation	Hand dexterity and strength	Large diameter knobs; textured knob surfaces; and controls with low resistance

Three Case Studies of Medical Device Design

The case studies that follow highlight some of the medical device design challenges. In addition, they constitute examples of how these challenges are not being addressed with respect to many existing products and provide opportunities for the human factors specialist to significantly contribute to the design of medical devices.

Home-Based Blood Glucometer

The Pacific Science and Engineering Group (Kelly, Callan, & Meadows, 1991) was charged by the U.S. Food and Drug Administration (FDA) to study all relevant human factors design issues for the blood glucometer. The ability of elderly diabetic patients to monitor their blood glucose allows better control of diabetes through medication (e.g., insulin), exercise, and diet. Errors using home glucometers were the number one problem identified in the FDA's device error registry. Most of the errors involved higher or lower values, which resulted in under- or overdosing of diabetes medication. Almost three-quarters of the errors were attributed to improper user technique. Examples of crucial errors were (1) failure to place enough blood on the test strip; (2) input of incorrect calibration codes; and (3) improper removal of the test strip. Not surprisingly, these errors were more likely for those models that had relatively lower tolerances or required a relatively high degree of user coordination and timing.

The investigation consisted of system evaluations of many of the popular home glucometers, associated training literature, and user manuals. Techniques included task analysis, user analysis, and usability studies. Several human factors design problems were cited. First, many visual displays were difficult to read due to font size and viewing angle. Reading these displays may have been impossible for patients with minor visual impairments. Second, many auditory cues could not be distinguished in a room with 60 dB of background noise. Third, some controls did not conform to human factors guidelines, and psychomotor coordination needed for some operations, like battery replacement, was substantial. Fourth, task analysis revealed several steps requiring very complex hand dexterity and cognitive processing, which they suggested were the route of many user errors. Finally, written instructions and training material were found wanting in the use of graphics, the presentation of information in a logical sequence, and the inclusion of warnings and cautions at the point of need in each task.

Home-Based Intravenous Perfusion Pump

As noted in Table 1, there is a push to shorten hospital stays, as well as utilize the patient or family members to deliver self-care. The tool (device) that provides controlled and direct medication delivery is the intravenous (IV) pump. The installation, operation, and maintenance of IV pumps are not trivial tasks. Errors can lead to illness or death with many of the medications that are delivered via IV. For example, the adverse effects of overdosing the drug Terbutaline cited in the following study, range from minor nausea to cardiac arrest.

Obradovich and Woods (1994) studied the operation and design of a computer-based IV pump and noted several design flaws that could lead to errors by older adults using the pump for home care. Interviews and usability lab tests revealed several deficiencies in the computer-based patient interface that would affect operation by *all* users, and it could be argued that the elderly user would be the most severely impacted by these deficiencies. Complex and arbitrary sequences of operation were accomplished through the four multifunction buttons. Different operating modes were hard to determine due to inadequate and confusing feedback from the 3/4 in. by 1 in. display and audible beep. Ambiguous alarms were a problem, including seven that were signaled by the same auditory alarm and cryptic alphanumeric displays. Poor feedback contributed to operators often getting lost in the complex arbitrary sequences of operation and troubleshooting.

Attempts to circumvent many of these design problems included procedural constraints imposed by nurses managing the situation, as well as a job aid (patient guide) developed by them. The job aid was likely printed and constructed to be readable by nurses without acuity or color deficits.

Blood Glucose Strips

Patients with Type II noninsulin dependent diabetes are likely to be elderly, and many will have diabetic retinopathy. As noted previously, visual acuity and color vision decrease steadily with age. Laux (1994) evaluated the readability of indicator strips used by diabetics to monitor their blood sugar at home, with special attention to the extent to which visual characteristics of the elderly can lead to problems in their use.

Three groups of 20 healthy subjects (ages 21–30, 40–59, and 60–78) were asked to interpret the color of the glucose color test strips under various lighting conditions. Performance overall was poor, with readings being incorrect 26% of the time. Age was not correlated with poorer performance, but corrected visual acuity was. Worse yet, the errors across all ages and lighting conditions were highest when an accurate reading was most important—when glucose levels were high, but read as normal. Though not considered in this study, dexterity and cognitive performance are also important in handling and using these color test strips.

REHABILITATION

The Elderly in the Rehabilitation Context

For many older adults, the rehabilitation context begins and ends with inpatient rehabilitation services. Unlike children, whose rehabilitation can continue through the educational system, and working adults, who benefit from back-to-work programs and the Americans with Disabilities Act, adults who are or will be no longer working benefit from few directed rehabilitation services outside the inpatient setting. Unless they have significant amounts of private funding, their rehabilitation options are limited. There is an obvious breach in the continuum of care.

In addition, inpatient rehabilitation services, until recently, have followed the medical model, which dictates that rehabilitation constitutes "fixing" the individual, if possible, otherwise teaching him or her to adapt to the disability (i.e., to learn to live with it). This, of course, is antithetical to a human factors approach, as well as to the independent living (IL) model (Enders, 1991), which dictates that the environment—both the physical environment and the attitudinal environment—be changed to accommodate the disability. In this model, the relevant rehabilitation outcomes are defined in terms of control over one's environment, *not* in terms of the number of tasks that can be carried out without technological or personal assistance.

Rehabilitation programs for the older adult, unless they are progressive and follow an IL approach, do not consider the environmental context beyond the hospital. As a consequence, assistive technology solutions that are effectively employed in the hospital, for example, may no longer be used or usable when the patient returns home (Mann, Hurren, & Tomita, 1993; Mann, Karuza, & Hurren, 1992). As Enders (1991) has noted, it is not the technology that fails but the delivery system.

Another aspect of the rehabilitation context relevant to this discussion is the third party reimbursement situation. Whether we like it or not, decisions about and provision of both rehabilitation services and assistive technology are determined, to a great extent, by third party reimbursement rules.

Assistive Technology Issues in Rehabilitation

In the process of rehabilitation, there are three levels of outcomes (Holm & Rogers, 1991): (1) restoration of previous capabilities; (2) compensation for remaining sensorimotor, cognitive, and psychosocial impairments; and (3) substitution of performance by human or technology proxies. The assistive technology-related human factors issues fall under outcomes (2) and

(3). One of the biggest of these issues is the reasons for and the prevention of abandonment of assistive technology by the elderly.

We have already noted that one genesis of the nonuse problem may be the failure of the delivery system to assess the older adult's home environment during inpatient rehabilitation. There are many other potential explanations, some related to human factors, some not. Page, Galer, Fitzgerald, and Feeney (1980) cited inappropriate prescriptions, inadequate training on device use, mismatches within the person–task–environment triad, and poorly designed devices as causes. Gitlin, Levine, and Geiger (1993), more than 10 years later, cited (1) cumbersomeness of devices; (2) other people taking over performance of the task for which the device was being used; (3) equipment loss or failure; (4) lack of knowledge concerning the appropriate use of the device or how to fix a broken device; (4) denial of need or embarrassment over the disability; (5) equipment inappropriate to the environment; (6) poor aesthetic quality of the devices; (7) embarrassment or awkwardness associated with device use; and (8) difficulties in using the device.

A number of studies have also assessed whether older adults felt they needed additional assistive technology (Mann et al., 1992, 1993). These studies have shown that older adults felt they had unmet needs, but *all* of the articulated needs represented items commercially available already. This suggests that information about the availability of assistive technology is not always reaching the elderly.

The preceding discussion indicates that at least three factors—person-centered characteristics, environmental conditions, and device characteristics—interact to determine device use and that all of these elements must be considered when prescribing rehabilitation technologies for the older adult (Gitlin et al., 1993), as shown in Figure 2.

The figure suggests several strategies for improving the delivery of rehabilitation services and assistive technology to the elderly. First, it suggests that complete environmental assessments be done to understand the environment in which the person will be using the technology and the constraints it imposes on the technology and its use. Second, it suggests that there is much room for improvement in instructional strategies, both for learning how to use the devices and learning how to proceed with respect to maintaining and repairing them. Third, it suggests strongly that the client must be involved in the decision-making process by being empowered through education and by having the opportunity to articulate his or her needs and values during the rehabilitation process. In other words, *it is imperative that a systems approach, applying human factors throughout the continuum of rehabilitation contexts relevant to each patient, be employed in rehabilitation service delivery.*

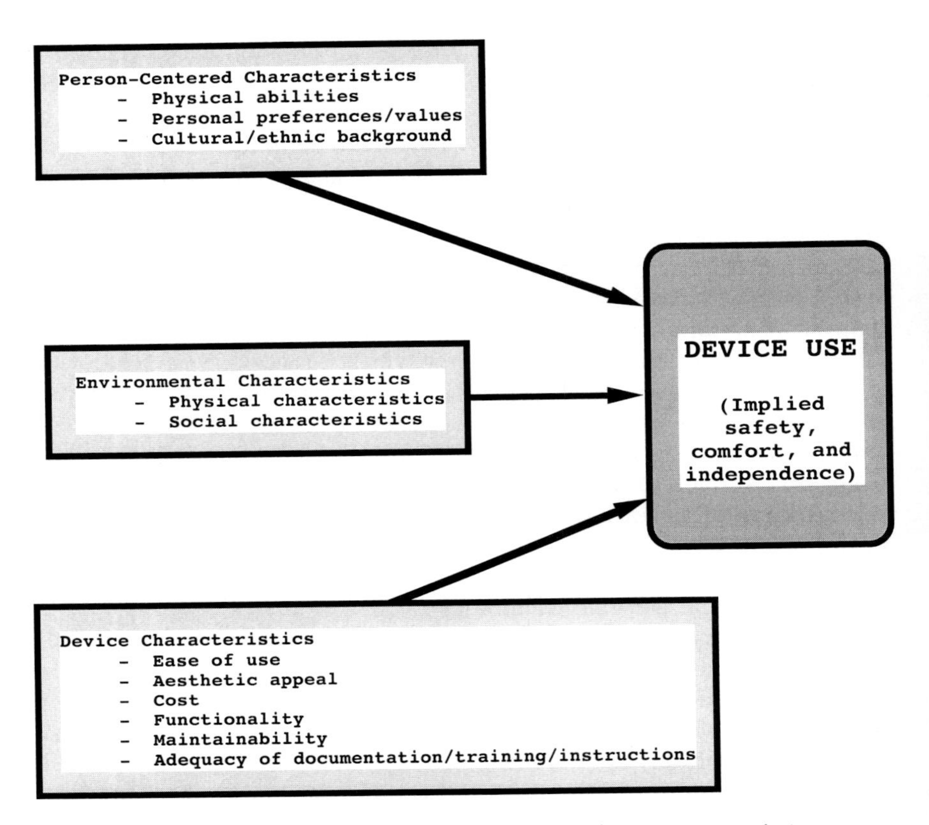

FIGURE 2 Impact of person, environment, and device characteristics on device use.

With respect to device design, specifically, the figure points to a need for devices that are aesthetically appealing and not clinical looking. It also suggests that devices need to be easy to operate, to maintain, and if possible, to repair. It suggests that device manufacturers should provide documentation suitable for use by the elderly, and materials for rehabilitation therapists that can be used to instruct clients adequately. Finally, it suggests that devices must be selected or designed to meet specific client needs.

Wheelchair Design

Nothing spells disability like W-H-E-E-L-C-H-A-I-R. The simple fact of having to carry on conversations with people while looking up at them wrestles control and freedom away from the individual in the wheelchair. Furthermore, scant attention has been given to the seating needs of the elderly, although they constitute a large proportion of wheelchair users (Redford, 1993). Why does this situation exist? According to Redford (1993), Medicaid and Medicare look only at the cost of devices; manufacturers employ mass specifications; dealers stock only a few designs; and too few people understand the importance of adequate seating. As an example, Redford notes that the most widely available chair has a vinyl hammock-type seat and back and fixed arm and leg rests, none of which is conducive to adequate seating. In addition, even those involved with the prescription of wheelchairs tend to think in terms of "seating and positioning" or "wheeled mobility," not in terms of the wheelchair's design as it relates to *task completion* or *meeting the goals of independent living*. Epstein (1990) has noted, moreover, that failure to employ a coordinated approach to wheelchair management has been shown to (1) decrease user independence, (2) increase costs, (3) inhibit safety control measures, and (4) contribute to deterioration in the user's physical condition.

Redford's paper is one of the few devoted to the selection and design of wheelchairs for elderly clients and for that it is notable. However, it, too, fails to go beyond a classification of the elderly into four groups: (1) nonmobile and dependent, (2) mobile and nonambulatory, (3) ambulatory with special wheelchair needs, and (4) frail but ambulatory. There is no discussion of user goals, user tasks, or chair functionality beyond that required for providing postural stability or mobility. Hence, if the older adult client would like to be able to interact with a computer while seated in a wheelchair, there is virtually no guidance as to the chair's design. Luckily, some articles, most notably one by O'Leary, Mann, and Perkash (1991) that is aimed at older adults, address the computer access problem.

Redford sums up the elderly seating problem as follows: "too many old people who are sitting too many hours a day in wheelchairs that provide too little postural support or mechanisms for pressure relief over vulnerable skin surfaces" (1993, p. 884). This statement exemplifies the lack of attention to the user's view concerning the *functionality* of the chair. Postural support and pressure relief are laudable goals, but is it a wonder that people in nursing homes are *simply sitting*, and sitting poorly, when poorly designed chairs are used with little or no regard to the tasks and activities the user might need or like to perform?

One of the more insidious problems with wheelchairs is their almost complete lack of aesthetic appeal. Not that this problem could not be solved. A most innovative design was developed by a relative of the first author who suffered from arthritis. His wheelchair, fabricated from plastic pipe, was both pleasant to look at and functional in ways most chairs are not (you could take it into the shower with you). Certainly, more needs to be done in this area, which is one of significant importance to the elderly.

Rehabilitation services must be oriented toward improving the independence and control of clients and enabling them to function, as closely as possible, in the manner they did prior to events that necessitated prescription of the wheelchair.

Falls

The most hazardous and likely accident problem for the elderly is falling (Smith, 1990). The frequency of falls increases as people advance from middle to old age and is a special problem among those who are institutionalized. There are many risk factors for falls (Tiderksaar [1989] identified 50; Nevitt, Cummings, Kidd, & Black [1989] identified 35); therefore, design solutions to prevent falls must be based on those risk factors deemed to exist in particular situations.

A Walker Comparison

A study by Mahoney, Euhardy, and Carnes (1992) is one of the few we found that employs older adults as subjects, evaluates real products, and employs tasks or activities relevant to the older adult in the evaluation. We use it as an example of the kinds of studies that should be conducted to evaluate and improve both medical care and rehabilitation technologies for this population.

Both short stride lengths and slow gait speeds are associated with falling in older adults (e.g., Wolfson, Whipple, Amerman, & Tobin, 1990). Therefore, assistive technologies that can increase stride lengths and gait speeds should be helpful to rehabilitation clients. In their study, Mahoney et al. compared the usability of the standard wheeled walker, which has four legs, with wheels on the front two, with a three-wheeled walker, which has the front wheel pivoting freely. Subjects in their study were 65 and older with no walker experience. However, all were candidates for a walker because of gait instability. Subjects used each walker to navigate a 15 ft walkway and a 60 ft obstacle course, after they had completed each task without the aid of any walker, to provide baseline measurements. The dependent measures were the stride length on the walkway and time to complete the walk, the time to complete the obstacle course, the number of bumps made on the obstacle course (i.e., the number of times the user bumped an obstacle), and walker preference. After the initial testing, the subjects were allowed to take one of the walkers home with them for a three-week trial. After this trial adjustment period, the tests were conducted again.

The results showed that, during the initial testing for the walkway task, stride length increased over the baseline measurement for the three-wheeled but not the two-wheeled walker and that the gait speed was higher for the three-wheeled than for the two-wheeled walker. The differences between the groups disappeared, however, by the three-week follow-up testing. In the initial testing for the obstacle course, time to complete the course was greater for the two-wheeled walker than for the three-wheeled walker. This difference persisted at the three-week follow-up. Interestingly, however, the number of bumps for the three-wheeled walker was much greater than for the two-wheeled walker in the initial testing, although it dissipated somewhat during subsequent testing. The authors also noted that the number of bumps was significantly negatively correlated with subject performance on the Mini-Mental State Examination, which assesses cognitive impairment and was administered at the beginning of the experiment. Finally, subject preference was overwhelmingly in favor of the three-wheeled walker.

In this case, although the three-wheeled walker was preferred and, generally, outperformed the two-wheeled walker, it had its problems, which increased the number of bumps experienced by subjects on the obstacle course. The investigators reasoned that the triangular design of the walker was such that the rear two wheels were out of the subject's field of vision, thus the reason for the significant number of bumps. Nevertheless, the follow-up data indicated that practice could alleviate some of these effects.

These types of studies provide useful data to both manufacturers and potential product users alike. Furthermore, the act of participating in such studies is a positive experience for older adults (Nayak, 1995), who relish this opportunity both to provide data and to contribute to the design process. The need for such studies should be obvious, given the current lack of design data on older adults, and the number of new devices that are being marketed for both home health care and rehabilitation.

WHERE DO WE GO FROM HERE?

The answer to this question, to some extent, depends on whether you are a research scientist, a designer, or a student. In the following paragraphs, we provide some guidance for those human factors professionals who want to become more involved in work in the rehabilitation and health care arena.

Becoming Comfortable with the Subject Matter

Several scientific and technical organizations related to human factors and medicine are addressing the many issues outlined in this chapter. However, most are not using human factors methodology, applying human factors principles, or even aware of the human factors standards that exist. Some are familiar with human factors engineering but have relegated it to a science that measures toilet seats or theorizes about cognitive models. Becoming involved in these organizations can benefit you in two ways: (1) you can begin to learn the terminology in use in their field, essential if you're to become and "insider"; and (2) you can improve their members' perceptions of the human factors field by engaging in activities like presenting papers at their meetings or serving on their committees.

In addition to the Human Factors and Ergonomics Society (P. O. Box 1369, Santa Monica, CA 90406, (310) 394-1811) and its Technical Group on Medical Systems and Rehabilitation, some of the relevant organizations are as follows:

American College of Medical Quality
9005 Congressional Court
Potomac, MD 20854
(301) 365-3570

Society for Medical Decision Making
1 Main Street
P. O. Box 447
West Lebanon, NH 03784

American Medical Informatics Association
4915 St. Elmo Avenue
Suite 302
Bethesda, MD 20814

Anesthesia Patient Safety Foundation
515 Busse Highway
Park Ridge, IL 60068
(708) 825-5586

Healthcare Information and Management Systems Society (HIMSS)
Division of the American Hospital Association
840 N. Lake Shore Drive
Chicago, IL 60611

Society for Health Systems: A Society of the Institute of Industrial Engineers (IIE)
25 Technology Park
Norcross, GA 30092
(404) 449-0460

Association for the Advancement of Medical Instrumentation (AAMI)
3330 Washington Boulevard, Suite 400
Arlington, VA 22201

There has never been a better time to become involved in AAMI, not only because of the Food and Drug Administration's recently announced Human Factors Plan, mandating the application of human factors in the design of medical equipment and devices, but because AAMI is currently beginning the process of revising *Human Factors Engineering Guidelines and Preferred Practices for the Design of Medical Devices* (Association for the Advancement of Medical Instrumentation, 1993). This American National Standards Institute (ANSI) guidelines document was developed with limited input from the human factors community, a situation that, we hope, will be remedied in this revision.

The appreciation of human factors engineering is somewhat greater within the rehabilitation and assistive technology community, possibly because of the increasing employment of computer technology in assistive devices and the regulatory impact of the Americans with Disabilities Act (ADA). RESNA is the premier organization serving rehabilitation engineering professionals in the United States and offers several special interest groups (SIGs) that should be of interest to human factors professionals. These include (1) personal transportation, (2) sensory aids, (3) wheeled mobility and seating, (4) computer applications, (5) job accommodation, (6) gerontology, and (7) universal access. You can contact RESNA at

RESNA
1700 N. Moore Street
Suite 1540
Arlington, VA 22209-1903
(703) 524-6686

There are also organizations specifically devoted to issues involving augmentative and alternative communication (techniques and assistive technology for people who cannot speak or who have speech impairments), as follows:

International Society for Augmentative and Alternative Communication (ISAAC)
P. O. Box 1762, Station R
Toronto, Ontario M4G 4A3 Canada
(905) 737-0624

United States Society for Augmentative and Alternative Communication (USSAAC)
P. O. Box 5271
Evanston, IL 60204-5271
(708) 869-2122
e-mail: USSAAC@aol.com

A quick and easy way to familiarize yourself with issues related to rehabilitation and assistive technology is to subscribe to one of the Internet discussion groups to discover the current issues and problems in this area. A few of the more illuminating groups include the following:

- *Disability research*—subscribers discuss, primarily, social research issues with respect to disabilities. To subscribe, send an e-mail message with a blank subject line to mailbase@mailbase.ac.uk. In the body of the message type only "join disability-research ⟨Firstname Lastname⟩".
- *RESNA*—subscribers are limited, at this time, to members of RESNA SIGs 9 and 11, wheeled mobility and seating and computer applications, respectively. To subscribe, send an e-mail message with a blank subject line to LISTSERV@SJUVM.STJOHNS.EDU. In the body of the message, type only "SUBSCRIBE RESNA ⟨Firstname Lastname⟩".
- *UACCESS-L*—subscribers discuss all aspects of universal access to technology for individuals with disabilities. To subscribe, send an e-mail message with a blank subject line to LISTPROC@TRACE.WISC.EDU. In the body of the message, type only "SUBSCRIBE UACCESS-L ⟨Firstname Lastname⟩".

It is important to recognize that, particularly in the medical arena, human factors work often occurs "in disguise" in various organizations and units of hospitals and other health care facilities. Many of the individuals doing this work would never think of calling it a human factors activity. For those searching for the means of entry into this field, it is important to know some of the relevant job titles and positions.

Both medical and nursing informatics positions exist in some hospitals. The former are involved with the design and use of information systems in the medical setting; the latter often gather the needs of users and translate these for technical specialists. Those involved in medical and nursing informatics have domain knowledge in both the health care and computer areas. Probably all but the smallest hospitals have information systems (IS) departments, which analyze staff needs for information, provide user training, and implement all changes in the hospital's information systems. These departments currently hold volumes of data that could be used effectively in human factors investigations.

Most hospitals and other health care facilities have industrial engineering functions, but they are often buried within hospital departments like systems analysis, continuous quality improvement (CQI), quality assurance, and finance. Often, the people carrying out these functions are termed *management engineers.*

In medical device companies, human factors functions are sometimes performed by individuals whose positions are titled *clinical engineer, quality engineer,* or *industrial designer.* In addition, in some hospitals and medical device companies, human factors is considered as part of the company's marketing function.

The Role of Human Factors Research Scientists

The research scientist's charge is to add to the knowledge base with respect to health care, rehabilitation, and the elderly. The following are some ideas for enriching the contributions of research scientists.

Performing Research in Context

There is a definite need to learn more about the performance capabilities and limitations of older adults in real-world settings as opposed to the contrived situations of the laboratory. To best understand the performance issues related to the use of medical and assistive technology by the elderly in the home, for example, one should be conducting research in that setting. In no other way can we really understand the performance challenges to the elderly posed by the *combined* effects of the home environment, the technology, and the capabilities and limitations of the individual user.

Communicating with Designers

For your research to have an impact on the lives and performance of the elderly in health care and rehabilitation settings, your results must be quantifiable and communicated to designers in such a way that they can use the information. That is, designers need the information packaged to facilitate their development of design requirements. Therefore, they need not only the results but some indication of the generalizability of the results and any situational or human constraints that limit their applicability. Knowing the implications of your results for designers and communicating that information in an effective manner is an often forgotten step in moving from knowledge to practice.

Taking a Systems Approach to Problems across the Continuum of Care

Health care and rehabilitation involve service delivery systems that are, by and large, very inefficient and, unfortunately, sometimes ineffective as well. Research that studies the aging individual in the context of the entire delivery system can help us to improve the overall quality of care for the elderly, and the ability of each elderly individual to take advantage of opportunities for self-care. More studies should, therefore, take a systems approach to studying the human factors issues faced by the elderly in health care and rehabilitation.

In medicine, the concept of a *clinical path* is being considered as a means of decreasing the variability in the health care process, as well as its outcomes, for various diseases. A clinical path, simply put, is typically a detailed set of instructions for the care of patients with a particular problem (e.g., diabetes, depression). It is possible, given today's information technology, to evaluate, across all involved hospital units, the quality of care an individual receives by doing detailed monitoring at various points (sometimes many of them) along the clinical path. As a result, the researcher can find out where errors occur in the care of the patient and exactly how they occurred. Detailed analyses of such data can be used to improve the clinical path and patient care. We initiated an in-depth analysis of the pneumonia clinical pathway being used at one of our local Kalamazoo hospitals (Barber et al., 1995). The design changes resulting from such analysis may range from administrative and procedural changes to equipment improvements.

To take an example from the rehabilitation context, consider the elderly person for whom the clinical need for an assistive technology has been identified. Let us say the device is a wheelchair. The human factors issues are many and extend quite a ways beyond the user–wheelchair interface. What barriers must the elderly person eliminate to *acquire* the wheelchair? What training requirements for wheelchair use are unique to elderly users? What causes elderly users to maintain use of the wheelchair vs. to abandon it after a period of time? What problems does the system impose on the elderly user with respect to maintenance and repair of the device? These issues may reflect user–system problems, the system being the rehabilitation services delivery system.

We would urge human factors researchers to devote more attention to user–system issues. Developing new tools, techniques, and methodologies for obtaining basic knowledge of the human factors issues in distributed, fragmented health care and rehabilitation services delivery systems would move us a long way toward solutions to human factors problems. Expanding the knowledge base only as it relates to improving the user–device interface for an elderly user, for example, will not be useful if the many other relevant user–system interfaces are ignored.

The Role of Designers

Designers can both improve the medical devices and delivery systems currently used by the elderly and develop new systems and devices, based on user needs. Designers can benefit in a number of ways, as follows, from the information in this chapter.

Making Use of Guidelines and Standards

Designers can benefit from the guidelines and standards that are available and can help to improve them. The Safe Medical Devices Act of 1990 speaks to the requirement to adhere to quality design principles, including human factors engineering methods and guidelines (Kahan, 1991). The AAMI/ANSI standard, described previously in this chapter, is one source of guidelines in this area. For facilities, the Health Care Facility Guidelines (American Institute of Architects, 1987) provide recommendations for the design of building layouts and were developed with input from the human factors community.

Developing Participant Groups for Usability Testing

The information in this chapter provides some practical information that should assist designers in recruiting participants for the usability testing of medical and rehabilitation devices. However, even those who are in the health care and rehabilitation domains often encounter difficulty identifying reasonable cross-sections of the elderly population for testing purposes, especially if they are not looking for individuals who are extremely sick. For devices used for particular diseases or chronic conditions, one can look to community support groups, particularly in larger cities. Participants, as well as sites, for usability testing can often be found at senior centers that offer a variety of health rehabilitation, and wellness-related activities. If you are looking for participants from the general medical population, many health care organizations have patient advisory boards that assist in quality assessment and patient education efforts.

Taking a Systems Approach to Design

Just as researchers are encouraged to consider health care and rehabilitation as service delivery systems, the designer is encouraged to look beyond the design of the device or equipment to the system in which it must function. Devices designed in a vacuum, with no attention to the operating environment, are going to be problematic in practice. A most telling example, described at a panel session on warnings in medicine at the 1995 Annual Meeting of the Human Factors and Ergonomics Society (Bogner, Weinger, Laughery, Amundson, & Haas, 1995) is that of multiple warnings from multiple pieces of equipment being indistinguishable and uninterpretable in operating rooms and intensive care units. As long as device designers and manufacturers fail to consider the environmental contexts in which their products operate, these problems will continue to exist. An integrated approach—a systems approach—is needed. Designers, in addition, should be at the forefront of standardization efforts that will prevent these types of problems.

Guidance for Students

How can today's students become active in human factors work involving medicine, rehabilitation, and the older adult? Our advice is that students take course work that will give them some basic understanding of the language and content of these subject domains. Classes in medical terminology, basic human anatomy and physiology, medical systems (both micro and macro), epidemiology, and public health would be helpful for those interested in pursuing work in the medical domain. Courses in rehabilitation subspecialties—physical therapy, occupational therapy, speech pathology, and audiology—and rehabilitation engineering would be helpful to those who want to work in this domain. Once students feel comfortable with the content areas, they should try to gain real-world experience through an industry-based internship or volunteer work in a local medical or rehabilitation facility or school. A final piece of advice is that students should attend at least one conference at which human factors issues will be discussed—but *not* from a human factors perspective—so they can see what they will be up against, observe the zeitgeist, get an idea of who might be willing to hire them, and so forth.

CONCLUSIONS

In this chapter, we have attempted to outline some of the more pressing *process* issues that exist in health care and rehabilitation contexts of the older adult. Applied literature is particularly sparse in this area, and it is our view that significant applied research efforts are needed to understand the health care and rehabilitation systems existing in the United States, so that the human factors issues in those systems, as they apply to the nation's elderly, can be better addressed. Among the goals and objectives of such applied work are the following:

- To describe those characteristics of the diseases and injuries of the older adult most relevant to the design of medical devices, medical communication systems, and rehabilitation devices and systems.
- To identify and characterize the specific problems encountered by the elderly using medical and rehabilitation devices, including medical communications systems, within all medical or rehabilitation contexts.
- To develop and test the reliability and validity of human factors field techniques for developing medical and rehabilitation systems and devices for older adults living in both rural and nonrural environments.
- To determine the impact of managed care on health care and rehabilitation services delivery to the elderly, and to develop strategies for implementing human factors approaches to medical or rehabilitation device design and selection within the context of managed care.

The application of human factors to health care and rehabilitation has a short history and, with respect to specific issues relevant to older clients, almost no history. However, with the advent of managed care and its emphasis on better treatment results with decreased costs, we have an opportunity to affect the quality of care through the employment of human factors methodologies and approaches to medical and rehabilitation problems. It is an opportunity not to be missed.

References

Allen, A. (1995). Home health care via telemedicine. *Telemedicine Today, 3*(2), 26–27.

American Institute of Architects. (1987). *Health Care Facility Guidelines*. Washington, DC: Author.

Association for the Advancement of Medical Instrumentation. (1993). *Human factors engineering guidelines and preferred practices for the design of medical devices* (ANSI/AAMI HE48-1993). Arlington, VA: Author.

Barber, M., Barnes, R., Barr, C., Gardner-Bonneau, D., Paska, K., & Rogers, G. (1995). *Protocol: Randomized controlled trial of the Borgess clinical path for pneumonia*. Kalamazoo, MI: Borgess Medical Center. (Contact Daryle Gardner-Bonneau for additional information)

Bocker, M., & Muhlbach, L. (1993). Communicative presence in videocommunications. In *Proceedings of the Human Factors and Ergonomics Society 37th annual meeting* (pp. 249–253). Santa Monica, CA: Human Factors and Ergonomics Society.

Bogner, M. S., Weinger, M. B., Laughery, K. R., Amundson, D. E., & Haas, E. (1995, October 9–13). *Warnings in medicine*. Panel presentation at the 39th annual meeting of the Human Factors and Ergonomics Society, San Diego, CA.

Coward, R. T., & Cutler, S. J. (1989). Informal and formal health care systems for the rural elderly. *HSR: Health Services Research, 23*(6), 785–806.

Enders, A. (1991). Rehabilitation and technology—Self-help approaches to technology: An independent living (IL) model for rehabilitation. *International Journal of Technology and Aging, 4*(2), 141–152.

Epstein, C. F. (1990). Wheelchair management: Developing a system for long term care facilities. *Journal of Long Term Care Administration, 8,* 1–12.

Gitlin, L. N., Levine, R., & Geiger, C. (1993). Adaptive device use by older adults with mixed disabilities. *Archives of Physical Medicine and Rehabilitation, 74,* 149–152.

Gosbee, J. W. (1996 in press). *Human factors engineering and telemedicine.* (a Technical Report). Rockville, MD: U. S. Office of Rural Health Policy.

Greenberger, M., & Puffer, J. C. (1989). Telemedicine: Toward better health care for the elderly. *Journal of Communication, 39*(3), 137–144.

Grigsby, J., Sandberg, E. J., Kaehny, M. M., Kramer, A. M., Schlenker, R. E., & Shaughnessy, P. W. (1994, May). *Analysis of expansion of access to care through use of telemedicine and mobile health services.* Denver, CO: Center for Health Policy Research.

Holm, M. B., & Rogers, J. C. (1991). High, low, or no assistive technology devices for older adults undergoing rehabilitation. *International Journal of Technology and Aging, 4*(2), 153–162.

Hubble, J. P., Pahwa, R., Michalek, D. K., Thomas, C., & Koller, W. C. (1993). Interactive video conferencing: A means of providing interim care to Parkinson's Disease patients. *Movement Disorders, 8*(3), 380–382.

Kahan, J. S. (1991, January). The Safe Medical Devices Act of 1990. *Medical Device and Diagnostic Industry,* pp. 30–38.

Kelly, R. T., Callan, J. R., & Meadows, S. K. (1991). Impact of new medical technology on user performance. In *Proceedings of the Human Factors Society 32nd annual meeting* (pp. 699–702). Santa Monica, CA: Human Factors Society.

Koncelik, J. (1982). *Aging and the product environment.* Florence, KY: Scientific and Academic Additions.

Kovar, M. G., & La Croix, A. Z. (1987). Aging in the eighties: Ability to perform work-related activities. In *Advance data from vital and health statistics* (No. 136, DHHS Publication No. PHS87-1250). Hyattsville, MD: National Center for Health Statistics.

Lassey, W. R., & Lassey, M. L. (1985). Physical health status of the rural elderly. In R. T. Coward & G. R. Lee (Eds.), *The elderly in rural society: Every fourth elder* (pp. 83–104). New York: Springer.

Laux, L. (1994). Visual interpretation of blood glucose test strips. *The Diabetes Educator, 20*(1), 41–44.

Lonergan, E. T., & Krevans, J. R. (1991). Special report: A national agenda for research on aging. *New England Journal of Medicine, 324*(25), 1825–1828.

Mahoney, J., Euhardy, R., & Carnes, M. (1992). A comparison of a two-wheeled walker and a three-wheeled walker in a geriatric population. *Journal of the American Geriatric Society, 40,* 208–212.

Mann, W. C., Hurren, D., & Tomita, M. (1993). Comparison of assistive device use and needs of home-based older persons with different impairments. *American Journal of Occupational Therapy, 47*(11), 980–987.

Mann, W. C., Karuza, J., & Hurren, D. (1992, December). Assistive devices for home-based elderly persons with stroke. *Topics in Geriatric Rehabilitation, 8*(2), 35–52.

Nayak, U. S. L. (1995, January). Elders-led design. *Ergonomics in design* (pp. 8–13).

Nevitt, M. C., Cummings, S. R., Kidd, S., & Black, D. (1989). Risk factors for recurrent nonsyncopal falls: A prospective study. *JAMA, Journal of the American Medical Association, 261,* 2663–2668.

Norton, C. H., & McManus, M. A. (1989). Background tables on demographic characteristics, health status, and health services utilization. *Health Services Research, 23,* 726–755.

Obradovich, J. H., & Woods, D. D. (1994). Users as designers: How people cope with poor HCI design in computer-based medical devices. In *Proceedings of the Human Factors and Ergonomics Society 38th annual meeting* (pp. 710–714). Santa Monica, CA: Human Factors and Ergonomics Society.

O'Leary, S., Mann, C., & Perkash, I. (1991). Access to computers for older adults: Problems and solutions. *American Journal of Occupational Therapy, 45*(7), 636–642.

Page, M., Galer, M., Fitzgerald, J., & Feeney, R. J. (1980). Problems of the selection, provision, and use of aids. In J. Bray & S. Wright (Eds.), *The use of technology in the care of the elderly and the disabled* (pp. 119–129). London: Frances Pinter.

Redford, J. B. (1993). Seating and wheeled mobility in the disabled elderly population. *Archives of Physical Medicine and Rehabilitation, 74,* 877–885.

Regnier, V., & Pynoos, J. (Eds.). (1987). *Housing the aged: Design directives and policy considerations.* New York: Elsevier.

Small, A. (1987). Design for older people. In G. Salvendy (Ed.), *Handbook of human factors* (pp. 495–504). New York: Wiley.

Smith, D. B. D. (1990). Human factors and aging: An overview of research needs and application opportunities. *Human Factors, 32*(5), 509–526.

Soldo, B. J., & Longino, C. F., Jr. (1988). Social and physical environments. In *The social and built environment in an older society* (pp. 103–183). Washington, DC: National Academy Press, National Research Council, Institute of Medicine.

Stahl, S. M. (1984). Health. In D. J. Mangen & W. A. Peterson (Eds.), *Research instruments in social gerontology: Vol. 3. Health, program evaluation, and demography* (pp. 85–116). Minneapolis: University of Minnesota Press.

Tiderksaar, R. (1989). *Falling in old age: Its prevention and treatment.* New York: Springer.

Wiklund, M. E. (1992, August). Designing medical devices for older users. *Medical Device & Diagnostic Industry,* pp. 78–83.

Wolfson, L., Whipple, R., Amerman, P., & Tobin, J. N. (1990, January). Gait assessment in the elderly: A gait abnormality rating scale and its relation to falls. *Journal of Gerontology, 45*(1), M12–M19.

Chapter 11

Medication Adherence and Aging

Denise C. Park
Timothy R. Jones

INTRODUCTION

Much of the current focus of health research is on the development of treatments and medications to treat various disorders. Many common health problems—heart disease, hypertension, some forms of arthritis, and a broad range of mental disorders to name a few—can be treated very successfully with medication. An obvious aspect of a successful treatment is that the individual being treated takes the medication as prescribed. The failure to take medicine as prescribed is termed *medication nonadherence* or *medication noncompliance*. Medication nonadherence can take a variety of forms. Individuals may not take the medication at all; they may omit some doses; they may take extra doses or extra quantities within a dose; or they may take it at improper times, in the wrong combination, or without following special instructions associated with the medication (Park, 1992).

There is little doubt that medication nonadherence is a serious problem, particularly for older adults, because they consume the greatest proportion of prescription medications in this country. Gryfe and Gryfe (1984) found that 84% of elderly Medi-Cal patients took at least one prescription drug,

Handbook of Human Factors and the Older Adult

whereas Kiernan and Isaacs (1981) reported that elderly adults living independently took an average of 2.9 medications per individual. The accurate usage of medications is a particular concern for older adults, not only because of the high medication usage by this age group but also because older adults are considerably more susceptible to side effects and drug interactions from medications than younger adults, as medications metabolize far less rapidly in this population (Jernigan, 1984).

Robbins (1990) stated in a recent Schering report that nonadherence to medications is a $100 billion a year problem for the United States in terms of lost productivity and extra annual medical costs. Given this figure, it is not surprising that nonadherence appears to be a significant contributor to hospital admissions, particularly for older adults. Col, Fanale, and Kronholm (1990) reported that 11.4% of elderly hospital admissions for acute care were due directly to noncompliance, and an additional 16.8% were admitted due to adverse drug reactions. Similarly, Grymonpre, Mitenko, Sitar, Aoki, and Montgomery (1988) reported that 19% of hospital admissions of older adults were drug-related admissions. Of these, they reported that 27% were due to intentional nonadherence and an additional 10% to inadvertent medication errors.

An extensive literature documents the problem of nonadherence. Also dozens of studies have attempted to determine causes of nonadherence and potential interventions to improve it. Most of this work has been conducted within a medical model framework by health care professionals. It is becoming increasingly clear that medication adherence is an extraordinarily complex behavior and that effective interventions to improve adherence can be developed only to the extent that we understand mechanisms underlying the behavior. Recently, behavioral models of adherence have been developed (Park, 1992, 1994) that include a range of constructs hypothesized to predict adherence. A proposed hypothetical model for adherence appears in Figure 1.

This model suggests that three key constructs predict medication adherence: (1) the patient's representation of his or her illness, (2) the patient's cognitive function, and (3) external cues or strategies used by the patient to enhance medication-taking behavior. For example, the model might predict that the adherence of an elderly man with severe hypertension might be predicted by the following three factors: how seriously ill he thought he was and whether he understood that taking the medication might prevent a stroke (illness representation), whether he comprehended and remembered the instructions associated with the medication (cognitive function), and whether he developed a strategy of placing his medications in an organizer for memory assistance (external aid). This model is a revision of one presented earlier by Park (1992) and will be used as the organizational basis for

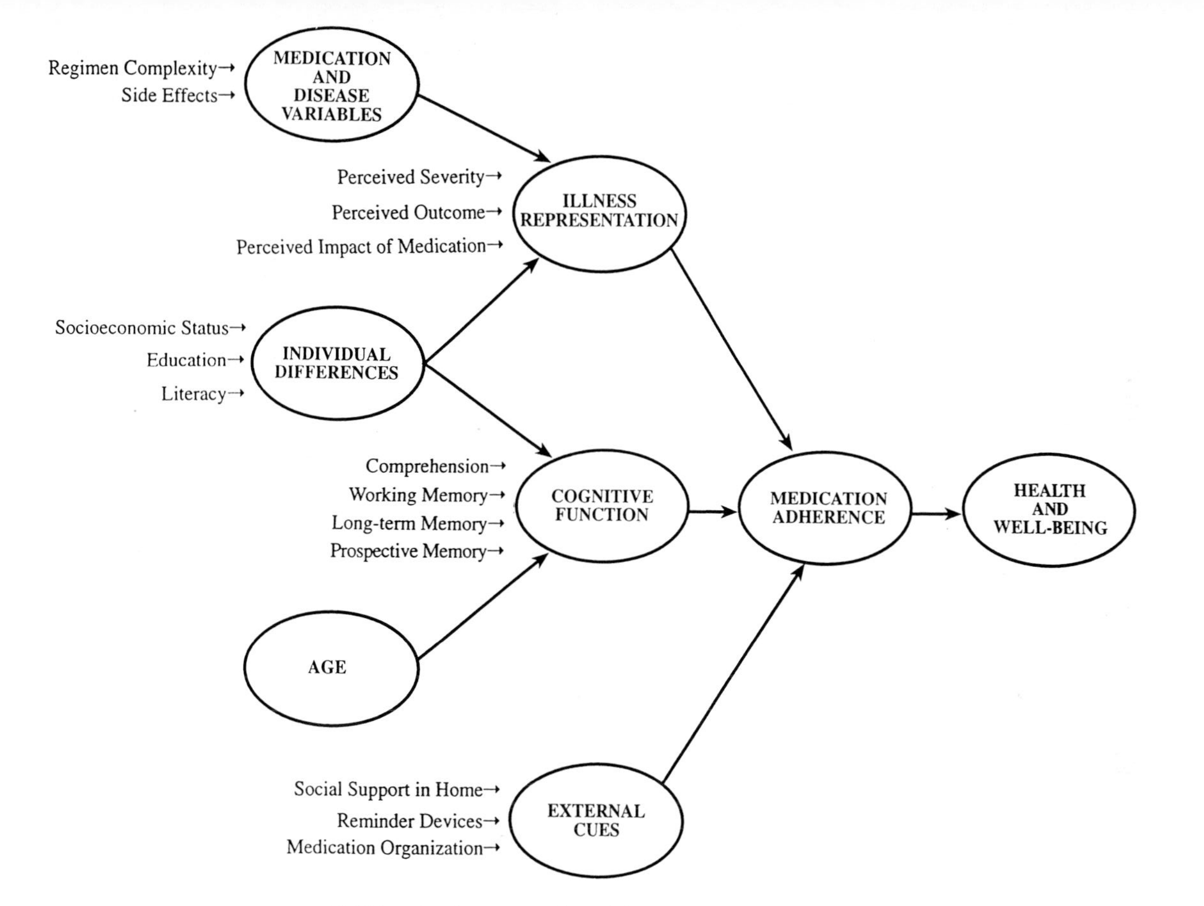

FIGURE 1 A conceptual model of medication adherence.

the present chapter and for reviewing and discussing human factors interventions to improve adherence.

In the proposed model, illness representation—that is, the patient's perception of his or her illness—is hypothesized to play a much more important role in determining medication adherence than objective disease variables. This is consistent with the earlier views of Leventhal and Cameron (1987). The severity of an illness, actual side effects from a drug, and the objective limits an illness may place on one's desired activity are hypothesized to shape an individual's perceptions and beliefs about an illness. Beliefs about the illness rather than objective symptoms and severity predict adherence behavior (Park & Mayhom, in press). If an individual does not believe he or she is ill or if the medication prescribed for the illness is perceived to be ineffective, nonadherence is likely to occur regardless of objective symptoms. Individual difference variables such as socioeconomic status, literacy, and education will also shape the individual's beliefs about illness and medications and may contribute to nonadherence indirectly through the illness representation. Illness representation is typically measured indirectly by preparing a battery of questionnaires that address the indicators presented in Figure 1, such as how seriously ill an individual perceives himself or herself to be, what he or she expects the trajectory of the disorder will be, and how the individual perceives adherence to medication will affect disease course and physical function.

Age is expected to function primarily through cognitive factors, as age-related decline in processing ability is a well-documented phenomenon (Salthouse, 1991). The amount of cognitive resources available to an individual, in some circumstances, will determine whether he or she is able to comprehend and remember a complex medication regimen. An individual who does not understand or remember a medication regimen cannot adhere to it. Compensatory strategies and external cues for taking medications are also viewed as an important component of medication adherence in the model. Social support in the home is included as an external cue because partners frequently play a role in reminding an individual to take medications (Doherty, Schrott, Metcalf, & Iasiello-Vailas, 1983; Lorence & Branthewaite, 1993; Schwartz, Wand, Zeitz, & Goss, 1962). It should be recognized that the model assumes that medication adherence is a good thing and leads to health and well-being, although there are many disorders, such as osteoarthritis, for which it has never been determined that adherence to prescribed medications improves outcomes (Park, 1994).

Finally, it is important to recognize in the present discussion that medication adherence is not necessarily a global behavior. In other words, an individual may be selectively nonadherent; that is, an individual may take one medication with a high degree of accuracy but behave in an extremely nonadherent fashion with another (Park, Morrell, Frieske, Gaines, & Lautenschlager, 1993; Park, Willis, Morrow, Diehl, & Gaines, 1994). We hypothesize that this occurs because individuals with multiple disorders have unique illness representations for each disorder they are experiencing (Park & Mayhorn, in press). Thus, a medication prescribed for a perceived serious disorder (e.g., heart disease) might have a high rate of adherence; while the same individual might be extraordinarily nonadherent with a medication for another disorder he or she perceives to be less serious or for which they believe the medication is less effective.

From the preceding discussion, it should be evident that effective interventions that improve adherence may differ depending on what component of the conceptual model is contributing to the nonadherence. The model is congruent with a human factors approach as human factors specialists typically are very concerned with designing materials and interventions specific to the mechanism that results in suboptimal performance. Until recently, researchers have typically approached the problem of nonadherence in an either/or fashion—assuming that it was primarily a beliefs problem and examining the role of education and counseling interventions or assuming that it was primarily a cognitive problem and examining the role of memory aids and other supports. We have used a holistic approach congruent with the Figure 1 model in our laboratory to understand and improve medication adherence, thus encompassing all aspects of the model. The focus of this chapter will be primarily on how devices and design can improve medication adherence, with an emphasis on what mechanism displayed in Figure 1 the recommended design or device operates. We will initially discuss measurement of adherence behaviors, an area where great strides have been made, and then discuss causes of nonadherence. This will be followed by a detailed review of human factors-based interventions designed to improve adherence.

MEASUREMENT OF ADHERENCE

The study of medication adherence is complicated by a number of factors. First, taking medication is essentially a private behavior that cannot be observed in a laboratory setting. Hence, all techniques for measuring the behavior have some degree of inaccuracy. Second, medication adherence may be a reactive behavior, such that the awareness that medication events are being monitored may change the behavior. Even when devices that permit surreptitious measurement are available, human subject committees generally require that subjects be told their medication-taking behavior is being monitored, so this is a concern permeating all recent medication adherence research. Third, it is not clear what constitutes a meaningful operationalization of nonadherence or nonadherence errors. Are subjects nonadherent if they take medication a few hours late? Should subjects be classified as nonadherent if they take 85% of their medication correctly, when only 80% adherence is required for the drug to have a clinical effect? Fourth, nonadherence is a dynamic behavior that occurs over time. In a typical adherence study, a large quantity of data is aggregated and the statistical techniques used in analysis are not necessarily well suited to capturing the dynamic nature and changes in the behavior over time. A detailed discussion of the measurement of adherence is presented by Rudd and Marshall (1990), Dunbar (1980), and Park et al. (1993).

There are a number of techniques for recording or estimating adherence behavior. All have problems. As Rudd (1979, p. 627) noted, "The ideal standard would be simultaneously unobtrusive (to avoid patient sensitization and maximize cooperation), objective (to produce discrete and reproducible data for each subject), and practical (to maximize portability and minimize cost)." One option for measuring adherence is to use biological assays to detect traces of a medication in the blood or urine, but this measure falls short on the grounds that it does not permit a very accurate assessment of adherence and is also intrusive. Such measures typically provide only evidence that some unknown quantity of a drug was taken within some broad time frame. Thus, they do not permit precise estimates of adherence behavior (Deyo, 1982; Dunbar, 1980).

Another widely used technique is that of pill counts, in which the amount of medication remaining in a bottle is used to estimate how many doses subjects took relative to the prescribed dosage. Rudd et al. (1989) consider this measure problematic, reporting evidence of pill-dumping just prior to appointments, a finding also reported by Rand et al. (1992). Moreover, this technique does not permit accurate measurement of the time course of adherence.

A third technique is self-report. Dunbar, Dunning, and Dwyer (1989) argue that self-reports of adherence can be accurate if interviews are carefully structured, but this view is disputed by Paulson, Krause, and Iber (1977), who compared biological markers to verbal reports and found gross discrepancies, with subjects reporting more adherence than actually occurred. Rand et al. (1992) reported a similar finding when pill counts were compared to verbal reports.

Park, Morrell, Frieske, and Kincaid (1992) used bar-coding technology to measure adherence, a technique suggested by Leirer, Morrow, Pariante, and Sheikh (1988). With this technique, subjects are given a small, credit-card size "time wand" and each medication is assigned a bar code. Subjects scan with the time wand each time they take a medication, recording the date and time that the medication is taken. The data are uploaded by the experimenter after the subject returns the wand. This provides accurate data, but does not meet the Rudd (1979) gold standard for an unobtrusive measure.

The most exciting advance in the measurement of adherence has been the introduction of microelectronic monitors housed invisibly in medication bottle caps. The date and time are recorded each time the medication bottle is opened, providing unobtrusive, accurate adherence data. The best known example of this is the medication event monitoring system (MEMS) distributed by the Aprex Corporation in Fremont, California. A comparison of MEMS to pill counts and verbal reports indicated rates of adherence of 69.85, 92.00, and 98.99%, respectively (Waterhouse, Calzone, Mele, & Brenna, 1993). This suggests that both verbal reports and pill counts provide underestimates of rates of nonadherence. Rudd, Ahmed, Zachary, Barton, and Bonduelle (1992) also reported evidence that pill counts provided gross underestimates of nonadherence relative to the accuracy of monitors. In contrast to this finding, however, Matsui et al. (1994) reported equivalent findings when comparing MEMS to pill counts. Based on patients' verbal reports about their use of MEMS, the researchers were particularly concerned that patients removed pills from the MEMS system in quantity and then took them at a later time. In a recent study just completed in our laboratory, we found that the MEMS system and the bar-code based time wand system yielded equivalent rates of nonadherence in a group of osteoarthritis patients (Park, Morrell et al., 1994), suggesting the general accuracy and comparability of the two microelectronic monitoring devices to one another.

Although the microelectronic systems are not without problems, they have yielded detailed information about patterns of medication-taking behavior over time that have been difficult to document to date. Feinstein (1990) coined the term *white coat adherence,* based on MEMS data. That is, patients tend to take medication accurately just before or after a visit to a physician, with adherence declining in the interim. This phenomenon was also documented by Cramer, Scheyer, and Mattson (1990). As a result of data from MEMS, Urquhart and Chevalley (1988) discuss the construct of a "drug holiday." This is a complete absence of medication-taking behavior for three days or more, which they suggest occurs in about 20% of patients. Kruse, Rampmaier, Ullrich, and Weber (1994) reported that subjects were more likely to omit doses on weekends, perhaps isolating the most likely time for a drug holiday. Kruse et al. (1994) also noted better adherence for morning compared to evening doses. This time-of-day effect was demonstrated by Leirer, Tanke, and Morrow (1994) in a study of prospective memory for simulated medication and appointment adherence, with memory reported to be better in the morning rather than later in the day. It is possible that the cognitive system of older adults functions better in the morning. May, Hasher, and Stoltzfus (1993) found that the vast majority of older adults rate themselves as being morning people, and that these subjects performed better on a recognition memory task when tested in the morning. Finally, in our own lab, we have found evidence for "selective adherence," where patients accurately take one medication but are highly nonadherent with another (Park, Willis et al., 1994).

More in-depth discussions of the measurement of adherence can be found from other sources. Nevertheless, it is important to note that these advances in the measurement of adherence behavior are important to the study of human factors related to the behavior. Previously, it was difficult to document reliably the impact of an intervention or design improvement proposed to facilitate adherence. With the advent of precise monitoring techniques, we can now measure the impact not only on global levels of adherence but also on specific behavioral configurations that are problematic, such as the drug holiday or omissions primarily in the evening hours. The precision with which the behavior can now be measured lends itself to the development of refined interventions.

FACTORS AFFECTING ADHERENCE

Medication and Disease Variables

As shown in Figure 1, variables such as regimen complexity and medication side effects are hypothesized to operate indirectly by affecting the illness representation. In a medical model view of adherence, factors such as these are believed to affect adherence directly, and hence, a considerable amount of work has been done on these topics, particularly regimen complexity.

Regimen Complexity

Regimen complexity can be defined as how many medication events are prescribed for a patient in a day, and it can be a function of either taking many medications or taking only a few medications that have complex schedules and must be taken three or four times a day. Also some medications have very odd dosing schedules, where large quantities of pills are taken only once or twice a week (e.g., methotrexate for rheumatoid arthritis), which result in complex rules regarding the medication schedule. It is widely believed that nonadherence increases with regimen complexity and that the elderly are particularly susceptible to these effects. The mechanism by which elderly adults are believed to be susceptible to regimen effects is primarily cognitive—as there are more medication events to integrate and remember, performance deteriorates due to the high cognitive load associated with complexity.

The evidence with respect to the interaction of aging with complexity is mixed but generally is not strongly supportive of the hypothesis that older adults are particularly susceptible to complexity effects. Using verbal reports, Bergman and Wilholm (1981) found that reported nonadherence increased with regimen complexity for elderly adults but not for young adults. Blackwell (1979) reviewed the literature on adherence and complexity and concluded that increased dosing (up to three times a day) did not affect adherence but that an increased number of medications beyond a total of three caused nonadherence to increase sharply. Law and Chalmers (1976) suggested that the elderly have particular problems developing strategies for taking medications when the medication load becomes complex. Shimp and Ascione (1985) also suggest that complexity increases noncompliance, particularly for the elderly, when multiple illnesses may also play a role, but do not present data.

Despite the inconclusive findings associated with aging, it does appear that complexity exerts an overall effect. In perhaps the most convincing study to date, Kruse, Eggert-Kruse, Rampmaier, Runnebaum, and Weber (1991) studied adherence to estradiol in a group of female outpatients being treated for primary infertility. Patients were prescribed the medications twice or four times daily, and the MEMS system was used for precise recording of behavior. Kruse et al. (1991) reported that compliance was 85% for those prescribed two daily doses, but 67% for those with four daily doses. Similarly, Botelho and Dudrak (1992) found that adherence in an elderly sample for those prescribed once or twice daily medications was 72%, in contrast to 54% for drugs to be taken three or four times daily. Because young adults were not tested in this study, whether or not age is interactive with complexity was not determined.

Overall, relatively scant data are available on the role of regimen complexity and adherence. It is an appealing hypothesis that older adults will have more problems as regimen complexity increases due to declines in cognitive function, but this is not our own observation. In our own laboratory, we do not find strong effects of regimen complexity when MEMS or time wands are used, particularly with the elderly. We have noted that older adults taking a very large number of prescriptions (6 to 12) frequently organize their lives around taking the medications. These individuals usually have substantial health problems and management of their healthy may be a primary task for them, as most of these individuals do not work. One might expect complexity to be an important factor only when strategies are not used to take medications, when a medication regimen is new, or when an illness representation is not compatible with taking medications.

Side Effects

Little is known about the role perceived side effects play in medication adherence. Maddox, Levi, and Thompson (1994) reported that significant amounts of nonadherence occurred for antidepressants, both tricyclics and selective seratonin reuptake inhibitors (SSRIs). A total of 52% of the patients ceased treatment after 10–12 weeks, and of these, 30% reported unpleasant side effects as the primary reason. In our laboratory, we interview patients for perceived side effects of medications. Preliminary data indicate that arthritis patients do not frequently report the occurrence of side effects, even when probed for more information. To date, we have been unable to get enough variance in reported side effects to use this as a predictor in regression equations for nonadherence. It may be that patients stop taking medications relatively quickly if they have unacceptable side effects and that only prospective studies of the sort conducted by Maddox et al. (1994) will permit a determination of their role in adherence.

Illness and Medication Representation

This is a complex topic, which was introduced at the beginning of this chapter. As Figure 1 suggests, beliefs about illness and medications have a strong impact on medication adherence. In a recent study, we found that the belief that an individual is not likely to get sick in the future was a strong predictor of nonadherence in hypertensives (Morrell, Park, & Kidder, 1995). We have also found that in addition to beliefs about illness, beliefs about medications are important in predicting adherence. For example, subjects who endorsed the statement "My doctor should have prescribed less of this medication for me" were found to be significantly nonadherent, although these same subjects reported, when asked directly, that they accurately took the medication in question (Park, Morrell et al., 1994). A detailed discussion of the role of illness and medication representation are well beyond the scope of this chapter but are treated extensively in Park (1994) and Park and Kidder (1996). Also, the relationship of cognitive variables to belief systems and adherence is discussed in detail in Park and Mayhorn (in press). For the purposes of the present chapter, it is important to keep in mind the role of the patient's beliefs system in conjunction with the human factors perspective. Devices based on a human factors approach that improve ease of use of the medication by modifying instructions or labels, adding reminders, organizing information, and the like will be of little value if the individual's illness and medication representations are not consistent with taking the medication. A great deal of emphasis is placed on patient education, designed to shape an illness representation that will motivate the patient to adhere. More discussion of this issue will occur later in this chapter when interventions are discussed.

Individual Difference Variables

Individual difference variables that have frequently been hypothesized to affect medication adherence relate to education and socioeconomic status, as shown in Figure 1. The premise here is that, with lower education and poor literacy, individuals will have illness representations inconsistent with adherence, due to poor understanding of their disorder, and will also be limited in their ability to comprehend and remember medication information. Although age is traditionally considered an individual difference variable, and could be displayed in Figure 1 as such, due to the centrality of interest in this topic and the potentially large effect associated with age, it is treated as a separate construct in the model.

Socioeconomic Status, Illiteracy, and Education

The data are not entirely clear with respect to the impact of socioeconomic status and education (with the concomitant factor of illiteracy in cases of limited education) on medication adherence. LeSage and Zwygart-Stauffacher (1988) reported an impact of financial difficulties on nonadherence. The failure of Medicare to cover the cost of prescription drugs is widely perceived to be a primary factor in nonadherence and is frequently brought up as a concern about causes of nonadherence in our conversations with practicing physicians. The impact of low socioeconomic status on adherence is likely to have been underestimated in many of the adherence studies, because subjects would not be admitted to most of the studies described here if they had not initially filled their prescriptions. At the same time, failure to fill prescriptions for socioeconomic reasons is not something that can be remedied by a human factors approach, so this will not be treated in great detail here.

Of greater concern to the human factors specialist is the potential that illiteracy and low education contribute to difficulties in following a prescription regimen. For example, Levy, Mermelstein, and Hemo (1982) reported that a low level of education and nonprofessional employment were significant predictors of hospital admissions that occurred due to nonadherence. They hypothesized that this is due to a poor understanding of the consequences of nonadherence as well as an incorrect understanding of how to take the medications. Illiteracy is a particular concern for adherence behaviors, as illiteracy results in decreased access to the information about when and how to take medications. Interventions that address the issue of illiteracy will be discussed later in this chapter.

Age

Despite the commonly held belief that older adults are more nonadherent than young adults, little evidence actually supports this perspective. Many studies on adherence focus only on elderly subjects, partially because the elderly are easily isolated as a group using many medications. However, this focus on the elderly does not permit age-graded comparisons of adherence. Absolute rates of nonadherence for elderly adults taking multiple medications appear to be high. Using a pill count procedure, Botelho and Dudrak (1992) found that 54.7% of a mixed group of elderly outpatients were nonadherent to their medication regimen at an overall compliance level of 80%. Neely and Patrick (1968), measured adherence in the elderly with self-reports and arrived at a nonadherence rate of 54% for a combination of commission, omission, dosage, time, and reason errors. Similarly, White (1980) used pill counts for psychoactive drugs taken by elderly subjects and reported nonadherence rates of 48% at an overall compliance level of 85%. These relatively high rates of nonadherence suggest that older adults not only fail to take a significant amount of their medication but also commit a significant number of commission, dosage, time, and reason errors.

A few studies make age comparisons. Bergman and Wilholm (1981) interviewed subjects prior to hospital admission who were taking three or more drugs on a regular basis. They found that elderly adults on multiple medications reported higher levels of nonadherence than young adults. Green, Mullen, and Stainbrook (1986, p. 59) reviewed 10 studies of the effect of age on adherence and concluded that there is "no conclusive or consistent evidence that the elderly (over 65) are less compliant than younger cohorts of patients." Richardson, Simons-Morton, and Annegers (1993) reported that nonadherence to a hypertension regimen was predicted by age, but that the young subjects were more nonadherent. In our own laboratory, we have found that age can predict nonadherence, but only at the extreme end. Park et al. (1992), used bar-code technology to measure adherence in old adults taking three or more medications and reported that old-old adults (over age 77) were significantly more nonadherent than young-old adults (ages 60–76). Congruent with this finding, Park, Morrell et al. (1994) found that with a group of hypertensive adults, the old-old adults were the most nonadherent. However, the next most nonadherent group was middle-aged adults. We have consistently found that young-old adults (ages 60–75) are among the most adherent of all subjects. We believe this is because young-old adults have both the cognitive function and the motivation (e.g., perceived vulnerability to disability and death), as well as the time, to take steps to see that medications are taken accurately (Park, 1994).

Therefore, it seems likely that age is not necessarily a strong predictor of nonadherence except at the extreme end. From a human factors perspective, however, age is quite relevant to designing interventions. The types of interventions that will support adherence in a very old population may be quite different from those that will support adherence in a younger population, as it is more likely that declining cognitive and sensory function is the basis for nonadherence in the very old compared to other age groups.

Sensorimotor Function

Although not presented in Figure 1, sensory function is an important construct in medication adherence that would be hypothesized to operate through aging and cognitive function. It is well documented that there are declines in the visual and auditory system associated with normal aging (Botwinick, 1984). With age, there is a decrease of visual acuity, a decrease in pupil size, and a clouding and loss of elasticity of the lens. These changes result in a number of difficulties for the elderly, including increased sensitivity to glare, difficulty focusing on near objects, loss of contrast sensitivity, diminished color vision, and slowed dark adaptation. All of these changes have implications for the use of medications and undoubtedly contribute to adherence errors. For example, the elderly may have problems reading information presented on a prescription label due to glare or problems with contrast sensitivity and focus. Moreover, difficulty in making color or shape discriminations may be a particular problem that contributes to nonadherence in older adults (LeSage & Zwygart-Stauffacher, 1988). Shimp and Ascione (1988) suggested that older adults are most likely to confuse blue and green tablets and yellow and white tablets and that, if possible, these colors should not be mixed in a prescription regimen. Kendrick and Bayne (1982) studied the ability of older adults to discriminate tablets of different colors and found older adults were often unable to see a difference among pills that were different shades of yellow. Similarly, Hurd and Butkovich (1986) found that older adults made more color discrimination errors of pills than young adults and that 6 of 14 subjects had difficulty discriminating capsule sizes. However, Botelho and Dudrak (1992) have reported that visual acuity did not predict nonadherence in a group of elderly patients, although they did not collect complete measures of visual function. Thus, the relationship of poor visual function to nonadherence seems plausible; but to date, there is strong evidence for a relationship, mainly because little data exist on the topic.

In addition to visual difficulties, older adults may also experience motor difficulties that may be problematic with respect to adherence. Nearly all older adults suffer from some degree of osteoarthritis, and this may limit hand strength and ability to manipulate fingers. Several researchers have found that older adults have difficulty opening containers with childproof lids (Hurd & Butkovich, 1986; Kendrick & Bayne, 1982). This problem can be surmounted by requesting screw-off caps when prescriptions are filled. Gallez, Bird, Wright, and Bennett (1984) found that a bottle with a wing-shaped cap on an undulated base was easiest to open for arthritis patients, and this design likely would be an improvement over traditional medication caps.

Cognitive Processing of Medication Information

Perhaps the area where human factors specialists can have the greatest impact is on the information processing aspects of medication adherence. As Park (1992) notes and as shown in Figure 1, accurate medication adherence has a number of cognitive components, including (1) the comprehension of the medication instructions, (2) organization of the individual medication instructions into a medication plan, that is, a temporal sequence that integrates multiple medications and doses, (3) retention of the medication plan, and (4) remembering to take the medication at the planned time. Much of the age-related variance that occurs in medication adherence is likely mediated through cognitive function, a relationship displayed in Figure 1.

Considerable evidence shows that comprehension declines with age, particularly information that is inferential in nature (Cohen, 1981). This is an important issue with respect to medication adherence since the failure to understand what one is to do with medications precludes accurate adherence (Blackwell, 1979). Kendrick and Bayne (1982) asked elderly adults to interpret what *take every six hours* means and found that only 22% could translate this into an accurate medication plan. Hurd and Butkovich (1986) reported that 10 of 14 older adults made one or more errors when asked to interpret four medication labels, with half of the adults making seven errors. Morrell, Park, and Poon (1988) presented community-dwelling older adults with medication instructions for an actual elderly patient and asked them to develop a plan for taking the medications. They reported that about 25% of the information was incorrectly comprehended when translated into a medication plan. Diehl, Willis, and Schaie (1995) report a similar finding. They have developed a drug label comprehension test and report that older adult subjects answer about 80% of the questions correctly, with the biggest problems relating to information requiring inferences, such as the need for refills and how long medications will last. Education, family income, and cognitive ability scores predicted comprehension. In addition, the number of days hospitalized was a negative predictor of comprehension, so that those individuals who were hospitalized the most had the poorest understanding of their medication regimen, although comprehension was not related to adherence, as measured by pill counts. Levy et al. (1982) reported that both poor comprehension and forgetfulness played a significant role in drug-related hospitalization among less educated elderly patients. Overall, there is some evidence that comprehension of their medication regimen is poor among older adults; and limited data suggest that this poor comprehension is related to nonadherence.

Other research, however, has suggested that older adults have a similar schema for taking medications when compared to young adults. Morrow,

Leirer, Andrassy, Tanke, and Stine (in press) and Morrow, Leirer, Altieri, and Tanke (1991) reported that older adults' schema for organizing medication information and taking medications is the same as that for young adults. They reported that instructions organized in a manner compatible with subjects' mental models for taking medication were better comprehended than those that were inconsistent. Overall, more research is warranted in the area of comprehension and medication adherence, particularly in less-educated samples, as this may be the high risk group where effects of poor comprehension on adherence are likely to emerge.

It is well documented that many aspects of memory declines with age (Light, 1991; Salthouse, 1991). Deficits in working-memory function (the ability to simultaneously store and process information on-line) may contribute to problems in organizing complex medication information, resulting in what is apparently poor comprehension of a regimen (Park, 1992; Park & Kidder, 1996). Declines in long-term memory may affect older adults' ability to remember what they are to do with a medication plan once they have developed one. Ley et al. (1976) reported that age did correlate with increased forgetting of information. Morrell et al. (1988) found that older adults remembered less information about a medication regimen presented for study than young adults, even when they received unlimited study time. These data suggest that older adults are disadvantaged in their ability to remember prescription information and that they do not compensate for deficits by increasing study time. More naturalistic studies are needed that examine what patients remember from encounters in physicians' offices and from instructions given to them that are directly relevant to their own health. Page, Verstraete, Robb, and Etzwiler (1981) found that of seven recommendations made to diabetic patients about their health, an average of only two was remembered. A greater understanding of the mental models (illness representation) older adults have regarding their medications would permit effective interventions and supports for declining cognition.

Another type of memory that has a critical impact on medication adherence is prospective memory; that is, remembering to perform planned actions in the future. Remembering to take medication at the appropriate time is an example of a prospective memory task. Prospective memory tied to a contextual cue or an event (such as taking medication with breakfast) does not appear to decline as much with age when compared to prospective memory that is time based, when a response must occur at a specific time, but is not cued by an event (Einstein & McDaniel, 1990; Park, Hertzog, Morrell, Kidder, & Mayhorn, 1994). Park and Kidder (1996) discuss the prospective aspects of medication-taking behavior in detail. They conclude that the retrospective aspects of taking medication (understanding and remembering the regimen) may influence subjects' prospective performance with respect to medication taking. Because of the time-based nature of medication adherence, this aspect of adherence may be a particularly difficult task for older adults that can be mitigated to some extent by tying the time-based task to an event. They also note that there is evidence that more salient prospective tasks are more likely to be remembered than less salient tasks (Kvavilashvili, 1987), so that in evaluating prospective behavior it becomes important to understand how concerned the individual is that the medication be taken accurately. Also, some illnesses provide internal cues (e.g., joint pain from arthritis), which may serve as an internal event-based cue that reminds subjects to take medication. For this reason, one would expect that painful conditions would have a higher adherence rate for medications than less painful conditions. Park and Mayhorn (in press) also note that the prospective aspect of medication adherence has a reality monitoring component to it. Subjects must remember if they actually took a medication at a given time or if they merely thought about taking it, a documented problem in taking medication accurately (Morse, Simon, & Balson, 1993). Hashtroudi, Johnson, and Chrosniak (1990) have demonstrated that older adults are less effective than young adults at reality monitoring, so this little-studied aspect of adherence could also contribute to poorer adherence rates in older adults.

Overall, there is substantial reason to believe that the cognitive aspects of medication adherence are an important element of this complex behavior. Given that older adults do evidence decline in a number of cognitive domains and that they do appear to comprehend and remember less about medication information than young adults, cognitive interventions would seem to be of importance for the elderly. Credibility is added to this conclusion when one considers that we have found in two field studies of adherence that the oldest old were the most nonadherent subjects (Park et al., 1992; Park, Morrell et al., 1994). Much of the human factors approach to medication adherence has focused on supporting and improving the cognitive aspects of adherence. We turn now to a discussion of intervention techniques for improving medication adherence. Although the primary focus will be on cognitive aspects of adherence, the interaction of these factors with interventions that operate on illness representation and other important components of adherence will not be neglected.

INTERVENTIONS OF IMPROVING MEDICATION ADHERENCE

Timing of Intervention

A small but emerging literature suggests that the time at which an adherence intervention occurs is important and that there may be different rates of adherence for acute versus chronic disorders. Haynes, Wang, and Gomes (1987) argue that adherence to short-term treatments such as antibiotics can be improved with clear instructions, reminders, and calendars, but suggest that it is much more difficult to improve adherence for chronic disorders. It would appear that patients who seek treatment for acute, short-term disorders such as an infection would be motivated to maintain medication adherence but may not be able to remember to do so, resulting in memory aids being an effective intervention. In contrast, patients with chronic disorders should be highly skilled in the development of workable strategies to remember medications, but may develop beliefs about their illness and medications over time that are inconsistent with adherence. Haynes et al. (1987) suggest that interventions for chronic disorders need to focus on the provision of feedback to patients, rewards, social support, and counseling. Essentially, Haynes et al. (1987) are arguing that interventions for acute disorders may need to be primarily cognitive, but for chronic disorders, operating on the illness representation component of Figure 1 may be more important. Kruse et al. (1994) suggest that interventions may be particularly critical for chronic patients at the beginning of treatment. They reported that an intervention in the form of feedback about blood pressure to hypertensive patients had a greater impact when it occurred at the time treatment was initiated than when administered to existing patients. In support of this point, Richardson et al. (1993) reported that longer duration of treatment was associated with higher rates of nonadherence in a group of hypertensive patients. In contrast to this finding, Lorence and Branthwaite (1993) found no difference in adherence rates as a function of short- versus long-term treatments, when comparing a group of subjects on antibiotics to a group of subjects who were primarily taking diuretics and hypertension medications. To date, the timing of an intervention has not received substantial attention. The studies recently conducted suggest that an intervention is likely to be more effective at the time of diagnosis, although the lack of adequate control conditions clouds this conclusion somewhat. More research is needed here, and the likelihood that different types of intervention may interact with disease course and chronicity must also be considered in future research.

Social Support

Although social support is not an intervention that can easily be provided to improve adherence in an individual, it is important that it be recognized that this can be an important aid to medication adherence. Specifically, growing evidence indicates that living with another individual—a spouse, partner, or family member—enhances medication adherence when compared to individuals living alone (Doherty et al., 1983; Lorence and Branthwaite, 1993;

Schwartz et al., 1962). It is not clear whether the improvement occurs because the presence of another individual helps to shape an illness representation that is more consonant with a desire to adhere or due to the reminder function that the presence of another can serve in helping the individual to adhere. We are systematically investigating the effects of social support in our laboratory and believe that it is more likely that it operates as a form of collaborative cognition, providing event-based prospective cues to take medication (Park & Mayhorn, in press).

Restructuring Beliefs

A discussion of how to restructure patient beliefs about disease and medications is well beyond the scope of the present chapter, which is focused primarily on human factors interventions. Nevertheless, a detailed literature examines the role of patient education and counseling in affecting outcomes of illness, and perhaps a few caveats should be noted. First, patient education, per se, will not necessarily improve adherence. Parker et al. (1984) presented arthritis patients with an intensive patient education program and noted increased reported pain and disability in the education group relative to a control group. They concluded that the education had sensitized patients to potential pain and disability. It is essential to recognize that any intervention must focus on creating an illness representation consonant with adherence and that the provision of more information and education to patients will not necessarily ensure this outcome without specific planning and structuring toward this goal. The work of Lorig and colleagues (1989) with arthritis patients provided strong evidence that counseling and education may improve the general construct of self-efficacy and subsequent adherence. Thus, the belief that an individual can manage a disorder may be an important underlying construct in an appropriate illness representation and successful medication adherence. Second, it appears that presenting patients with information inconsistent with existing beliefs may require detailed elaboration and explanation. Rice and Okun (1994) presented elderly arthritis patients with educational interventions that either affirmed or disconfirmed the patients' existing illness representations. Older patients were more likely to recognize and recall medical information congruent with their beliefs. Rice and Okun conclude that identification and understanding of a patients' prior beliefs is an important component of educational interventions. A more complete discussion of the role of self-regulation of disease and illness representation can be found in Leventhal and Cameron (1987) and Park (1994).

Feedback about the Impact of Adherence

Another intervention that may favorably affect adherence for some disorders is patient feedback. For a disorder like hypertension, where adherence to medication yields control of the disorder and where feedback about the patient's disease state is readily available, feedback appears to be a very effective way to maintain medication adherence (Marks & Malinowski, 1994). Kruse et al. (1994) reported that providing subjects with feedback about hypertension control improved adherence among hypertension patients. McKenney, Munroe, and Wright (1992) reported a similar finding except that they tested the improvement in adherence in conjunction with a digital cap that displayed the last time the cap was removed, so the effect of feedback was not assessed independently. In general, the use of feedback would appear to be a potent tool to develop a medication and illness representation consonant with adherence, but it needs to be recognized that feedback is often not possible. In fact, for some progressive chronic disorders (e.g., Parkinson's disease, rheumatoid arthritis), medications may slow continuing decline. Providing patients with evidence that function and disease are getting worse in the face of medication adherence might have a negative impact. Moreover, in other disorders, such as osteoarthritis, medication has no known impact on disease progression but instead controls symptoms, so no external feedback regarding the impact of adherence is available to the patient. Of course, in many instances the patient will receive internal feedback when medication successfully controls obvious symptoms such as pain, itching, or heart palpitations.

Information Processing Interventions

Information processing interventions designed to improve adherence may (1) involve a restructuring of medication information to make it easier to process, (2) take the form of a device that reorganizes the medications themselves, or (3) serve some type of reminder function to take medication. Initially we will discuss information restructuring interventions that improve comprehension of the regimen through improved instructions or labels. Then, interventions in the form of devices designed to improve comprehension as well as help organize the medication regimen in a temporal sequence will be presented. These include special packaging, calendars, and medication organizers. Finally, devices such as voice mail, digital caps, and beeping caps that focus primarily on serving as external reminders for the prospective act of taking medication will be discussed.

Design of Medication Labels and Instructions

The design of medication labels and instructions has received considerable attention lately. Morrow, Leirer, and Sheikh (1988) presented a systematic review of design principles for medication instructions based on findings from the cognitive aging literature. They suggested that instructions should be designed to be compatible with older adults' existing mental models for taking medication and advocate the dissemination of expanded instructions to older adults along with the limited information available from the prescription label. In general, they suggest that well-structured instructions that require the subject to make no inferences about medication usage are preferred, as older adults are particularly disadvantaged in this domain. Morrell, Park, and Poon (1989) presented older and younger adults with well-structured labels designed in a manner similar to that advocated by Morrow et al. (1988). They reported better comprehension and memory for the labels by both old and young adults when compared to labels presented as written for an actual patient.

Following up on these recommendations, Morrow et al. (1991) reported that older adults did have a common medication schema for taking medications and that memory for medication information improved as it became more compatible with the schema, a finding also reported by Morrow, Leirer, Andrassy, Tanke, and Stine (in press). In other work, Morrow, Leirer, and Altieri (1995) reported that a highly structured, organized list format for medication instructions facilitated comprehension in older adults and was also preferred by them. Although at present, no research directly links improved instructions or expanded instructions to actual adherence behaviors, Wogalter and Young (1994) have reported that young subjects were more likely than control subjects to follow instructions to wear plastic gloves when using glue to make a model airplane if these special instructions were displayed on a tag protruding from the glue bottle. Control subjects received only standard labels on the bottle. This finding suggests that labeling might improve adherence behaviors. Nevertheless, there is insufficient data and this remains an important research question that needs to be addressed.

Other research on instructions has focused on presenting label information in a pictorial format. It is a well-documented finding that picture recognition does not decline with age (Park, Puglisi, & Smith, 1986), so Morrell et al. (1989) investigated the possibility that pictorially based medication labels might facilitate memory for medication information. The labels are displayed in Figure 2. Results indicated that the pictorial labels did improve the memory of the information for young adults but older adults did better with highly structured verbal labels. Meisel and Kiely (1981) designed and used pictorial labels for an illiterate Native American sample and reported

Mixed Label

Pharmacy
No. 3014
M. Griffin

390 Broad Street
Athens, GA 30602
(404) 555-8888
Dr. Morrell
4/17/88

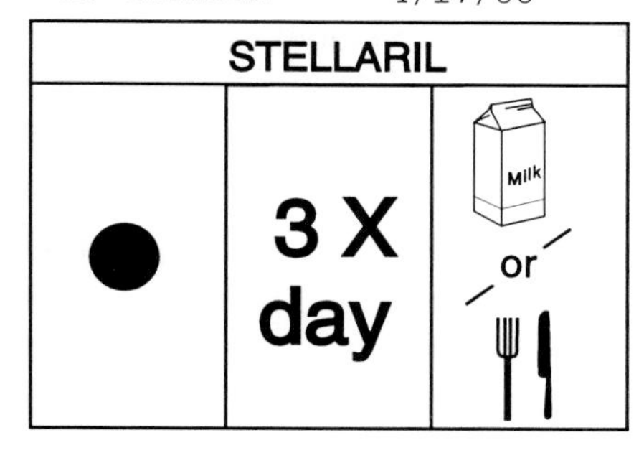

Verbal Label

Pharmacy
No. 3014
M. Griffin

390 Broad Street
Athens, GA 30602
(404) 555-8888
Dr. Morrell
4/17/88

Take 1 capsule
3 times a day
with milk or food
for blood pressure

Stellaril Refill 2

FIGURE 2 Examples of types of labels used in Morrell, Park, and Poon (1988).

the labels to be successful in an anecdotal account. Eustace, Johnson, and Gault (1982) designed nonverbal, symbol-based medication labels and reported them to be successful for patients with low vision or who were illiterate, but their account of improved adherence is also anecdotal. Other researchers have color-coded medications for illiterate patients in an effort to enhance adherence, and both Abel and Blackstone (1981) and Ow-Wing and Kerner (1981) report some success in this area. In general, the notion of redesigning labels with explicit pictorial symbols appears promising and worthy of further research, but data are insufficient to propose this as a successful support for adherence at this time.

Packaging

Packaging is a potentially innovative solution for problems of comprehension related to medication adherence. In addition to improving comprehension, packaging may also provide the patient with information about whether or not a prescribed dose has been taken if the individual is not sure. One common packaging solution is the use of blister packages that are cards or strips on which pills are placed and covered with clear plastic. The patient pushes the pill through to gain access to it. Detailed information can be provided on the blister pack about when the medication has been or should be taken, thus enhancing adherence. Linkewich, Catalano, and Flack (1974) examined the effects of blister packaging on adherence among young participants with a four-dose-per-day antibiotic and found that subjects receiving blister packs or blister packs along with a reminder calendar adhered better than those in a control condition. Extending this research to include elderly participants, Wong and Norman (1987) examined adherence rates for calendar blister packs compared to screw bottles over a three month period and then utilized a crossover design at the end of three months. They found strong evidence that blister packaging not only enhanced adherence, but also was considered easier to use than tamper-resistant containers. None of the elderly participants reported difficulties in using the blister packs. Both authors noted problems with portability of the strips as a potential barrier to adherence. This problem, of coarse, becomes exacerbated when multiple medications are required. Moreover, the advantages of blister packaging would seem to decline as numbers of medications increase, because the individual packages do not permit integration of different medications' dosing schedules. Thus, blister packaging may be a good solution for individuals taking one or at most two medications, but the support they provide for comprehension of the regimen is lost beyond that number.

Calendars and Medication Organizers

A number of investigators have examined the role that calendars and medications organizers can play in relieving the cognitive burden associated with comprehending and integrating multiple medication schedules to adhere to a medication regimen. Calendars alone restructure the medication information in a written form, typically along the temporal dimension, day by day, hour by hour, whereas medication organizers actually involve restructuring the locations of the medications themselves. When organizers are used, the medications are placed in a single container that has compartments structured to be congruent with times the medications are to be taken.

The use of calendars and related restructuring techniques has generally proven to be helpful. Moulding (1961) stapled pill packets to a calendar for Native Americans and reported enhanced adherence. Ascione and Shimp (1984) reported that a calendar was an effective reminder for improving adherence in the elderly, operating by improving knowledge about medication. MacDonald, MacDonald, and Phoenix (1977) found little evidence that a pill wheel or a tablet identification card improved adherence but found evidence that a tear-off calendar produced modest benefits. Gabriel, Gagnon, and Bryan (1977) also reported that providing geriatric hypertensive patients with a drug reminder chart improved adherence. Park et al. (1992), however, used electronic monitors and found no significant improvement in adherence in elderly adults relative to control subjects when the adherence aid was a calendar checkoff list that the individual could elect to receive in either poster or booklet form. One obvious problem with calendars is maintaining the proximity of the calendar to the medications to be taken.

Medication organizers circumvent this problem because the medications are placed in it. As a visit to any pharmacy counter will suggest, quite a range of secondary containers or medications organizers are designed presumably to enhance adherence. Some of the organizers may be quite confusing. To improve an individual's adherence, it is necessary that the organizer be loaded correctly. Park, Morrell, Frieske, Blackburn, and Birchmore (1991) examined the ability of arthritis patients to load three types of medication organizers accurately. They reported that the simplest container—one that merely had seven compartments, one for each day of the week—had the greatest number of loading errors. In contrast, a highly structured organizer that had 28 compartments created by crossing the seven days of the week with four times a day was loaded with a high degree of accuracy. In a later study, Park, Morrell et al. (1994) found that very old adults who received both this highly structured organizer (loaded with the subjects' medications by the experimenter) along with a calendar were significantly more adherent than control subjects. Young-old adults (ages 60–77) were not facilitated by these interventions because their initial level of adherence was nearly perfect. Moulding (1989) reviews a range of different types of organizers and medication dispensers and suggests that these devices can indeed be facilitative of adherence and even suggests that devices should be developed that can serve as electronic pill dispensers at the appointed time, removing all aspects of cognition from the adherence behavior. Although there may be great enthusiasm for the use of medication organizers to facilitate adherence, a number of caveats must be issued. First, they are not particularly well suited to highly mobile individuals, as the organizers can be quite cumbersome and difficult to carry on one's person. Second, once the medications are removed from their initial containers, information about the identity of the medications, as well as instructions for taking them are unavailable to the patient, and this lack may pose a hazard. Finally, as should be obvious, if the medication organizers are not loaded correctly, the net effect will be confusion of medications and increased nonadherence. Thus, these devices have the potential to be quite dangerous if used improperly. It seems likely that they are most facilitative for the very elderly who have more limited cognitive resources and need assistance in the comprehension and organizational function, as the work of Park, Morrell et al. (1994) suggests. For this reason it is recommended that some oversight be used by a pharmacist, medical staff member, or family member in the loading operation, to prevent a catastrophic result.

Prospective Reminders

Calendars and organizers are supportive primarily of the comprehension, working memory, and long-term memory components of adherence (Park et al., 1992). They address only peripherally the prospective aspect of medication adherence; that is, remembering to take a medication at the appointed time. Although the sight of a medication organizer, a calendar, or even a pill bottle may remind one to take a medication, devices and interventions have been explicitly designed to address the prospective component of adherence. Some devices are designed merely to provide the individual with the information that the medication was actually taken, a problem in reality monitoring noted by Park and Kidder (1996). McKenney et al. (1992) provided hypertensive subjects with a digital cap that presented patients with information about when the bottle was last opened. They reported improvement in adherence from 78% for control subjects to 95% for those receiving the cap, as well as a decrease in blood pressure for those evidencing higher adherence. Nides et al. (1993) also noted a marked increase in adherence for patients using bronchodilators who received feedback as to time of last use. Thus, knowing with certainty that a medication has been taken or not appears to be a subtle but important factor in adherence behavior.

Perhaps the most explicit program of research to improve the prospective aspect of adherence has been developed by Leirer and colleagues. Initially, Leirer et al. (1988) reported that older adults given a pseudo-drug regimen that was monitored microelectronically showed substantial forgetting for taking the medications, although they did show some improvement as a result of memory instruction. Later, Leirer, Morrow, Tanke, and Pariante (1991) demonstrated that adherence to such a regimen was improved when subjects received telephone voice reminders about performing the prospective medication-taking task. In later work they have also demonstrated that influenza vaccine rates increased if older adults received a voice mail reminder (Leirer, Morrow, Pariante, & Doksum, 1989) and that tuberculosis patients were more likely to keep clinic appointments with a voice reminder (Tanke & Leirer, 1993). Leirer, Tanke, and Morrow (1993) describe critical aspects of development of effective reminding systems.

In our laboratory, we are currently investigating the role of personal prospective reminding devices on medication adherence, an area about which little is known. The devices include personal wrist watches programmed to beep at appropriate intervals, medication bottle caps that beep insistently when it is time to take the medication, and combinations of prospective and organizational devices. In general, given the explosion of microelectronic technology available in our society, there is likely to be increased interest in the development of various devices to improve medication adherence (see Bond & Hussar, 1991, for a review of emerging technology beyond that reported here).

Training

The development of effective training modules to improve performance has always been an important aspect of a human factors approach to performance. Although the substantial literature on the role of patient education in improving adherence is well beyond the scope of the present chapter, very little work has been done in developing training techniques to improve the information processing aspects of medication adherence behavior. In one noteworthy study, Leirer et al. (1988) provided subjects with a medication recall training module that was designed to improve subjects' motivation to take medications, enhance comprehension and organization of the information, and improve prospective remembering. Leirer et al. (1988) found that subjects who received the training showed less forgetting for a pseudo-drug regimen that closely simulated an actual sequence of medication-taking behavior. This is an important finding that suggests that training programs with specific targeted objectives might be effective in improving actual medication adherence, although such a demonstration has not yet occurred. Training modules could be developed to address many of the components of nonadherence presented in Figure 1 and could be selectively applied to patients, depending on the locus of their nonadherence problem. More work needs to be done in this important area.

SUMMARY

The primary point that is emphasized in the present chapter is the complexity of adherence behavior and the importance of tailoring an intervention that addresses the underlying causes of the nonadherence. Complex memory aids will not improve adherence in an older adult who believes that the medications prescribed are ineffective or that he or she has a disorder for which there is no effective treatment. Similarly, providing patients with elaborate counseling about their illness when the fundamental cause of nonadherence is that their medication regimen is too complex for them to manage will prove futile. When information processing interventions do appear to be in order, the human factors specialist, nevertheless, must determine what component of medication cognition is in need of support. Human factors experts need to focus not only on designing devices that will support medication cognition and improve adherence, but also must be aware of techniques and instruments that permit them to determine what types of interventions will be effective for a particular subject relative to the constructs presented in Figure 1. Human factors experts must also be sensitive to the possibility that multiple factors account for nonadherence and that more than one of the constructs represented in the model can be a combined source of nonadherence in a particular person. Scientists now have available to them relatively accurate techniques for measuring nonadherence. The challenge of adherence work remains to determine the causes of nonadherence in any given individual and to select interventions accordingly.

Acknowledgments

The authors have engaged in numerous discussions with an interdisciplinary team consisting of Chris Hertzog, Roger Morrell, Howard Leventhal, Danny Birchmore, and Elaine Leventhal. The contributions of these colleagues to our thinking is gratefully acknowledged.

The authors gratefully acknowledge the support of the National Institute on Aging for this work. Support was provided by grants to the first author including AGO6265-08, AGO9868-02, and P5011715-01.

References

Abel, S., & Blackstone, M. (1981). Color-keyed patient medication counseling system. *American Journal of Hospital Pharmacy, 38,* 704–705.

Ascione, F., & Shimp, L. (1984). The effectiveness of four education strategies in the elderly. *Drug Intelligence and Clinical Pharmacy, 18,* 926–931.

Bergman, U., & Wilholm, B. E. (1981). Patient medicine on admission to a medical clinic. *European Journal of Pharmacology, 20,* 185–191.

Blackwell, B. (1979). The drug regimen and treatment compliance. In R. B. Haynes, D. W. Taylor, & D. L. Sackett (Eds.), *Compliance in health care* (pp. 144–156). Baltimore: Johns Hopkins University Press.

Bond, W. S., & Hussar, D. A. (1991). Detection methods and strategies for improving medication compliance. *American Journal of Hospital Pharmacy, 48,* 1978–1988.

Botelho, R. J., & Dudrak, R., II. (1992). Home assessment of adherence to long-term medication in the elderly. *Journal of Family Practice, 35*(1), 61–65.

Botwinick, J. (1984). *Aging and behavior.* New York: Springer.

Cohen, G. (1981). Inferential reasoning in old age. *Cognitive Psychology, 9,* 59–72.

Col, N., Fanale, J. E., & Kronholm, P. (1990). The role of medication noncompliance and adverse drug reactions in hospitalizations of the elderly. *Archives of Internal Medicine, 150,* 841–845.

Cramer, J. A., Scheyer, R. D., & Mattson, R. H. (1990). Compliance declines between clinic visits. *Archives of Internal Medicine, 150,* 1509–1510.

Deyo, R. A. (1982). Compliance with therapeutic regimens in arthritis: Issues, current status, and a future agenda. *Seminars in Arthritis and Rheumatism, 12*(2), 233–244.

Diehl, M., Willis, S. L., & Schaie, W. (1995). Everyday problem solving in older adults: Observational assessment and cognitive correlates. *Psychology and Aging, 10*(3), 478–491.

Doherty, W. J., Schrott, H. B., Metcalf, L., & Iasiello-Vailas, L. (1983). The effects of spouse support and health beliefs in medication adherence. *Journal of Family Practice, 17,* 837–841.

Dunbar, J. M. (1980). Assessment of medication compliance: A review. In R. B. Haynes, M. E. Mattson, & T. D. Engebretson, Jr. (Eds.), *Patient compliance to prescribed antihypertensive medication regimens: A report to the National Heart, Lung, and Blood Institute.* Washington, DC: U.S. Department of Health and Human Services, 59–82.

Dunbar, J. M., Dunning, E. J., & Dwyer, K. (1989). Compliance measurement with arthritis regimen. *Arthritis Care and Research, 2*(3), 8–16.

Einstein, G. O., & McDaniel, M. A. (1990). Normal aging and prospective memory. *Journal of Experimental Psychology: Learning, Memory, and Cognition, 16,* 717–726.

Eustace, C. A., Johnson, G. J., & Gault, M. H. (1982). Improvements in drug prescription labels for patients with limited education or vision. *Canadian Medical Association Journal, 127,* 301–302.

Feinstein, A. R. (1990). On white-coat effects and the electronic monitoring of compliance. *Archives of Internal Medicine, 150,* 1377–1378.

Gabriel, M., Gagnon, J. P., & Bryan, C. K. (1977). Improved patient compliance through use of a daily drug reminder chart. *American Journal of Public Health, 67*(10), 968–969.

Gallez, P., Bird, H. A., Wright, V., & Bennett, A. P. (1984). Comparison of 12 different containers for dispensing anti-inflammatory drugs. *British Medical Journal, 288,* 699–701.

Green, L. W., Mullen, P. D., & Stainbrook, G. L. (1986). Programs to reduce drug errors in the elderly: Direct and indirect evidence from patient education. *Journal of Geriatric Drug Therapy, 1*(1), 59–70.

Gryfe, C. I., & Gryfe, B. (1984). Drug therapy of the aged: The problem of compliance and the roles of physicians and pharmacists. *Journal of the American Geriatrics Society, 32*(8), 301–307.

Grymonpre, R. E., Mitenko, P. A., Sitar, D. S., Aoki, F. Y., & Montgomery, P. A. (1988). Drug-associated hospital admissions in older medical patients. *Journal of the American Geriatrics Society, 36,* 1092–1098.

Hashtroudi, S., Johnson, M. K., & Chrosniak, L. D. (1990). Aging and qualitative characteristics for memories for perceived and imagined complex events. *Psychology and Aging, 5,* 119–126.

Haynes, R. B., Wang, E., & Gomes, D. M. (1987). A critical review of interventions to improve compliance with prescribed medications. *Patient Education and Counseling, 10,* 155–166.

Hurd, P. D., & Butkovich, S. L. (1986). Compliance problems and the older patient: Assessing functional limitations. *Drug Intelligence and Clinical Pharmacy, 20,* 228–231.

Jernigan, J. A. (1984). Update on drugs and the elderly. *American Family Physician, 29*(4), 238–247.

Kendrick, R., & Bayne, J. R. (1982). Compliance with prescribed medication by elderly patients. *Journal of the Canadian Medical Association, 127,* 961.

Kiernan, P. J., & Isaacs, J. B. (1981). Use of drugs by the elderly. *Journal of Research in Sociological Medicine, 74,* 196.

Kruse, W., Eggert-Kruse, W., Rampmaier, J., Runnebaum, B., & Weber, E. (1991). Dosage frequency and drug-compliance behavior—A comparative study on compliance with a medication to be taken twice or four times daily. *European Journal of Clinical Pharmacology, 41,* 589–592.

Kruse, W., Rampmaier, J., Ullrich, G., & Weber, E. (1994). Patterns of drug compliance with medications to be taken once and twice daily assessed by continuous electronic monitoring in primary care. *International Journal of Clinical Pharmacology and Therapeutics, 32*(9), 452–457.

Kvavilashvili, L. (1987). Remembering intention as a distinct form of memory. *British Journal of Psychology, 78,* 507–518.

Law, R., & Chalmers, C. (1976). Medicines and elderly people: A general practice survey, *British Medical Journal, 1,* 565–568.

Leirer, V. O., Morrow, D. G., Pariante, G. M., & Doksum, T. (1989). Increasing influenza vaccination adherence through voice mail. *Journal of the American Geriatrics Society, 37,* 1147–1150.

Leirer, V. O., Morrow, D. G., Pariante, G. M., & Sheikh, J. I. (1988). Elders' nonadherence, its assessment, and computer assisted instruction for medication recall training. *Journal of the American Geriatrics Society, 36,* 877–884.

Leirer, V. O., Tanke, E. D., & Morrow, D. G. (1994). Time of day and naturalistic prospective memory. *Experimental Aging Research, 20,* 127–134.

Leirer, V. O., Morrow, D. G., Tanke, E. D., & Pariante, G. M. (1991). Elders' nonadherence: Its assessment and medication reminding by voice mail. *Gerontologist, 31*(4), 514–520.

Leirer, V. O., Tanke, E. D., & Morrow, D. G. (1993). Commercial cognitive/memory systems: A case study. *Applied Cognitive Psychology, 7,* 675–689.

LeSage, J., & Zwygart-Stauffacher, M. (1988). Detection of medication misuse in elders. *Generations, 12*(4), 32–36.

Leventhal, H., & Cameron, L. (1987). Behavioral theories and the problem of compliance. *Patient Education and Counseling, 10,* 117–138.

Levy, M., Mermelstein, L., & Hemo, D. (1982). Medical admissions due to noncompliance with drug therapy. *International Journal of Clinical Pharmacology, Therapy and Toxicology, 20*(12), 600–604.

Ley, P., Whitworth, M. A., Skilbeck, C. E., Woodward, R., Pinsent, R. J., Pike, L. A., Clarkson, M. E., & Blark, P. B. (1976). Improving doctor-patient communication in general practice. *Journal of Royal College of General Practitioners, 26,* 720–724.

Light, L. L. (1991). Memory and aging: Four hypotheses in search of data. *Annual Review of Psychology, 42,* 333–376.

Linkewich, J. A., Catalano, R. B., & Flack, H. L. (1974). The effect of packaging and instruction on outpatient compliance with medication regimens. *Drug Intelligence and Clinical Pharmacy, 8,* 10–15.

Lorence, L., & Branthwaite, A. (1993). Are older adults less compliant with prescribed medication than younger adults? *British Journal of Clinical Psychology, 32,* 485–492.

Lorig, K., Seleznick, M., Lubeck, D., Ung, E., Chastain, R. L., & Holman, H. R. (1989). The beneficial outcomes of the arthritis self-management course are not adequately explained by behavior change. *Arthritis and Rheumatism, 32*(1), 91–95.

MacDonald, E. T., MacDonald, J. B., & Phoenix, M. (1977). Improving drug compliance after hospital discharge. *British Medical Journal, 2,* 618–621.

Maddox, J. C., Levi, M., & Thompson, C. (1994). The compliance with antidepressants in general practice. *Journal of Psychopharmacology, 8*(1), 48–53.

Marks, E. A., & Malinowski, J. M. (1994, December). Pro bono publico: Pharmacist involvement in patient monitoring. *American Druggist,* pp. 59–66.

Matsui, D., Hermann, C., Klein, J., Berkovitch, M., Olivieri, N., & Koren, G. (1994). Critical comparison of novel and existing methods of compliance assessment during a clinical trial of an oral iron chelator. *Journal of Clinical Pharmacology, 34,* 944–949.

May, C. P., Hasher, L., & Stoltzfus, E. R. (1993). Optimal time of day and the magnitude of age differences in memory. *Psychological Science, 4*(5), 326–330.

McKenney, J. M., Munroe, W. P., & Wright, J. T., Jr. (1992). Impact of an electronic medication compliance aid on long-term blood pressure control. *Journal of Clinical Pharmacology, 32,* 277–283.

Meisel, S., & Kiely, K. (1981). Graphic prescription labels. *American Journal of Hospital Pharmacy, 38,* 1116.

Morrell, R. W., Park, D. C., & Kidder, D. P. (1995). *Hypertension and medication adherence across the life span.* Unpublished manuscript, University of Georgia, Athens.

Morrell, R. W., Park, D. C., & Poon, L. W. (1988, November). *Effects of differing labeling techniques on memory and comprehension of prescription information in young and old adults.* Paper presented at the annual meeting of the Gerontological Society of America, San Francisco.

Morrell, R. W., Park, D. C., & Poon, L. W. (1989). Quality of instruction on prescription drug labels: Effects on memory and comprehension in young and old adults. *Gerontologist, 29*(3), 345–354.

Morrow, D. G., Leirer, V., & Altieri, P. (1995). List formats improve medication instructions for older adults. *Educational Gerontology, 21,* 163–178.

Morrow, D. G., Leirer, V., Altieri, P., & Tanke, E. (1991). Elders' schema for taking medication: Implications for instruction design. *Journal of Gerontology: Psychological Sciences, 46*(6), 378–385.

Morrow, D. G., Leirer, V., Andrassy, J. M., & Tanke, E. D. (1994). Designing health service appointment reminder messages for older adults. *Journal of Clinical Geropsychology,* (Volume 1) (pp. 293–304).

Morrow, D. G., Leirer, V. O., Andrassy, J. M., Tanke, E. D., & Stine, E. A. L. (in press). Medication Instruction design: Younger and older adult schemes for taking medicine. *Human Factors.*

Morrow, D. G., Leirer, V., & Sheikh, J. (1988). Adherence and medication instructions review and recommendations. *Journal of the American Geriatrics Society, 36,* 1147–1160.

Morse, E. V., Simon, P. M., & Balson, P. M. (1993). Using experimental training to enhance health professionals' awareness of patient compliance issues. *Academic Medicine, 68,* 693–697.

Moulding, T. (1961). Preliminary study of the pill calendar as a method of improving the self-administration of drugs. *American Review of Respiratory Disease, 84,* 284–287.

Moulding, T. (1989). The development of pill calendars and medication monitors from one participant's perspective. *Journal of Compliance in Health Care, 4*(1), 9–21.

Neely, E., & Patrick, M. L. (1968). Problems of aged persons taking medications at home. *Nursing Research, 17,* 52–55.

Nides, M. A., Tashkin, D. P., Simmons, M. S., Wise, R. A., Li, V. C., & Rand, C. S. (1993). Improving inhaler adherence in a clinical trial through the use of the nebulizer chronolog. *Chest, 104,* 501–507.

Ow-Wing, S. D., & Kerner, J. A. (1981). Color-coded prescription labeling. *American Journal of Hospital Pharmacy, 38,* 631.

Page, P., Verstraete, D., Robb, J., & Etzwiler, D. (1981). Patient recall of self-care recommendations in diabetes. *Diabetes Care, 4,* 9698.

Park, D. C. (1992). Applied cognitive aging research. In F. I. M. Craik & T. A. Salthouse (Eds.), *Handbook of cognition and aging* (pp. 449–493). Hillsdale, NJ: Erlbaum.

Park, D. C. (1994). Self-regulation and control of rheumatic disorders. In S. Maes, H. Leventhal, & M. Johnston (Eds.), *International handbook of health psychology* (pp. 189–217). New York: Wiley.

Park, D. C., Hertzog, C., Morrell, R. W., Kidder, D. P., & Mayhorn, C. B. (1994, August). *Event-based and time-based prospective memory: Effects of age and frequency of prospective tasks.* Paper presented at the Third Practical Aspects of Memory Conference, College Park, MD.

Park, D. C., & Kidder, D. P. (1996). Prospective memory and medication adherence. In M. Brandimonte, G. Einstein, & M. McDaniel (Eds.), *Prospective memory: Theory and applications.* (pp. 369–390). Hillsdale, NJ: Erlbaum.

Park, D. C., & Mayhorn, C. B. (in press). Remembering to take medications: The importance of nonmemory variables. In D. Hermann, M. Johnson, M. McEvoy, C. Hertzog, & P. Hertel (Eds.), *Research on practical aspects of memory* (Vol. 2). Hillsdale, NJ: Erlbaum.

Park, D. C., Morrell, R. W., Frieske, D., Blackburn, A. B., & Birchmore, D. (1991). Cognitive factors and the use of over-the-counter medication organizers by arthritis patients. *Human Factors, 31*(3), 57–67.

Park, D. C., Morrell, R. W., Frieske, D., Gaines, C. L., & Lautenschlager, G. (1993). Measurement techniques and level of analysis of medication adherence behavior across the life span. In *Proceedings of the Human Factors and Ergonomics Society 37th annual meeting* (pp. 188–192). Santa Monica, CA: Human Factors and Ergonomics Society.

Park, D. C., Morrell, R. W., Frieske, D., & Kincaid, D. (1992). Medication adherence behaviors in older adults: Effects of external cognitive supports. *Psychology and Aging, 7,* 252–256.

Park, D. C., Morrell, R. W., Hertzog, C., Leventhal, H., Birchmore, D., Kidder, D. P., & Jones, T. R. (1994, July). *Psychosocial and cognitive predictors of medication adherence in early osteoarthritis patients.* Paper presented at the meeting of the Third International Conference of Behavioral Medicine, Amsterdam, The Netherlands.

Park, D. C., Puglisi, J. T., & Smith, A. D. (1986). Memory for pictures: Does an age-related decline exist? *Journal of Psychology and Aging, 1,* 11–17.

Park, D. C., Willis, S. L., Morrow, D., Diehl, M., & Gaines, C. L. (1994). Cognitive function and medication usage in older adults. *Journal of Applied Gerontology, 13,* 39–57.

Parker, J. C., Singsen, B. H., Hewett, J. E., Walker, S. E., Hazelwood, S. E., Hall, P. J., Holsten, D. J., & Rodon, C. M. (1984). *Archives of Physical Medicine and Rehabilitation, 65,* 771–774.

Paulson, S. M., Krause, S., & Iber, F. L. (1977). Development and evaluation of a compliance test for patients taking disulfiram. *Johns Hopkins Medical Journal, 141,* 119–125.

Rand, C. S., Wise, R. A., Nides, M., Simmons, M. S., Bleeker, E. R., Kusek, J. W., Li, V. C., & Tashkin, D. P. (1992). Metered-dose inhaler adherence in a clinical trial. *American Review of Respiratory Disease, 146,* 1559–1564.

Rice, G. E., & Okun, M. A. (1994). Older readers' processing of medical information that contradicts their beliefs. *Journal of Gerontology: Psychological Sciences, 49*(3), 119–128.

Richardson, M. A., Simons-Morton, B., & Annegers, J. F. (1993). Effect of perceived barriers on compliance with antihypertensive medication. *Health Education Quarterly, 20*(4), 489–503.

Robbins, J. (1990). *Schering report XVI—"OBRA '90": Pharmacists not only count, but they also make a difference.* Kenilworth, NJ: Shering Laboratories.

Rudd, P. (1979). In search of the gold standard for compliance measurement. *Archives of Internal Medicine, 139*(6), 627–628.

Rudd, P., Ahmed, S., Zachary, V., Barton, C., & Bonduelle, D. (1992). Compliance with medication timing: Implications from a medication trial for drug development and clinical practice. *Journal of Clinical Research and Pharmacoepidemiology, 6,* 15–27.

Rudd, P., Byyny, R. L., Zachary, V., LoVerde, M. E., Titus, C., Mitchell, W. D., & Marshall, G. (1989). The natural history of medication compliance in a drug trial: Limitations of pill counts. *Clinical Pharmachology and Therapeutics, 46*(2), 169–176.

Rudd, P., & Marshall, G. (1990). Medication-taking in hypertension. In J. H. Laragh & B. M. Brenner (Eds.), *Hypertension: Pathophysiology, diagnosis, and management* (pp. 2309–2327). New York: Raven Press.

Salthouse, T. A. (1991). *Theoretical perspective on cognitive aging.* Hillsdale, NJ: Erlbaum.

Schwartz, D., Wand, M., Zeitz, L., & Gross, M. E. (1962). Medication errors made by elderly chronically ill patients. *American Journal of Public Health, 52,* 2018–2029.

Shimp, L. A., & Ascione, F. J. (1985). Potential medication-related problems in noninstitutional elderly. *Drug Intelligence and Clinical Pharmacy, 19,* 766–772.

Shimp, L. A., & Ascione, F. J. (1988). Causes of medication misuse and error. *Generations, 12*(4), 17–21.

Tanke, E. D., & Leirer, V. O. (1993). Use of automated telephone reminders to increase elderly patients' adherence to tuberculosis medication appointments. In *Proceedings of the Human Factors and Ergonomics Society 37th Annual Meeting* (pp. 193–196). Santa Monica, CA: Human Factors and Ergonomics Society.

Urquhart, J., & Chevalley, C. (1988). Impact of unrecognized dosing errors on the cost and effectiveness of pharmaceuticals. *Drug Information Journal, 22,* 363–378.

Waterhouse, D. M., Calzone, K. A., Mele, C., & Brenna, D. E. (1993). Adherence to oral tamoxifen: A comparison of patient self-report, pill counts, and microelectronic monitoring. *Journal of Clinical Oncology, 11*(6), 1189–1197.

White, P. H. (1980). Psychoactive medication noncompliance in a geropsychiatric outpatient agency. *Journal of Gerontological Nursing, 6*(12), 729–734.

Wogalter, M. S., & Young, S. L. (1994). The effect of alternative product-label design on warning compliance. *Applied Ergonomics, 25*(1) 53–57.

Wong, B. S. M., & Norman, D. C. (1987). Evaluation of a novel medication aid, the calendar blister-pak, and its effect on drug compliance in a geriatric outpatient clinic. *Journal of the American Geriatrics Society, 35,* 21–26.

Chapter 12

Assistive Devices

Geoff Fernie

INTRODUCTION

We all have an opinion on how old one has to be to belong to the "elderly population." I am not sure that it really matters whether we choose 55, 65, or older for the purpose of this chapter. There are very important differences to be kept in mind, however, when considering the application of human factors to the design of assistive devices for the elderly population in contrast to the population of disabled people of all ages.

As we grow older, most of us will accumulate several relatively minor disabilities. We will probably have a little arthritis that may restrict movement, we will almost certainly need reading glasses and may have more difficulty driving at night. Our strength, endurance, balance, bladder control, and hearing may be somewhat compromised. We may even find ourselves to be a little more forgetful. The onset of these difficulties is likely to be gradual, and each of them may be relatively minor. However, in combination, they may threaten our ability to continue to live independently in our own homes and may reduce our enjoyment of life. Nevertheless it is likely that we will not perceive ourselves as belonging to the population of "disabled" or "handicapped" people.

In contrast, people who have been disabled since birth or who become disabled as a result of injury or disease before they are elderly are more

Handbook of Human Factors and the Older Adult

likely to identify themselves as disabled. Their impairments may be more severe but less diffuse. They are fewer in number. Of course, younger disabled also grow old but they have established their coping strategies and are experts in their disabilities. Their knowledge about assistive devices and their acceptance of the need for these devices is generally much greater.

This chapter begins with a discussion of the concepts of "universal design." If devices that we all use every day can be designed to continue to be usable as our abilities decline with age, then this is the most satisfying and effective way of addressing the needs of the vast majority of elderly. Unfortunately, there is often a trade-off of aesthetics against function. Both are important but a device that fails to meet the crucial functional needs of a person with a disability is useless. The chapter then proceeds to descriptions of the numbers and categories of devices used. The application of human factors is described through a discussion of some aspects of design in each of the most common categories of devices. These descriptions may lead the reader to believe that the field is well advanced and that there is little room for improvement. This is far from the case. This author believes that the design of assistive devices is generally still at quite a primitive stage. Surveys have shown that many assistive devices are abandoned. The notion that this is evidence of the inadequacy of design has been exaggerated, but clearly, there is a need for the incorporation of more human factors knowledge in design. The chapter concludes with a description of some of the tools available to provide the human factors data through laboratory testing and effective consumer interaction.

WHAT IS AN ASSISTIVE DEVICE?

Assistive devices are generally defined as devices that reduce functional limitations resulting from physical, sensory or cognitive impairment. There are two practical difficulties with this definition. The more minor difficulty is that not all technology in the information age takes the form of a physical device. For this reason, a broader term assistive technologies is often used. The second difficulty is that the definition is too inclusive. A food mixer could be considered to be assistive technology by this definition since it may overcome strength or agility impairments of some people to some degree.

Obviously it is not always helpful to include food mixers and all such devices within an operational definition of *assistive devices*. However, many products for general use are now being designed with features that make them more usable by people with impairments. The terms *universal* and *transgenerational design* are widely used to describe a concept where prod-

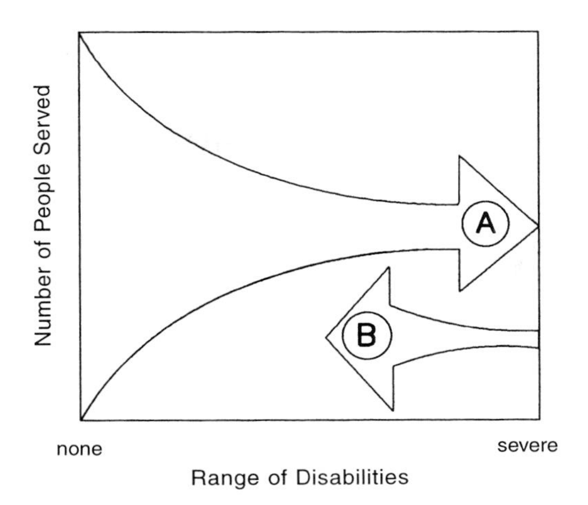

FIGURE 1 Arrow *A* symbolizes the thrust of a "universal" design to extend the usability of products from large numbers of ablebodied people to include people with disabilities. The arrow *B* symbolizes the alternative strategy of designing products that meet demanding specialized functional needs of people with more severe disabilities and presenting them with a more attractive and less stigmatizing appearance that appeals to larger numbers of users with more minor impairments.

ucts are designed to be usable by the people of all ages and functional abilities (Henry, 1993; Pirkl, 1994). Such features as larger push buttons are becoming more common as business recognizes the growing market segment of elderly with functional limitations and disposable income. Equal rights legislation, such as the Americans with Disabilities Act, is also promoting awareness of the need for universal design to increase the accessibility of products and environments.

The objective of universal design is shown schematically in the Figure 1. The target is to extend the arrow showing the distribution of the product across the range of abilities. In the case of transgenerational design, the horizontal axis would be labeled *age*.

Unfortunately, universal and transgenerational designs frequently compromise specific aspects of function. An attractive device with less than optimum function is of little use to a person who must depend heavily on the device to overcome a significant functional limitation. In these cases a less ambitious strategy may be more successful, whereby the assistive device is not designed to appeal to everyone but is targeted to be acceptable to people with a wider range of disabilities. The objective is to improve ("normalize") the appearance of the device so that people with minor functional limitations choose to use it without compromising performance for those with the most severe limitations. This alternative strategy is shown as the second arrow in Figure 1.

A person needing an assistive device often uses that device almost all of the day in the presence of others. It is, therefore, particularly important that it not be ugly. Embarrassment can be a reason for delaying or avoiding starting to use an assistive device. Self-concept and self-esteem are very important factors. Also, if an assistive device can be made attractive to a broader market and designed so that expert fitting or setup is not required, then the retail price can be greatly reduced by marketing in higher volumes through regular mass-marketing channels.

WHO NEEDS ASSISTIVE DEVICES?

The terms *impairment, disability,* and *handicap* have distinct meanings. An impairment is a decrease in physical or cognitive function. An impairment may prevent a person from performing an activity as quickly, as easily, or in a manner that is considered normal. If this is the case then the impairment has resulted in a disability. If the disability puts the individual at a competitive disadvantage compared to others in society, for example, by limiting employment opportunities, then the person is said to have a handicap. *Activity limitation* and *functional limitation* are often used as synonyms for *disability.*

Canada's Health Promotion Survey, conducted in 1985, found a total of 16.1% of the population over 15 years of age reported some level of limitation in their activities because of a long-term physical condition or health problem. The prevalence increased sharply with age. For the age range of 65 and over, 34.3% of people had an activity limitation, and these people constituted 26.6% of the total disabled population over 15 years old (Charette, 1988). Elderly people have expressed a desire to continue to live at home, and governments appear to believe that providing care in the community will be less expensive and provide a better quality of life. Assistive devices are essential to maintaining sufficient independence and to reducing the physical burden on familial caregivers if the community alternative is to be workable. Consequently, the need for assistive devices is growing as the population ages and with the trend away from institutional care.

In 1980, about 6% of the population of the world was 65 years and older. It was 11.9% in the United States (slightly greater than in Canada) and much higher in Europe (e.g., 15.1% in the United Kingdom and 16.8% in Sweden; Ontario Gerontology Association, 1988). In the United States, the elderly population constituted 31 million people (12% of the population) in 1994. This number will double by 2025. The rapid growth in the elderly population causes many observers to anticipate a corresponding rate of growth in the numbers of people with disabilities. However, Manton, Corder, and Stallard (1993) point out that the prevalence of chronic disability in the United States did not increase during the 1980s to the extent that might be predicted on the basis of this growth and the increasing average age of the elderly population. Reasons for this mismatch include improvements in prevention and treatment of strokes and heart disease.

Longino (1994) suggests that sharp rises in the use of assistive devices and housing modifications are partly responsible for the fact that the prevalence of disability is not rising in step with the growth of the elderly population. He comments that this is fortunate, since demographers warn of impending disaster because the supply of younger caregivers would not keep pace with the growth in the elderly population. Longino hypothesizes that the growing use of assistive technology is part of a "modern elderly person's long-term adaptive process" (see Longino, 1994, p. 41). He predicts that the market for assistive devices will grow, reducing the growth in personal assistance and institutional programs. Longino makes the point that the proportion of older Americans having difficulty or unable to use a phone or do their laundry actually decreased during the 1980s by 9.1% and 4.1%, respectively. One might suggest that these are examples of the impact of universal design; that is, telephones and washing machines have become easier for people with a wider range of abilities to operate. On the other hand, the proportion of the growing elderly population experiencing difficulties with outdoor mobility increased by 16% over the same period.

HOW MANY DEVICES ARE USED?

The global market for medical devices is huge—about CDN $86 billion—and is growing about 7% annually, almost triple the growth rate of the total world economy (Health Industries Advisory Committee, 1994). LaPlante, Hendershot, and Moss (1992) reported that in 1990, 5.3% of (13.1 million) Americans were using assistive devices to accommodate physical impairments. Users of assistive devices were divided almost equally between those under and over 65 years of age.

LaPlante's data on the usage of assistive devices were based on interviews in 46,476 households and extrapolated to the U.S. population. The largest category of assistive devices was canes and crutches (approximately 5 million). There were almost 4 million users of braces (orthoses) of various kinds. Similar numbers of people were users of hearing aids. However,

LaPlante states that more people use assistive devices to cope with mobility-related impairments than any other kind of impairment. The most common mobility related devices were handrails that were available for use by nearly 3.4 million people in their homes. Over 2 million people were living in homes equipped with ramps. More people were found to use walkers (1.7 million) than wheelchairs (1.4 million). Raised toilets were almost as common as wheelchairs (1.3 million).

LaPlante also noted that 2.5 million Americans in 1990 said that they needed assistive devices but could not afford them. Clearly the rate of growth in the market for assistive devices will be influenced by the cost of the devices and the ability of disabled people to purchase them. In contrast, it should be noted also that many people who become disabled in later years are not poor. For example, people over 50 in Canada make up 25% of the population and hold 55% of discretionary spending power and 80% of personal wealth (Prime Times Strategies, 1993).

CATEGORIES OF ASSISTIVE DEVICES

Assistive devices exist for almost every functional impairment. The most common age-related disabilities are mobility related. It just gets more difficult to move around and to transfer in and out and on and off for most of us as we age. In this chapter, we will focus on the categories that are most frequently used by people as they grow older. The reader is referred elsewhere for descriptions of other less-common mobility-related categories of assistive devices, such as orthoses (braces) and prostheses (artificial limbs) (American Academy of Orthopaedic Surgeons, 1985, 1992). Although the prevalence of sensory impairments increases with age, space limitations prevent inclusion of assistive devices for communication, hearing, and vision. The reader is referred to (Alm & Parnes, 1995; Jose, 1983; Nowakowski, 1994; Sandlin, 1988, 1990; Skinner, 1988), respectively, for reviews of these topics.

Now let us review some of the common categories of mobility-related assistive device.

Walkers

There are numerous designs of walkers but most fall into one of three categories: walking frames, two-wheeled walkers, and four-wheeled walkers, (otherwise known as rollators). Examples of the three categories are shown in Figure 2.

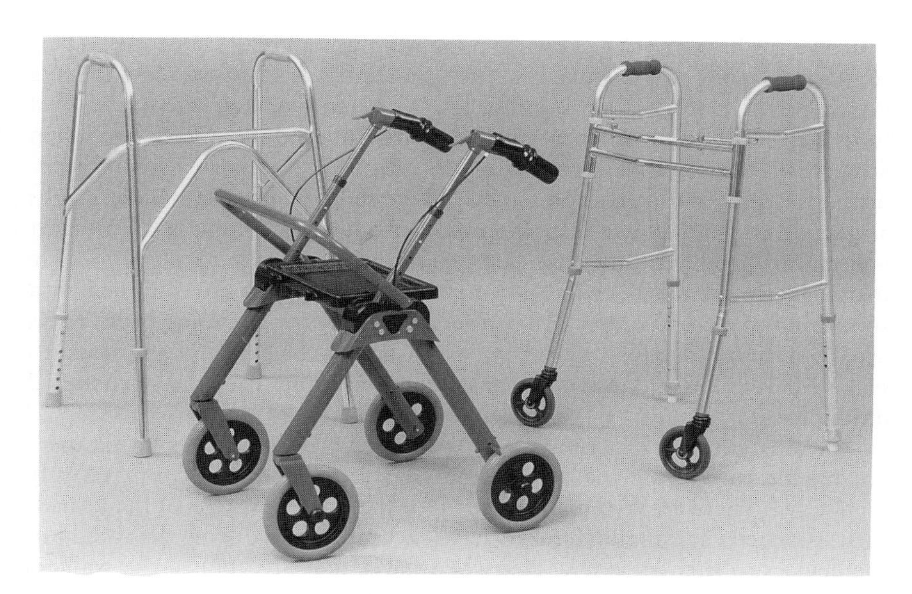

FIGURE 2 Examples of the three common styles of walker are shown: a walking frame with no wheels (back left), a two-wheeled walker (back right), and a high-quality indoor/outdoor four-wheeled walker (front center).

Walking frames have no wheels and are designed to assist with balance. They are used to help rise from a sitting surface. Movement requires lifting the frame and placing it on the floor ahead and then stepping up to the frame. This is a slow process and there is no opportunity for a rhythmic alternating gait to develop. However, the lack of wheels eliminates any possibilities of the walker rolling away and provides for greater security during transfers. The lifting and balance required to advance the frame are too difficult for many users.

Two-wheeled walkers are designed to eliminate the requirement to lift the walker from the floor. The two wheels on the front allow the walker to be slid forward fairly easily but when weight is applied the rubber feet at the back resist motion. These two-wheeled walkers also interrupt the smooth gait pattern. Let us remember that walking is really a succession of forward falls that are arrested by stepping ahead of the center of gravity with each stride. Some people, especially those with Parkinson's disease, appear to allow their center of gravity to travel too far forward to a point where they can no longer step quickly enough to stop a forward fall. A two-wheeled walker may be suitable for these people since there is a reduced tendency for the walker to roll forward too far ahead.

Rollators have rapidly growing popularity among elderly people. Their similarity to shopping buggies and their more attractive colors seem to have increased their acceptability. These four-wheeled walkers perform several functions in addition to increasing balance and stability. They are often fitted with seats so that it is possible to travel longer distances with intermediate resting periods. Almost all walkers have adjustable handle height and some have adjustable seat height. The average seat height is 23 in. but it is useful to be able to decrease that height by about 2 in. to accommodate many elderly users with reduced stature. Usually walkers are equipped with some kind of basket so they can be used effectively for shopping trips. Trays are often optional extras that can be clipped over the seat and are found to be particularly helpful indoors, transferring things between the kitchen and dining area.

The most often heard complaint about four-wheeled walkers is that users are unable to operate the brakes and that the brakes are comparatively ineffective. There are two main reasons for the ineffectiveness of the brakes. First, designers and manufacturers have succeeded in reducing the weight of the devices to such an extent that when the brakes are applied the walkers simply slide with the wheels locked across the floor. Second, average grip strength of people over 65 is lower than that needed to operate the brakes of typical walkers. Furthermore, arthritis is a common reason for an elderly person needing a walker and frequently reduces grip strength.

Wheelchairs

Every reader will be familiar with the common design of wheelchairs consisting of large diameter wheels at the back with rims that can be propelled by hand and smaller castor wheels at the front. In the most traditional form, these chairs have a fabric sling seat and sling back and are designed so that they fold by narrowing. We will outline some of the ways human factors have been applied to improve the comfort and maneuverability of wheelchairs.

The sling seat and back provide inadequate postural support and stress distribution. Improvements in seat and cushion design have the greatest impact on comfort. In its simplest form, better seating begins with a firm and flat surface suspended below the frame to allow room for the height of a stress-distributing cushion. A very large array of cushion designs exists. A simple flat foam cushion with sufficient depth to prevent "bottoming out" and a stretchable cover will often suffice to provide adequate comfort and stress distribution for elderly users. Sometimes cushions are assembled comprising layers of foam of different stiffness with sculptured areas to accommodated bony prominences (the ischial tuberosities and the sacrum) in attempts to distribute pressure. Some of these cushions incorporate a gel top layer with the intention of distributing shear stress. Yet another approach to wheelchair seating involves the use of modular shaped cushion components that are assembled to a custom shape by some means such as clipping to a substructure or adhering to each other.

The second area of wheelchair design improvement is the maneuverability and performance of the chairs. Developments in design and materials have made chairs lighter and stiffer. Such lighter and stiffer chairs have been associated mainly with younger wheelchair sports-oriented users. However, there is good reason to provide elderly users with these products since they can sometimes gain even greater benefit from reduced energy consumption and easier propulsion. The "X-braced" folding chair has remained popular because of convenience of storage especially for car transportation. However, it has been difficult to make wheelchairs with folding frames that are both stiff and light. Chairs with rigid, nonfolding frames have been popularized where transportability is achieved by removing the wheels using a quick release catch.

The key parameter affecting maneuverability is the positioning of the wheels (McLaurin and Brubaker, 1991). For the greatest mobility the axis of the wheels should fall under the center of gravity of the combined chair and user, which permits the user to perform a so-called wheelie. This maneuver involves tilting the chair backward and balancing on its two large wheels. Wheelies allow the front castors to be lifted up and over an obstacle such as a curb and allow the chair to be turned on the spot. Having the wheels aligned such that all of the weight is transmitted through the large wheels also creates two other advantages. The rolling resistance of the larger wheels is less, especially over softer surfaces or rough ground, than the castor wheels and therefore it is easier and less tiring to propel the chair. Second, when traversing a slope such as a curb cut or driveway entrance, if a proportion of the weight is applied to the castor wheels then there is a tendency for the chair to want to turn down the direction of the incline. This is not the case if all of the weight is over the large wheels. On the other hand, the risk of tipping backwards is increased. Backward tips can result from traveling up an incline or over an obstacle or from forward acceleration. The setting of the axis is therefore a compromise between stability and performance. Some chairs can be fitted with antitipping devices consisting of extensions protruding from behind the chair that come into contact with the ground if it tips beyond a certain point.

Elderly users who have limited lower limb function generally transfer on and off the chair by parking alongside and sliding sideways. Under ideal circumstances, the two surfaces are matched in height. Removable armrests allow this sideways or lateral movement. Other relevant design options include various styles of legrests, footrests, headrests, tilting and reclining seat mechanisms, brakes, and tires.

Powered Chairs

People with lower limb impairments but with the ability to use their upper body and arms are able to choose whether to use a manual or a powered chair. Sometimes they will elect to use a powered chair on occasions where fatigue is a concern. Frequently elderly people will choose a scooter because of its lower cost and less stigmatizing appearance than a full powered chair. Scooters have handle bar steering and simple seating and require the user to have good trunk balance and arm function. Scooters are usually designed so that they can be disassembled into two or three parts for ease with lifting, storing, and transporting in a vehicle. A variety of small compact hoists are available that can be fitted in the trunk of a car or to the rear of a van to ease the task of lifting the scooter in and out. For example, this set up allows an elderly wife with limited strength to be able to take her mobility-disabled husband on outings without the need for assistance.

There are many different manufacturers of powered scooters and many variations in design. However, scooters generally, fall into two categories: (1) those equipped with a motor powering the single steerable front wheel and (2) those driven through a differential to both rear wheels. The front-wheel drive scooters are generally the least expensive but are limited to travel over quite level and smooth ground. Principal features incorporated into scooters include an adjustable steering column that can be swung out of the way to provide greater clearance when entering or exiting the chair. Seats are usually adjustable in height and can swivel. The swivelling feature is important since the front wheel and steering configuration prevent a user pulling up to a table. Instead, the user parks parallel to the table and then swivels the seat. Some scooters have the additional feature of allowing the seat to swivel and slide closer to the table. Unfortunately, if the scooter user is sharing a table (e.g., at dinner) then the companion on one side will be some distance away separated by the steering column and the carrying bucket.

Elderly people with impairment to both upper and lower limb function have no choice but to use a powered wheelchair. Generally, powered chairs are four-wheeled with individually powered rear wheels and front idling castor wheels. Steering is achieved by applying different power to the two driven wheels. The usual method of control is a proportional joystick. Modern control systems are programmable so that parameters, such as maximum speed and acceleration, can be selected. Alternative forms of input are also available including head movement and sip and puff mouth control.

Other input modalities of speech, eye movement, and muscle and nerve electrical potentials have been implemented in research environments but have not gained wide acceptance.

Many wheelchair control systems also include interfaces for environmental control. The user can select between controlling the wheelchair and controlling communication aids, house lights, appliances, and so forth. Unfortunately, powered wheelchairs often have a tangle of wiring and experts are required to connect various of these input and output devices into the system—an example of poor human factors design. Standards are now being developed for interface buses that, one hopes, will eventually encourage manufacturers to produce components that can be interchanged easily.

Some chairs have the ability to raise and lower the height of the seat. Focus groups of elderly wheelchair users in our laboratory have emphasized the importance of being able to be lowered close to the floor to reach for dropped objects, clean the floor, and play with grandchildren. The ability to be raised to greater heights to provide comfortable access to standard kitchen counter tops and to reach higher shelves is rated as secondary to reaching the floor but still very desirable. Raising seat height makes conversation with others who are standing more comfortable and equal.

Options for backrest reclining and whole seat tilting are also often available. The tilting option is usually preferable with the elderly since reclining tends to accentuate the tendency for the user to slip forward out of the seat. This tendency to forward sliding induces potentially damaging shear forces on skin and soft tissues that may create decubitus ulcers (bedsores). A tilting seat is also helpful if the user is to be lifted in and out of the chair using a hoist since it matches the posture of the person suspended in the lifting sling. Backrest reclining options are valuable when the user must stay in the chair for prolonged periods and is at risk of developing flexion contractures at the hip.

Grab Bars and Handrails

Grab bars and handrails serve two purposes. They are there to enable people with good upper limb function and limited lower limb function to lift, pull, and push themselves usually when transferring from sitting to standing or to transfer between two surfaces such as a wheelchair and a toilet. The second purpose is to assist with balance and either prevent a fall or assist with recovery from a trip or a slip before falling to the ground.

Maki, Bartlett, and Fernie (1984) conducted biomechanical tests on a stairway using an apparatus that could measure the force applied to handrails. Various shapes and sizes of rail were tested at various heights. The optimum shape was circular with a diameter of $1\frac{1}{2}$ in. (38 mm). The study found that the higher the handrail, the more effective it was in preventing a fall, since more force could be generated and the force would be more effective in preventing either toppling forward or falling backward by creating a larger moment about the feet. The upper limit on the height of the handrail was the height at which the population would feel comfortable walking downstairs resting their hands on the rail. Obviously, we do not want to discourage people from using handrails by making them uncomfortable to any extent. For the North American population the recommended compromise was 36 in. from the center of the rail above the nose of the stair.

Interestingly, Cooper, Letts, and Rigby (1993) have found that coloring the handrails in a safety yellow was perceived as helpful by elderly users. These users reported that not only could they see the rail more easily but that they used the rail more frequently since the yellow color provided a functional reminding cue. It was found that elderly people would not have necessarily selected the color yellow at the time of purchase but when the researchers offered to remove the yellow units and replace them with the neutral gray option, they generally preferred to retain the yellow rails.

Lifts and Transfer Devices

Brown, Potter, and Foster (1990) have shown that caregiver burden is the most important factor determining the use of home support services and admission to a nursing home. The physical burden of having to lift someone into bed or onto the toilet sometimes becomes just too much for the family member. Nursing staff members have a higher rate of back injury than people in any other profession, including garbage collectors, truck drivers, and construction workers. Family often find the task of lifting elderly relatives impossible. The stresses involved on the lower back, shoulders, and elbows when lifting an adult are so great that injury with repeated lifting is an inevitable consequence for most caregivers. A range of assistive devices is available to reduce the effort required. We will focus on personal lifting devices. These can be divided into two broad categories.

The conventional lift is similar to hoists that are found in many workshops and garages. The subject is suspended in a sling from the end of a boom that is raised and lowered by means of a hand-pumped hydraulic cylinder. The mast that supports the boom is mounted on a wheeled base. Usually, the wheeled base is narrow enough to pass easily through doorways but is opened to provide a wider base of support when lifting the person. Garg, Owen, Beller, and Banaag (1991) have found that nurses perceive the effort involved in operating some of these devices to actually be greater than lifting the person manually. In particular, the action required to pump the hand-powered hydraulics and the effort required to maneuver the wheeled base around obstacles, especially when carrying a person, makes use of these lifts burdensome. The lifting action on more modern and expensive devices is electrically powered but the lifts are still very difficult to maneuver in the confined space of a home, especially by a lone caregiver or if narrow doorways and carpeted surfaces must be negotiated.

Overhead lifts are often more expensive since a track must be installed either attached directly to the ceiling or supported on a free-standing frame. Often the traversing motion is powered but even if this is not the case the effort required to move the rolling carriage along the smooth track is minimal. Other advantages of overhead lifts include avoidance of the need to store the often quite bulky floor lifts and the removal of the risk of tipping accidents that sometimes occur with wheeled lifts.

Stair Climbers, Wheelchair Elevators, and Passenger Elevators

Numerous stair climbing devices are on the market. Generally, a track is fixed to the wall on one side of the stairs. A seat or a platform is cantilevered from this track. The user either sits on the seat or wheels the wheelchair onto the platform and the system then climbs the track to the top of the stair. Installation of the track on a straight stairway is not difficult. Usually, the tracks can be installed only on the outside wall when negotiating a turn in the stairs.

One of the most practical ways of living at home with a mobility disability is to either move into a single level home or convert rooms in a multilevel house to allow the individual to live at ground level. However, the ground level of many single level homes in North America is raised above street level and there are several steps up to the entrance door. The most common way of addressing this problem is to build a ramp. Building codes allow for slopes of up to 1 in 12. This is actually a rather steep slope for most elderly wheelchair users. Sanford, Story, and Jones (1996) have shown that elderly people have the greatest difficulty walking down slopes. A shallower slope might be more appropriate. However, their test subjects emphasized the importance of good handrails more than they commented upon the gradient of the slope. The building and accessibility codes specify level resting points at intervals.

These ramps can become very long. For example, a five foot difference above street level could require as much as 100 feet of ramp length. The ramps are usually installed as switchbacks with level resting points at the turns. Some elderly people find steps to be easier and less tiring than long ramps. It is a good idea to provide both so that the user has a choice. The length of the ramps and the need to clear them of snow often makes an outdoor wheelchair elevator an attractive alternative. These elevators are usually platforms on scissor-jack mechanisms similar to the truck body lifting mechanisms at airports used to bring food trucks to the level of the plane door.

Seating

We already discussed some of the special seating systems available in the context of wheelchairs. However, human factors issues related to seat design for non-wheelchair users are also worthy of discussion. For an ambulatory person, the biggest concern is being able to rise from the chair. The principal factors affecting the ability to rise include seat height, armrest design, depth of cushioning, and seat rake (Holden, Fernie, & Lunau, 1988). Unfortunately, if the seat height is set such that it is still possible for the individual to rest the feet flat on the floor, then the height is not optimal for easing the process of standing up. Easiest egress is achieved when the height of the chair is set such that a foot rest is needed to support the feet when sitting. This presents a dilemma since foot rests can be hazardous, especially with elderly subjects who may have some memory or visual impairment. Accidents tend to occur when users forget that the foot rests are in place and attempt to stand on them. They also create a tripping hazard and can be expensive and unsightly since a mechanism is required to allow the user to swing them out of the way during sitting and standing maneuvers. Unlike wheelchairs, which can usually be adjusted to match an individual user's requirements, other forms of seating must often be shared by many different people. Since allowance must be made for elderly people who are short in stature, the problem of standing from the seat for average and taller individuals is further compromised unless a mix of seats of different heights is provided.

The design of the armrest has an important effect on the ease of ingress and egress. The height should be set so that the weight of the arm is supported with the shoulder in an anatomically neutral position. The top surface of the armrest should be parallel to the seat surface and should extend forward of the front edge of the seat. The armrest should be broad and lightly padded except for the forward end, which should be shaped to allow a good grip. The first use of the armrest during egress is to help the occupant pull herself or himself forward in the chair and the second is to push downward during rising and maintain stability through to standing. If the front of the armrest is too low then it will not be possible to provide support all the way to standing.

Although cushioning is required to minimize the occurrence of pressure sores, the ambulatory user presents fewer risks in this regard since she or he can frequently change position in the seat. A somewhat firmer seat cushion is therefore appropriate since it will be less restrictive on this movement and will facilitate easier standing.

Designers and marketers emphasize lumbar support as an important feature of chair design. Care must be taken when designing or selecting seating for use by elderly people to ensure that this feature is not exaggerated. Elderly spines appear to be stiffer in extension and the consequence of excessive lumbar support is that spine cannot achieve the lordosis required to fit the backrest. Instead, the lumbar support forces the pelvis to tilt anteriorly inducing a more slouched posture. This has the added disadvantage of exacerbating the already present tendency to slide forward in the seat. Elderly people also tend to develop fixed kyphotic deformities (hunchback). It is important to provide support for the head and neck and upper back that allows for this condition.

A number of devices are available that help a person rise from a seat by raising the seat surface in some manner. A common design of a unit that can be placed on top of a seat is similar to a clam shell with the hinge placed forward so that the clam opens up by means of a gas-powered strut. This can be useful in reducing the effort required to stand. The effectiveness is increased if the seat surface has a high coefficient of friction (Wretenberg, Arborelius, Weidenhielm, & Lindberg, 1993). Lounge chairs are also sold with electrically powered mechanisms that cause the whole chair to be raised.

Toilets, Bathtubs, and Showers

Rising from a toilet is particularly difficult for many elderly people. Most toilets in North America are 14 ½ in. high, whereas most other seats, including wheelchairs, are at about 19 in. Taller models of toilets are available but are not popular and therefore more expensive. The most common solution is a raised toilet seat that sits on, or is clamped to, the top of the toilet. The height increase ranges from as little as 1 ½ in. for an extra thick toilet seat to as much as 6 or 7 in. for some products. From the human factors perspective, raising the toilet seat level to the recommended height of chairs is generally helpful. However, many of the add-on raised toilet seats are not firmly fixed to the toilet and have resulted in falls. These products also tend to be visually stigmatizing. An alternative may be to raise the toilet on a plinth constructed using 2 by 4 in. wood studs on edge. Other more expensive options include the use of lifting seat mechanisms that are powered using water pressure or using a wheeled or overhead lift for transfers.

The easiest option for a nonambulatory person to bathe may be to wheel into a roll-in shower stall. This is simply a shower stall where there is no threshold to obstruct easy wheeled entry. However, many people enjoy soaking in a warm bathtub. Various special bathtubs and assistive devices have been devised to increase the accessibility of bathtubs. At the low end, these products include grab handles that clamp to the side of the tub,

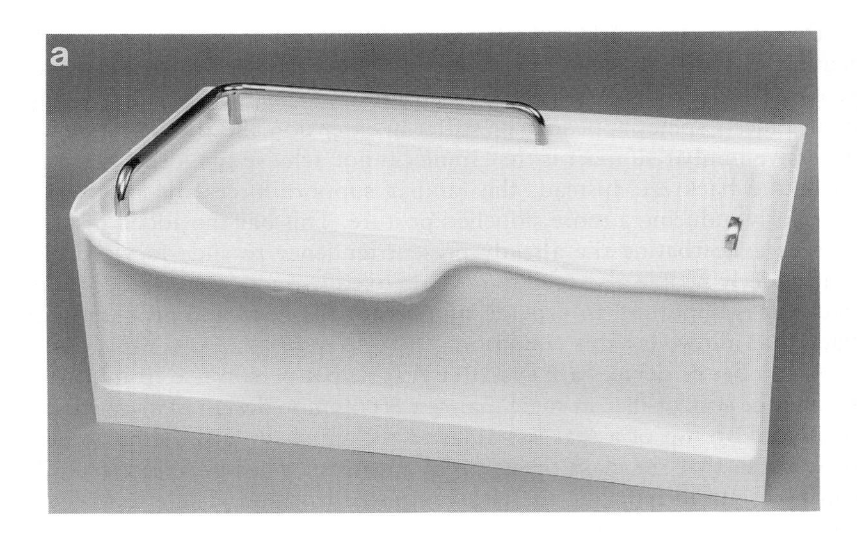

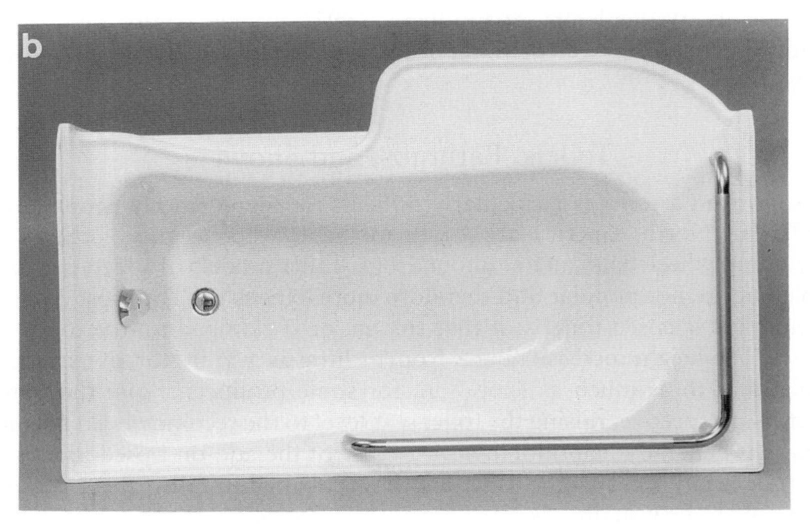

FIGURE 3 This accessible bathtub is an example of universal design. The user sits on the seat and pivots the legs over the narrower and slightly lower edge. A comfortable hand grip has been created along the total length of the near side of the tub. The handrail on the far side is an integral component of the tub. Accessories are available to increase accessibility by persons with major disabilities. The shape also provides a comfortable place for parents to sit and supervise their children and for bathtub readers to place their books.

nonslip rubber mats for inside the tub, stools and seats that are placed in the tub, and bathing benches that span the tub from edge to edge. More sophisticated options include a variety of designs of powered lifting seats that raise and lower the person in the tub. Many of these seats are water powered. Not only are falls a problem in bathtubs, we have also known people who have been stuck in tubs and have required assistance from emergency services. There are also reports, from time to time, of people being stuck in bathtubs for many days.

Several special bathtubs are marketed with various designs of doors to facilitate entry without having to step over the tub side. These doors usually have inflatable seals. Although they ease entry and exit, it is still necessary to be able to sit down in the tub and rise if the user wants to soak in the tub. Often these tubs are equipped with molded seats and are essentially intended for showering. One unfortunate disadvantage is that the user must sit in the tub waiting while it is being filled and the tub must be emptied before opening the door. The problem of the time spent waiting for a tub to fill and empty has been addressed in tipping designs of tub. These tubs can be prefilled to the height of the threshold in the door and the user transfers laterally onto the seat. The door is then shut and when the bath is tipped the user is put into a reclined position and is immersed in the water.

Special bathtubs with doors, tipping devices, elevating seats, and the like are often rather expensive. Landlords and homeowners tend to resist their installation because of fear that the home may become less attractive to future tenants or purchasers. Figure 3 shows a bathtub designed with the objective of meeting most of the accessibility and safety needs within a design that is affordable and with an appearance that is as close to a regular design of a bathtub as possible; that is, following the principles of universal design. The principal feature is a wider edge that acts as a seat. The user sits on this edge and swings the legs over the narrow, slightly lower section of the edge of the bathtub. The near side edge of the tub is rolled over with a radius of 1 ½ in. to allow grasping all the way along. This is in response to many comments by elderly people who found that they missed the old-fashioned tubs that stood on feet where they could grasp the exposed edge.

THE DEVICE ABANDONMENT ISSUE

Gitlin, Levine, and Geiger (1993) briefly summarized the literature on device abandonment. This literature indicates that between 50 and 80% of assistive devices are consistently used and that the remainder are either never used or abandoned after only a short period of use. They interviewed 31 therapists and found that 90% perceived mobility and bathroom equipment is used most frequently by elderly people, whereas 77% perceived grooming and hygiene equipment is seldom used. Brooks (1991) surveyed 595 scientists and engineers with disabilities. This group was chosen for study since they represent roles that are becoming increasingly available to people with disabilities. Overall assistive devices were viewed positively, although many of the devices were found to be inconvenient presumably as a result of poor human factors design. The subjects also felt that the public generally responded to the devices with acceptance rather than with rejection.

There has been much wringing of hands over the implication that public monies are being wasted by providing devices that are abandoned. Phillips and Zhao (1993) found that changes in the needs of the user were the most common reasons for abandonment. It surely is reasonable to expect the level of impairment of some individuals will either decrease as they recover from an injury causing them no longer to need a device or will increase as health or functional ability continues to deteriorate. On the other hand, this author, while placing the issue of abandonment in context, agrees with other authors that high cost and stigmatizing appearance can be barriers to acquisition of assistive devices and that poor function and inadequate incorporation of human factors in design are sometimes a reason for discontinuing the use of a device.

TECHNIQUES FOR APPLYING HUMAN FACTORS TO ASSISTIVE DEVICE DESIGN

There are significant opportunities at this time for human factors to contribute to improvements in the design of assistive devices in both function and appearance. In the past, designers have been in the habit of referring to standard texts on human factors. These reference tables tend to be based on ablebodied younger adults. Ablebodied, younger military personnel are the source of a high proportion of these data. Designers usually plan to meet the needs of 90 or 95% of the distribution of population characteristics. Assistive devices, on the other hand, may be targeted at the 5 to 10% of the population who, because of age and functional limitations, are in the tails of these distributions. Designers of assistive devices, therefore, often need to generate their own human factors data for their target population.

The principal laboratory tools used to gather the required human factors data for the design of assistive mobility devices are force plates and motion analysis systems. Force plates are measurement instruments that are usually a little less than 2 ft. square and generally installed flush with a walking surface. These force plates are strain gauged and measure all of the characteristics of the resultant force that is applied to their surface. For example, when a subject steps onto the plate it will provide the coordinates of the center of pressure under the foot, the magnitude and direction of the force components in all three planes, and the moment about all three planes. Motion analysis systems usually use some form of marker that can be attached to the subject or the assistive device. The markers are either reflective or are illuminated by a small light source. They may work with light in the visible or in the infrared range. A single camera is sufficient to collect data in two dimensions but two cameras, at least, are required for three-dimensional data collection. Sometimes, more than two cameras are required to provide redundancy, since markers may be obscured from the view of a camera during some part of a motion. The output from the video cameras is usually stored on videotape and then subsequently analyzed by a computer-controlled system that digitizes the video frames and identifies the markers.

Figure 4 shows an example of this technology being used to optimize the brake system design of a new walker. In this case the force plates have been mounted in a large platform that can be moved along any axis in the horizontal plane. The walking aid has been instrumented by the addition of load cells to measure the forces applied to the brakes. Reflective markers have been placed on the subject and the walker. The braked wheels of the walker are resting on two separate force plates to be able to record the shear force generated by the brakes. The platform is moved in an unpredictable direction at a random instance in time, disturbing the balance of the subject to assess the speed and effectiveness of postural adjustments and the use of the walker and the walker braking system to maintain stability.

Consumer input in the design process is as important as laboratory measurement to the success of the product. We have found a considerable willingness on the part of elderly consumers to participate in these activities, and there is no resistance from researchers and designers to this role. The amount and quality of feedback available increases if the concepts are presented clearly. In recent years computer graphics have allowed us to present realistic pictures depicting exactly how a product might look when manufactured. Consumers have commented that it is difficult to gain a full appreciation of product concepts from computer images without a sense of scale. We now include computer-rendered mannequins within concept drawings. Mannequins that are representative of the wide-ranging shapes and sizes of people with disabilities should be developed. These software mannequins must also mimic range of motion and postural limitations.

The growing sophistication of tools available to measure human factors data and model the interaction between assistive devices and users will enable designers to develop more functional and attractive assistive devices

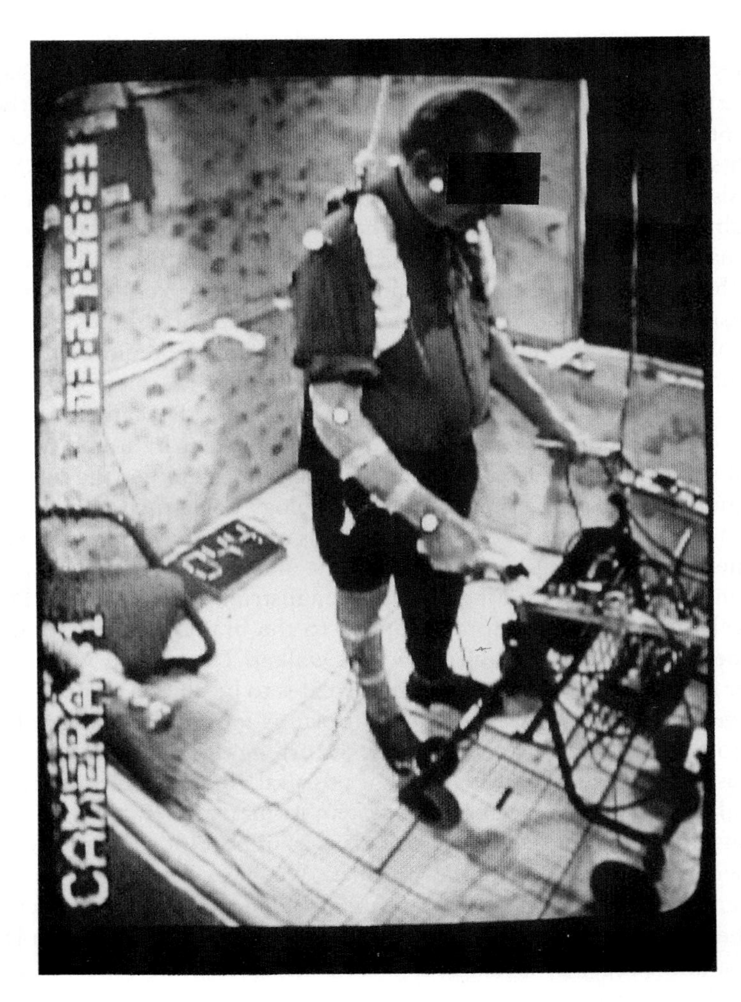

FIGURE 4 This figure shows an example of technology available in the laboratory to provide quantitative human factors data needed to design an improved assistive device. The image was taken from a video system that tracked the movement of light-reflective markers on a subject standing on a large multidirectional moving platform. Electrodes had been applied to the skin to measure the electrical activity of muscles and the subject was wearing a safety harness suspended from above. The walking aid was equipped with load cells to measure the force applied to the brake handles and the wheels were resting on force plates that measure all of the components of the floor contact forces. The platform was moved in an unpredictable direction and the efforts of the subject to maintain balance were recorded and analyzed.

incorporating effective consumer input. Wherever possible, designers who are attempting to meet the needs of the elderly should attempt to follow the principles of universal design. However, sometimes the pursuit of a universal solution may compromise function that is critical to the user. The challenge in these circumstances is to achieve that function in as attractive and affordable manner as possible.

References

Alm, N., & Parnes, P. (1995). Augmentative and alternative communication: Past, present and future. *Folia Phoniatrica et Logopaedica, 47*(3), 165–192.

American Academy of Orthopaedic Surgeons. (1985). *Atlas of orthotics: Biomechanical principles and application* (2nd ed.). St. Louis, MO: Mosby.

American Academy of Orthopaedic Surgeons. (1992). *Atlas of limb prosthetics: Surgical, prosthetic and rehabilitation principles* (2nd ed.). St. Louis, MO: Mosby.

Brooks, N. A. (1991). Users' responses to assistive devices for physical disability. *Social Science & Medicine, 32,* 1417–1424.

Brown, L. J., Potter, J. F., & Foster, B. G. (1990). Caregiver burden should be evaluated during geriatric assessment. *Journal of the American Geriatrics Society, 38,* 455–460.

Charette, A. (1988). *Canada's Health Promotion Survey: Special Study on Adults with an Activity Limitation.* Ottawa: Health Promotion Studies Unit, Health and Welfare Canada.

Cooper, B. A., Letts, L., & Rigby, P. (1993). Exploring the use of color cueing on an assistive device in the home: Six case studies. *Physical & Occupational Therapy in Geriatrics, 11,* 47–59.

Garg, A., Owen, B., Beller, D., & Banaag, J. (1991). A biomechanical and ergonomic evaluation of patient transferring tasks: Bed to wheelchair and wheelchair to bed. *Ergonomics, 34,* 289–312.

Gitlin, L. N., Levine, R., & Geiger, C. (1993). Adaptive device use by older adults with mixed disabilities. *Archives of Physical Medicine and Rehabilitation, 74,* 149–152.

Health Industries Advisory Committee. (1994). *Healthy & wealthy: A growth prescription for Ontario's health industries.* Toronto: Ontario Ministry of Health.

Henry, A. (1993, March). A universal approach to an ever-changing universe. *Appliance,* pp. 34–37.

Holden, J. M., Fernie, G. R., & Lunau, K. R. (1988). Chairs for the elderly—design considerations. *Applied Ergonomics, 19,* 281–288.

Jose, R. T. (1983). *Understanding low vision.* New York: American Foundation for the Blind.

LaPlante, M. P., Hendershot, G. E., & Moss, A. J. (1992). Assistive technology devices and home accessibility features: Prevalence, payment, need, and trends. *Advance Data: Centres for Disease Control, 217,* 1–11.

Longino, C. F. (1994, August). Myths of an aging America. *American Demographics,* pp. 36–42.

Maki, B. E., Bartlett, S. A., & Fernie, G. R. (1984). Influence of stairway handrail height on the ability to generate stabilizing forces and moments. *Human Factors, 26,* 705–714.

Manton, K. G., Corder, L. S., & Stallard, E. (1993). Estimates of change in chronic disability and institutional incidence and prevalence rates in the U.S. elderly population from the 1982, 1984, and 1989 National Long Term Care Survey. *Journal of Gerontology, 48,* S153–S166.

McLaurin, C. A., & Brubaker, C. E. (1991). Biomechanics and the wheelchair. *Prosthetics and Orthotics International, 15,* 24–37.
Nowakowski, R. W. (1994). *Primary low vision care.* Norwalk, CT: Appleton & Lange.
Ontario Gerontology Association. (1988). *Fact book on aging in Ontario.* Toronto: Office for Senior Citizens' Affairs.
Phillips, B., & Zhao, H. (1993). Predictors of assistive technology abandonment. *Assistive Technology, 5,* 36–45.
Pirkl, J. J. (1994). *Transgenerational design: Products for an aging population.* New York: Van Nostrand-Reinhold.
Prime Times Strategies. (1993). *Prime times: Success strategies to increase your share of the 50+ market.* Toronto: Ontario Ministry of Citizenship.
Sandlin, R. E. (1988). *Theoretical and technical consideration.* Boston: College Hill.
Sandlin, R. E. (1990). *Clinical considerations and fitting practices.* Boston: College Hill.
Sanford, J. A., Story, M. F., & Jones, M. L. (1996, June). Accessibility requirements for ramp slope: Results of human subjects testing. In A. Langton (Ed.), *Proceedings of the RESNA '96 annual conference* (Vol. 16). Arlington, VA: RESNA Press.
Skinner, M. W. (1988). *Hearing aid evaluation.* Englewood Cliffs, NJ: Prentice-Hall.
Wretenberg, P., Arborelius, U. P., Weidenhielm, L., & Lindberg, F. (1993). Rising from a chair by a spring-loaded flap seat: A biomechanical analysis. *Scandinavian Journal of Rehabilitation Medicine, 25,* 153–159.

Chapter 13

Using Technologies to Aid the Performance of Home Tasks

Sara J. Czaja

INTRODUCTION

One of the most important challenges facing researchers, policy makers, and designers is the need to develop strategies to effectively cope with an aging population. The number of elderly in the population has been growing in absolute and relative terms and will continue to increase in the next decade. Currently people over 65 represent 13% of the population and by the year 2000 they will represent about 23% (U.S. Senate Subcommittee, 1991). Not only are the number of older people in the population increasing but the aged population itself is growing older. By the year 2000 those aged 75–84 years will constitute one-third of the elderly population and those over 85 will represent about 15%. This means that there will be a greater number of very old people living in the United States. Given that the majority of older Americans live in the community, as opposed to institutional settings, an issue of critical importance is to what extent this population will be able to live independently and carry out activities and tasks essential to an acceptable quality of life.

Handbook of Human Factors and the Older Adult

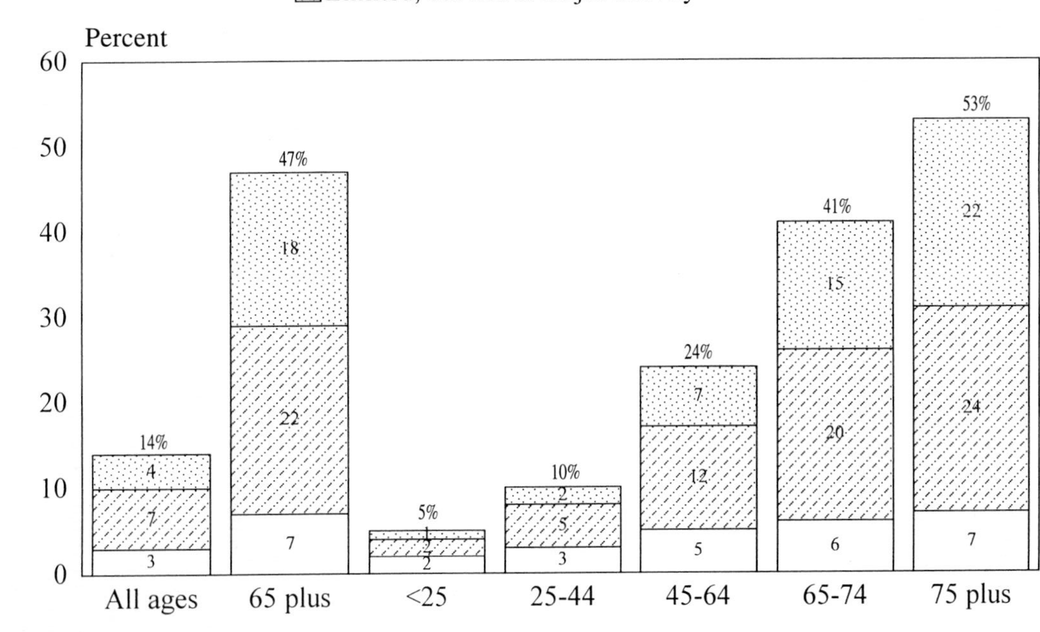

FIGURE 1 Limitation of activity due to chronic conditions by type of limitations and age, 1981. (*Adapted from Kart, 1989.*)

Most older people are self-sufficient and able to function independently or with minimal assistance. However, the prevalence of chronic conditions, such as hypertension, vision and hearing impairments, and arthritis, is higher among the elderly than among younger people. The presence of chronic conditions often has an impact on a person's ability to carry out routine activities. As shown in Figure 1, about 47% of persons over 65 have some limitation in activity performance and about 18% report being unable to carry out a major activity such as housekeeping (Kart, 1990). Further, the elderly use more health care services than younger people and their health care costs are higher than for younger people. Although the elderly represent only 13% of the population, they account for one-third of health-care expenditures because of their reliance on institutional services. As the elderly population increases and lives longer, larger number of older people will require help. It is projected that by the year 2040, if nursing home admissions continue to accelerate, the cost of nursing home care could increase between $84 and $134 billion (Kane, Ouslander, & Abrass, 1994). These demographic trends underscore the need to develop strategies, which maximize the ability of older people to live and function independently.

In this regard, a number of technologies can be used to enhance the independence of older people. For example, personal computers can be used to facilitate health care, communication, and the performance of home maintenance tasks such as banking and shopping. Simple technologies such as grab bars and walkers can aid mobility and magnifying glasses and illuminated telephones can help compensate for sensory deficits. The success of these technologies in fostering independence among older people is dependent on the awareness of their existence by older people and the willingness and ability of older people to use the various devices. The cost of the technology is also of critical importance. Currently, despite the availability of a myriad of products, the integration of technology into the homes of older persons has been limited. For example, only about 1% of people aged 65+ yrs regularly use computers (Swartz, 1988).

This chapter will discuss the potential use of technology in fostering the ability of older adults to live independently at home. The focus will be on "high-tech" products such as computers and communication technologies. Assistive technologies are discussed elsewhere in the handbook. The intent is to demonstrate how technology can be used to enhance the quality of life of older people and to summarize existing knowledge regarding the factors that affect the extent to which the benefits of technology are realized by the older population. Finally, the role of human factors engineering in the design and evaluation of home and health care technologies will be discussed.

HOME LIFE AND THE ELDERLY

Where and How Do Older People Live?

A discussion of the use of home technologies by older people must begin with some understanding of the living arrangements and the activity patterns of the older population. This type of information helps identify the technological applications that would be most useful for older adults. For example, using technology to facilitate activities such as banking and shopping takes on added significance if the majority of older people live in environments where they must rely on automobiles to reach facilities outside the home. Similarly, the value of smart appliances depends on the extent to which older people engage in and need assistance with activities such as meal preparation. Generally research (Czaja, Guerrier, Nair, & Landauer, 1993) has shown that older people are more receptive to technology if they perceive it as useful.

The majority of older adults live in independent households in the community. Only about 5% of the elderly population reside in nursing homes. However, the rate of nursing home residence increases with age. Among persons 65–74 years, the rate is less than 2%, whereas for persons 75–84 and 85+ years the rates increase to 7 and 20%, respectively (Kane et al., 1994). Estimates indicate that the rate of institutionalization among the elderly will increase and that, by the year 2000, 6% of persons 65+ years will be living in nursing homes. An important factor determining whether or not someone needs a nursing home is the extent to which support is available.

The living arrangements of older adults, who live in the community, vary as a function of age and gender. Elderly women are more likely to live alone than men. In 1980, 39% of women aged 65+ lived alone as compared to 14% of men in this age group. The likelihood of living alone increases with age for both men and women. The proportion of men, aged 65–69, living alone in 1980 was 10.9% as compared to 16.4% for men aged 75–79 years and 20% for men aged 80–84. Similarly, for women aged 65–69, 29% lived alone as compared to 44% for women aged 75–79 and 80–84 years (Office of Technology Assessment, 1985). As the number of people in the older decades increases, the proportion of older people, especially older women, living alone will also increase. This has vast societal implications, as people living alone are more likely to need some type of support. Recent data (Norburn et al., 1995) from a national sample of community dwelling older adults indicates that people who live alone are more likely to use assistive devices and make changes in their environments in response to difficulty performing activities than those who live with others. These findings suggest that in the future, as the number of older people living alone increases, the need for assistive technologies will also increase.

With respect to housing, the majority of older people own their own homes and live in single family dwellings. In 1980, among the 16.5 million elderly households, about 12.3 million were owner occupied and only 4.2 million were renter occupied. Older people also tend to live in housing that is older than that occupied by younger people. Generally, older homes tend to be less efficient and require more repairs than newer housing. Therefore, problems with household maintenance and household repairs are more likely for older than younger homeowners. Struyk and Soldo (1980), in their study of the quality of the housing of the elderly, found that homes owned by the elderly were more likely to have incomplete plumbing and kitchen facilities and more maintenance deficiencies than homes owned by the non-elderly. Mann (1994a) reports that older adults have an average of four environmental problems in their homes, with the kitchen and bathroom having the most problems. Housing deficiencies not only reduce the quality of life for occupants and increase the burden associated with household maintenance tasks, they also pose a threat to safety and security. The rate of home accidents among older people is high and the most common types of accidents are falls and burns or scalds. Hence, technologies that reduce problems associated with housing deficiencies, such as systems that monitor temperature, ventilation, and appliances are likely to be especially beneficial for older adults.

Data also indicates that an increasing trend among older adults to live in the suburbs of major cities. In 1980, 28% of older adults lived in the suburbs as compared to 17% in 1960. Because of inadequate public transportation and difficulty driving, problems with mobility are becoming increasingly common among older people. These problems are exacerbated by distances required to travel to services and shopping areas. Recent estimates indicate that about 1 million older people have mobility problems and difficulty reaching facilities and services outside their immediate neighborhoods (Office of Technology Assessment, 1985). Older people frequently report problems with tasks such as grocery shopping because of restricted mobility (Nair, 1989). Access to services, family, friends, and leisure activities is critical to quality of life. Maintaining the independence of older people requires attention to mobility and transportation problems. Technology can play a role in alleviating some of these problems. For example, on-line banking and shopping services allow older people to perform tasks independently and electronic links to physicians and caregivers fosters social support.

The Performance of Home Activities

Determination of the types of home technologies that might be useful for older adults requires understanding what types of activities older people engage in while at home, what types of home activities are difficult for older people to perform, and what difficulties they encounter when performing them. Household behaviors are complex and involve an interaction between the person and the environment. Many researchers (e.g., Faletti, 1984) have suggested that an older person's difficulty functioning effectively in residential environments can be linked to disparities between demands generated by the design and structure of the environment and home tasks and the ability of the older person to meet those demands. This view suggests that the functional independence of older adults might be improved by changing the demands of home tasks so that they are more congruent with the capabilities of older people. For example, adjustable shelves in kitchens may minimize the need for reaching and bending or a voice mail remainder might reduce the memory demands associated with medication compliance. To ensure that demands are commensurate with capabilities a quantification of task demands and relevant person capabilities is required.

In this context it is useful to distinguish between basic activities of daily living (ADLs) and instrumental activities of daily living (IADLs), as this dichotomy is commonly used in the literature. Basic activities of daily living include bathing, dressing, toiletting, eating, and ambulating. Instrumental activities include cooking, shopping, money management, using medication, housework, laundry, using the telephone and driving (Lawton, 1990). These tasks vary in complexity and in physiological and cognitive demands. For example, household tasks such as cleaning and laundry are characterized more by physical demands than tasks such as money management and using medication. To effectively use assistive technology it is important to understand the demands associated with household activities and which demands prove difficult for older people. Medication compliance may be difficult because a person is unable to manipulate the medication container or because that person is unable to remember the medication schedule. Interventions aimed at ameliorating problems with medication compliance must address both of these issues.

Generally data indicate that older people allocate a great deal of time to the performance of ADL and IADL activities. Also, as people age, they tend to spend more time at home, so the design of the home environment is a critical issue with respect to maintaining independence. Currently, data reflecting the amount of time older people spend performing specific household tasks is limited to a relatively small sample of older people. Moss and Lawton (1982) collected time-budget data from samples of independent (*N*

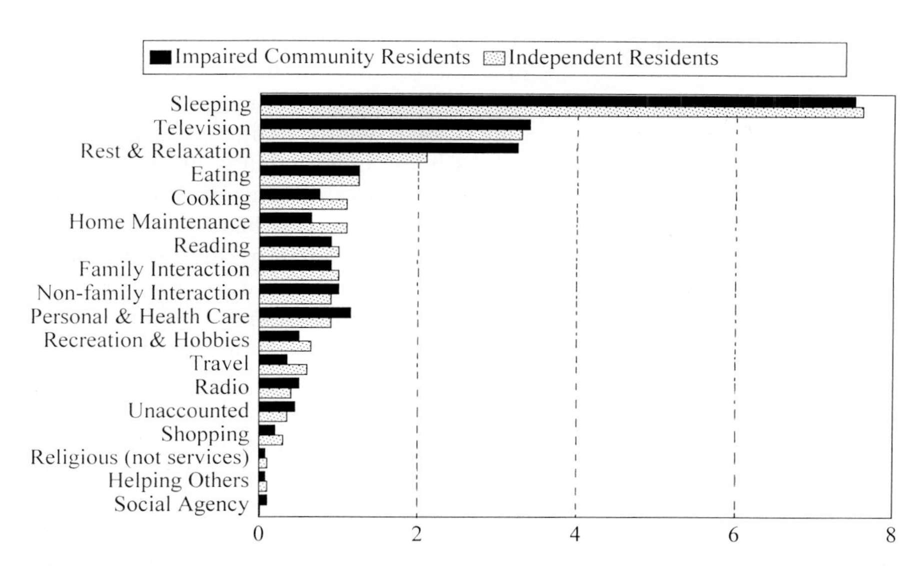

FIGURE 2 Mean hours in an activity for independent residents (N = 426, mean age = 75 years) and impaired community residents (N = 164, Mean age = 79). (*Adapted from Craik and Salthouse, 1992.*)

= 426) and nonindependent (N = 164) elderly people. They found that 82% of all waking behaviors occurred in the home and about one-third of the day was spent on ADLs. Comparison of the time budgets of the independent and nonindependent samples indicated that the latter group's activities were heavily weighted toward personal care and away from instrumental activities. As shown in Figure 2, among the independent sample, large amounts of time were allocated to eating and cooking, housework, and home maintenance. Interestingly, both groups allocated large amounts of time to watching TV. This implies that designers of remote control units, televisions and VCRs must ensure that their products are usable by older adults.

It is reasonably well established that older people often have difficulty performing home tasks such as cooking and cleaning. Data from the National Health Interview Survey (Dawson, Hendershot, & Fulton, 1987) indicates that about 23% of people 65+ living at home have difficulty in performing personal care activities such as bathing and dressing, and about 10% require help with these activities. Further about 27% of persons in this age group require help with instrumental activities such as meal preparation and shopping. Prevalence of problems with these tasks was found to increase with age. The tasks reported as most problematic were bathing, transferring, shopping, meal preparation, and housework. The sample also reported difficulty walking, reaching and bending, maintaining postures for extended periods, and carrying heavy objects. Data from a study conducted at the Stein Gerontological Institute (Czaja, Weber, Nair, & Clark, 1993), based on a sample of 244 older adults living independently in the community, also indicated that home tasks often prove difficult for older adults. Similar to the results of the National Interview Survey the tasks reported as most problematic included meal preparation, grocery shopping, house cleaning, and dressing. Problems with task performance were largely related to the physical demands of the tasks and included bending, reaching, carrying or lifting, and fatigue. Overall, women reported more problems with task performance than men. This is a significant finding as the rate of older women living alone in the community is increasing.

Further evidence for difficulty performing home tasks among older persons is that the rate of home accidents among older persons is high, accounting for 43% of all home fatalities. The most common causes of accidental injury for older people are (1) falls on stairways, floors and bathtubs; (2) burns or scalds from cooking, hot water, and fires; and (3) poisoning from gases and vapors (Sterns, Barrett, & Alexander, 1985). The reasons for the high rate of home accidents among the elderly are complex but include the fact that age-related changes in functional abilities make it difficult to perform home tasks; and the demands of the home environment are often substantive, in that the homes of the elderly are often difficult to maintain and in need of repair. Falls are frequently related to environmental hazards such as throw rugs, poor lighting, and poorly designed stairways. Burns and scalds are related to cooking, smoking, and improper use of appliance and water controls. Poisoning is generally related to improper use of medication or poorly maintained ventilation systems. In essence, many home accidents occur because older people have difficulty with routine activities. Further fear of accidents can cause older people to decrease engaging in activities. Therefore, while people are living longer, many are experiencing a reduced quality of life.

The preceding discussion clearly points to a need to develop strategies that allow older people to live safely and comfortably at home and enjoy an active and independent life. This is a pressing concern as the number of households occupied by the elderly is increasing, and large numbers of older people live alone. Technology can play an important role in promoting independence for older people. The appropriate use of technology can reduce or eliminate demands associated with everyday tasks. As noted by Lawton (1990), a number of routes can be used to obtain the goal of successful task performance. An impairment or change in functional level does not necessarily mean an inability to perform a task successfully performed without the impairment. Instead, alternative routes of goal attainment can be used such as changing behavior or using an assistive device or the help of another person. The following section will discuss how technology can be considered as an alternative route and augment task performance.

THE APPLICATION OF TECHNOLOGY TO THE PERFORMANCE OF HOME TASKS

What Types of Technologies Are Available?

Much has been written about the implication of technology for older adults. Numerous articles and books focus on this issue, and national and international conferences have been organized around this topic. In fact, recently, the discipline of "gerontechnology" has emerged, which is defined as "the study of technology and aging for the improvement of the daily functioning of the elderly" (Bouma, 1993, p. 1). In addition, numerous products have been developed for the "mature market" with the intention of making life easier for this segment of the population. HyperAbleData, a computerized database of assistive devices, lists over 17,000 products. Assistive technologies are available for individuals with hearing, vision, memory, communication, and mobility impairments. Table 1 provides a list of examples of both low- and high-tech devices for various impairments. The National Institute on Disability and Rehabilitation Research (NIDRR), which has a major program in rehabilitation engineering, has made aging a high priority. NIDRR recently funded development by the State University of New York at Buffalo of a Rehabilitation Engineering Research Center (RERC) on Aging (Mann, 1995). The center's projects in aging encompass four major areas: research, device development, education, and service. However, as discussed by Wylde (1995), the use of technologies is not limited to older persons with specific disabilities, as many older individuals who encounter difficulties performing everyday tasks are not classified as having a disability. For example, the force required to open jars or operate controls may prove difficult for healthy older women due to age-related declines in strength. Therefore, devices intended for persons with hand or finger impairments would be beneficial to a large number of people.

The following sections will discuss technologies that might be useful to older adults. The discussion will be organized according to type of technology. The intent is not to provide an exhaustive catalog and description of assistive technologies but rather to demonstrate how technology might be used to improve the quality of life for older people.

Prior to this discussion a definition of *assistive technology* would be

TABLE 1
Examples of Assistive Devices for the Functionally Impaired Elderly

Impairment	Simple devices	Complex devices
Vision	Lighted magnifying glass Large print books	Electronic reading machine that converts printed material to speech
Hearing	Handheld speaking tube or horn	Infrared hearing system that transforms an audio signal via infrared light beam to a receiver worn by the listener, thus suppressing background noise that is a problem for hearing aid users
Speech	Manual communication board; the individual points to a symbol or what he or she wants to say	Electronic communication board with memory and print-out capability. The individual uses a switch to activate a cursor on the board to indicate words or messages Portable speech synthesizer
Memory	Pad to keep notes for reminders	Clock radio system that verbalizes reminders and automatically controls some appliances
Mobility	Braces and splints	Computerized electrical impulse device to stimulate muscles and allow paralized persons to work
	Canes, walkers, and wheelchairs	Voice-controlled, electric wheelchair that can open doors and manipulate switches
	Ramps	Electric chairlifts for stairs
Upper extremity weakness	Reachers and grippers Levers to facilitate turning door knobs and faucet handles	Prosthetic control system using electronic sensors and mechanical transducers to operate a prosthetic arm
Bathing	Shower or bathtub chair Long-handled soaper	Hydralic bath lift Horizontal shower
Dressing	Velcro fasteners Clothing that opens in front	No complex devices known
Eating	Utensils with built-up handles	Automatic feeding machine
Toileting	Bedside commode	Commode with automatic toilet flusher, warm water bidet and hot air drying in a push-button unit
Shopping	Shopping cart for a wheelchair user Prepackaged, freeze dried meals	Shopping by computer
Cooking	Suction gripper to hold a jar to be opened	Robot that can prepare meals
Environmental control	Switches and controls on extension cords that can be reached by the patient	Computerized remote environmental control system to allow a bed- or chairbound patient to adjust lights, radios, TVs, thermostats, and other electrically controlled appliances

Source: Adapted from the Office of Technology Assessment (1985).

useful. According to the Technology Related Assistance for Individuals with Disabilities Act of 1988 an assistive technology device is any item, piece of equipment, or product system that is used to increase, maintain, or improve the functional capacities of persons with disabilities. This includes "low-tech" devices such as reachers and adaptive silverware and "high-tech" devices that typically involve microprocessors and computers, print enlargement systems, and environmental control units (cited in Mann, 1994b, p. 324). The focus of this discussion will be on "high-tech" devices.

Computer Technologies

Computer technology can be used in a number of ways to improve the quality of life for older persons. It is now possible to use home computers to carry out routine errands such as shopping, bill paying, and financial management. Older people commonly report problems with these tasks because of restricted mobility, inconvenience, difficulty carrying items such as groceries, and fear of crime (Nair, 1989). Data from a recent national survey (Norburn et al., 1995) indicates that, while most older adults are able to perform instrumental tasks such as money management, housework, and shopping, those who tend to have problems with these tasks report the problems as severe. Of those who have difficulty with shopping and money management, 50% report not being able to perform the activity at all. Shopping and banking at home, via a computer, could alleviate these problems and allow seniors to perform these tasks independently. Many on-line services such as Prodigy and Compuserve provide a forum for activities such as shopping. Software is also available for balancing checkbooks, paying bills, and calculating taxes. Older people can also use computers for information retrieval. For example, information about community events, transportation, and support services is available on-line.

Computer technology can also facilitate social interaction and enhance the intellectual and leisure activities of older adults. Older people have more leisure time and spend the majority of their discretionary time at home. They often report problems with social isolation, boredom, and loneliness (Neugarten, 1977). The report of a recent survey of 400 persons aged 60+ who have a disability indicated that leisure activities ranked highest among the activities that they missed (cited in Mann, 1995). Computers can help alleviate this problem by providing opportunities for these activities in home settings. Electronic networks can make it easier for older people to maintain ties to family and friends and to form new friendships. Bulletin boards allow people with special interests to exchange information or request advice on issues such as health insurance or locating health care specialists. Text message systems may be especially beneficial for older people with hearing impairments or for persons with loss of speech such as stroke victims.

Furlong (1989) found substantial use of mail, conferencing, news and bulletin board use among users of SeniorNet. Hahm and Bikson (1989) found that electronic mail increased the social interactions among a group of retirees. Further the sample in their study found the computers to be "fun" and a "challenge." However, the authors report that the users required a large amount of technical support during the initial seven months of interaction with the system. Software and organizational issues dominated the support requests. Eilers (1989) found that older people who used computers reported the following benefits: social interaction, mental stimulation, and memory enhancement.

We (Czaja, Guerrier et al., 1993) recently completed a study that assessed the ability of older adults to use an electronic message system to perform communication tasks. The study involved installing a specially configured computer system in the homes of 36 community dwelling older women ranging in age from 55 to 95 years. The results indicated that the study participants were both willing and able to use the computer system. Moreover, they reported that they enjoyed using the system and found it valuable. Participants were asked what they liked and disliked about the system. They indicated that they liked using the system because it allowed them to communicate with others and because it was interesting and stimulating. Reasons for using the computer included socialization, the chance to meet new people, the opportunity to learn something new, and experiencing a mental challenge. However, the results also demonstrated the importance of designing computer systems to accommodate age changes in cognitive and perceptual abilities. During the course of the study several aspects of the hardware, such as the keyboard, and various aspects of the software interface, such as the on-screen messages, needed to be modified to make the system more usable for the study population.

Computers also hold the promise of making discretionary time more meaningful for older people. Computers can provide opportunities for continuing education and recreation within home settings. Software is available for a wide variety of topics and electronic links can be established between the home and universities. University-based continuing education programs for seniors are becoming common across the country, and participation rates of older people in continuing education programs have been steadily increasing. Electronic links between the university and an older person's home would enable many more seniors to participate in these programs. Currently many older people fail to participate in continuing education programs because of lack of transportation, inconvenience in scheduling, and physical restrictions (Willis, 1985).

Computer technology can also play an important role in health care management and disease prevention. Seniors can use computers to become more actively involved in the management of their own health care. For example, computers may be used for health instruction. A number of health related software programs are available on topics such as stress management, nutrition, and diet and specialized topics such as low back pain or arthritis management. Computers may also assist disease management by providing reminders of medication schedules and dietary or rehabilitation instructions. Leirer, Morrow, Tanke, and Pariante (1991) found that computerized voice mail, sent via a telephone, significantly reduced medication nonadherence among a sample of older adults. The voice mail system improved the accuracy of the exact time the participants took their medication and reduced instances of complete forgetting. Holmes, Teresi, and Holmes (1990) demonstrated that computer systems can provide effective interfaces between patients and health care providers. Computer-assisted health care may allow frail elderly or people who are chronically ill to remain in their homes. An estimated 15–20% of elderly people who are currently institutionalized could remain in their homes if home health services were available and reimbursable (Office of Technology Assessment, 1985). Caregivers can use e-mail to conduct a daily status check on patients or remind them of home health care regimes. The computer can "call" the patient and ask routine questions. In the future computer technology may be used for measurement of physical functioning such as blood pressure, pulse rate, and temperature. The elderly patients may also use the computer to communicate with health care professionals. They may ask health related questions or indicate if they are experiencing some type of a problem.

Computer communication may also be used to provide support for homebound caregivers of persons with Alzheimers disease by linking the caregiver to other caregivers, family members, or local support organizations. Gallienne, Moore and Brennan (1993) found that access to a computer network increased the amount of psychological support provided by nurses to a group of older homebound caregivers.

Computers may also be used to augment the memory functioning of the elderly. For example, computer messages can be sent to remind people of appointments, or personal databases can be constructed to provide reminders of important dates, medication schedules, and the like. Computers can also be used for cognitive rehabilitation and for the training and retraining of cognitive skills such as memory and attention (Chute & Bliss, 1994). Another alternative is to use the computer as a prosthetic device to augment deficiencies in cognitive or motor abilities. Chute and his colleagues (Chute & Bliss, 1994) are developing a microcomputer application, Prostheses-Ware, which is designed to augment the abilities of persons with cognitive and central nervous system limitations. For example, for a person with some type of memory limitation, the software could remind the person of the need for and the sequencing of a personal hygiene task such as bathing. Prosthesesware is specifically customized to offer assistance appropriate to the individual, environment, and context for any particular ADL. An example of a ProsthesesWare Module is Speechware, which is a speech prosthesis for individuals who have lost the ability to communicate and who may also have severe motor impairments. It would allow, for example, a person who has lost motor control of both arms and of his or her voice to engage in telephone communication. Prosthesesware is still in the developmental stages, and while it holds great promise for enhancing the independence of persons with functional impairments, there are some potential limitations of this technology for older persons, including cost and training.

Finally microcomputer systems can be used to enhance safety and security. Systems can be programmed to monitor electrical, heating and ventilation systems, and appliances and can be linked to the appropriate agency or service provider. These systems can also be used as a security device and monitor doors, windows and movements outside the house. As will be discussed in the next section computerized environmental control systems might also be used to allow persons with restricted mobility to control lights, radios, TVs, and appliances. The "smart house" concept is an example of an integrated system of these types of technologies. Essentially the smart house is a place where the appliances, telephone, lighting, heating and ventilation, and security systems are monitored and controlled through a central computer control system. While the smart house is still in the stage of development, "smart" products such as appliances are available. Sharp produces a "smart" microwave oven, Smart and Easy, which was recently evaluated by the RERC-Aging at SUNY at Buffalo. It was found to be very easy to use and an excellent product for older people (Mann, 1995).

Environmental Control Devices

Environmental control devices are designed for persons with physical or cognitive disabilities. The devices are designed to allow a person with a disability to operate lights, radios, TVs, and other electrically controlled appliances. Handheld remote controls are an example of an environmental control device. These types of devices vary in cost, from $24 to $10,000, and function, from simple on–off to control of the whole home (Mann, 1994b). Environmental control units allow a person independent control of his or her environment. A recent study (cited in Mann, 1994b) found that nursing home residents who were given handheld environmental control units used their TVs with significantly greater frequency than those residents who were not given the units and had to rely on the assistance of others. However, one problem with these types of devices is that typically they are designed for younger adults and do not take into account the needs of the elderly. For example, the labels are often difficult to read and the operating procedures are often complex. Parsons, Terner, and Kearsley (1994) recently conducted a study to improve the design of remote control units (RCU) for seniors. They found that a large percentage of their elderly participants made errors when attempting to operate a remote control unit. They also queried manufacturers to determine if they considered the elderly when designing the RCU. Of the manufacturers that responded, none indicated that it considered product design issues for older consumers. Parsons et al. (1994) concluded that there are a number of opportunities for human factors engineers with respect to the design of RCUs.

Robotics

Another "high-technology application" that has the potential of helping elderly people, especially those with disabilities, remain at home is service robotics. *Service robotics* is defined as "robotics systems that function as smart, programmable, tools, and that can sense, think, and act to enable or benefit human beings" (Engelhardt, 1989, p. 6). Engelhardt (1989) identified several major tasks augmentable or replaceable by robotics technology, including patient transport–lift–transfer, ambulation, housekeeping, physical therapy, surveillance and monitoring, vital signs monitoring, and mental stimulation, and cognitive rehabilitation. HANC (home assisted nursing care) is an example of a type of service robotics. HANC is designed to foster independence among persons who are mildly impaired. HANC, which is networked via central telephone lines to a central station, can assist with various health maintenance activities such as monitoring vital signs, reminding about and delivering medications, and emergency response. HANC manages these activities using a voice interactive system (Stewart & Kaufman, 1993).

While robotics holds the promise of enhancing the ability of older adults to live independently it appears that in the near future their use will be limited. Robotics technology is costly and requires considerable programming. Also, home activities need to be decomposed prior to program development. Further, a number of issues (e.g., type of control device, user acceptance, safety) need to be addressed before this type of technology can be successfully used in home environments by older people.

Telephone/Communication Technologies

A number of emerging and existing telephone technologies can be used to augment the performance of home activities. Among the obvious benefits of this type of technology is that most older people own a telephone and know how to use it. Collins, Bhatti, Dexter, and Rabbit (1993) surveyed over 2000 people aged 50+ in the United Kingdom regarding their use of technology and found that 97% of the sample owned a telephone and, of these, 82% rated the telephone as essential.

Voice mail is one type of telephone technology that might be beneficial to older people. As discussed, voice mail was found to be successful in increasing medication compliance among a sample of older adults (Leirer et al., 1991). In a more recent study Tanke and Leirer (1993) found that voice mail reminders significantly increased elderly patients' adherence to tuberculosis medication appointments. Voice mail technology allows human voice messages to be recorded and stored in a computer's memory. The computer phones the person at prescheduled times and delivers the message. Voice mail can be very cost effective in assisting with home health care in that it does not require extensive staff time.

Garbe, Stockler, and Wald (1993) present several examples of how telecommunications technology is used to enhance the quality of life for elderly people in Germany. These include Tele-Ring, which is a social support service and involves established networks of six to eight elderly people who communicate at prearranged times; and Tele-Link, which is an extended form of the Tele-Ring and allows for conference calls. As the authors point out for some older people this communication represents their only link with the outside world. Other applications include Alzheimer Telephone, which is a telephone support service for patients and their caregivers; Tele-Medicine, which provides information and contacts within the field of health care; and a lifeline type service that offers quick help for older people in emergency situations. The RACE project in Frankfurt is a pilot project designed to evaluate how videotelephony or interactive audiovisual telephone communication can be used to assist communication for people with hearing, visual, or motor impairments. The target population is the elderly or caregivers of elderly relatives. The system will establish a link between the client and a service center that will provide services such as emergency response, information and assistance, support groups, and remote access to expertise. Initial data from the pilot study are encouraging: the technology has been accepted and used successfully by both caregivers and elderly clients (Robinson, 1993). Many benefits are associated with videotelephones for people who are hard of hearing, as they are able to make use of visual cues in communication. Presbycusis affects 60% of people aged 65+ who live in the United States (Kane et al., 1994). AT&T has developed a low-bandwidth videotelephone system for the mass market. However, it has not been evaluated in terms of its effectiveness as a communication aid for the deaf, hard of hearing, or older adults (Harkins, Levitt, & Peltz-Strauss, 1994).

Telephone relay service (TRS) is a recently developed nationwide telecommunications service that allows any deaf, hard-of-hearing, or speech impaired person to communicate on the telephone network. TRS, which involves the use of a text telephone, is an operator-assisted interface between text terminals and voice terminals. The operator is contacted by the impaired person, contacts the intended party (voice party), speaks the typed message to the voice party, and types the spoken messages to the text telephone user. While there are issues surrounding privacy, this technology permits many people who were previously unable to communicate using the telephone system. The technology is still evolving and efforts are underway to improve TRS through the application of other technologies such as speech recognition and operator multiplexing (Harkins et al., 1994). A number of user interface issues need to be addressed in the design of these system, such as identification of the optimal procedure and input device for call setup. These issues are especially important for older consumers.

Other telephone technologies being developed (by Bellcore) for persons who have some type of impairment include DeskSet, an information system for people who are blind or visually impaired; VADEC (voice activated dialing and environmental control), a telephone system and environmental control for people with mobility impairments that involves the use of speech recognition; and INVOCA, a communication aid for persons who are speech impaired (Tobias, 1994). Remote reading systems, which involve the use of telecommunications technology such as a fax machine, are also being developed for people who are visually impaired. All of these technologies offer the promise of improving the lives of older people who live at home.

Technologies for Sensory Impairments

Other technologies are available to assist people with visual, hearing, or speech impairments. A brief discussion of these technologies is provided, as many older adults have difficulties hearing and seeing and these difficulties can have a substantial impact on their ability to perform routine tasks (for more detail, see Mann, 1994b).

Products to assist people with visual impairments include character enlargement systems for computer monitors, stand-alone print enlargement systems, Braille output systems, and voice output systems. For example, the Alladin Personal Reader (Telesensory Corporation) is an electronic magnifying device designed for people who have reading difficulties. The Alladin magnifies printed material up to 25 times its actual size and allows people with visual problems to read newspapers, magazines, and other printed material. This product was recently selected as a cowinner of the American Society on Aging annual design competition because of the attention given to the design needs of older adults (Harper, 1995). Also, the font size of book collections on CD-ROM can be increased.

In addition to the telecommunication technologies already discussed products for the hearing impaired include amplification aids and assistive listening devices. Other devices that may be useful for improving communication include visual alerting devices and television listening systems. Synthetic speech applications are also being used as sensory aids for the visually impaired. However, the design of these systems needs to be carefully evaluated for older adults. Smither (1993) recently completed a study to determine if age had an impact on the perception of synthetic speech. She compared the performance of both younger and older adults on a memory recall task under conditions of natural and synthetic speech. She found that, in general, the older people performed more poorly than the younger people and both groups performed worse with synthetic speech. These results suggest that voice response systems may be problematic for older persons. Smither concluded that consideration of older adults in the design of these types of systems is of critical importance.

User Acceptance of Technology

As illustrated in the previous section, a number of technologies hold the promise of improving the quality of life for older people. However, availability of technology does not guarantee its success. The degree to which technology improves the lives of the elderly is dependent on the willingness and ability of older people to use the various products and devices. A commonly held belief is that older people are "technophobic" and unwilling to interact with "high-tech" products. Available data, while limited, largely disputes this assumption. Data from the 1990 National Health Interview Survey (LaPlante, Hendershot, & Moss, 1992) indicated that more than 50% of the people who used assistive technology were over age 65. Mann (1995) interviewed a sample of 400 older people with some type of disability, and found that on average they owned 14 assistive devices and used about 10 devices. He also found that many people were unaware of available products and devices. In general, age per se does not influence whether or not technology will be adopted but rather the degree to which the technology meets the needs and desires of an individual.

For example, data from a survey, conducted by AARP, of older people who had visited the Technology Center at its biannual meeting indicated that the majority of respondents were willing to use a personal computer to perform routine tasks such as preparing taxes, budgeting, and accessing health or benefit information. The sample was well educated, and the technology was introduced at the center in a highly interactive, understandable manner (Edwards & Engelhardt, 1989). Collins et al. (1993) in their survey regarding elderly and their use of technology, found that current use of technology was a stronger predictor of the perceived usefulness of future technology than demographic variables such as gender and age. They also found that the design of the technology is of critical importance, so that if the equipment is difficult to use, either physically or cognitively, older people will be unlikely to use it. In our study of e-mail (Czaja, Guerrier et al., 1993), we found that all of our participants ($N = 36$) found it valuable to have a computer in their homes, and the majority found it acceptable as a means of communication. However, we also found that, for the system to be used, it must be perceived as useful and provide access to useful applications. The most commonly requested applications were word processing, continuing education, health and emergency services, and banking and shopping. Eilers (1989), in her study of older adults who participated in a computer education program, found that the study participants were eager to learn to use computers for tasks such as money management, continuing education, access to data banks, and word processing.

A number of studies have examined age differences in attitudes toward computer technology. Although the findings from these studies are somewhat mixed in general, the results indicate that older people have positive attitudes toward computer technology. In our study of text editing (Czaja, Hammond, Blascovich, & Swede, 1989), we found no age differences in attitudes toward computers before or after training. Dyck and Smither (1994) examined the relationships among computer anxiety, computer experience, gender, and level of education among a sample of younger and older adults. They also measured attitudes toward computers. They found age differences in attitudes, with the older participants having more positive attitudes toward computers and more liking for computers than the younger participants. However, the older people indicated less computer confidence than the younger people. They also found a relationship between computer experience and computer anxiety such that higher levels of experience were associated with less anxiety and more positive attitudes. Jay and Willis (1992) also found that experience with computers has an influence on computer attitudes. They found that the attitudes of a sample of older adults toward computers became more positive following participation in a two week computer training program. Brickfield (1984) surveyed 750 adults ranging in age from 45 to 65+ years and found that the older adults had less positive attitudes toward technologies such as computers and were less willing to use these technologies. However, the results were moderated by employment status, education, and income. People with more education and higher incomes had more positive attitudes and were more likely to use technology. Krauss and Hoyer (1984) found no age differences in attitudes toward computers but found gender differences. Men had more positive attitudes than women. They also found that experience with computers resulted in more positive attitudes. Danowski and Sacks (1980) examined effects of participation with computer-mediated communication among a sample of older adults on attitudes toward computers. They found that a positive experience with computers results in more positive attitudes. They also found that design factors are important with respect to a person's willingness to interact with computers. Large-size displays and characters and small group training facilitated interaction, whereas complex command names and operating procedures inhibited interaction.

In addition to receptivity toward technology, older adults need to be able to learn to successfully interact with technological systems. Several studies have examined the ability of older adults to learn to use computer technology. The results of these studies will not be discussed in detail as this issue is addressed in Chapter 14 by Morrell and Echt. Overall, the results of these studies are encouraging in that they demonstrate that older people are able to learn to use computer applications. However, the findings indicate that older people have more difficulty than younger people acquiring computer skills, and they achieve lower levels of performance. Clearly more work is needed to identify factors such as training method and interface design that affect skill acquisition.

Overall existing research suggests that older adults are willing to use computers and other forms of technology if they perceive the technology as useful, they are provided with adequate training, and the technology is simple to use and operate. Awareness of the existence of the various technological applications and cost is also important. Gitlin (1995) indicates that the decision to accept or reject assistive technology is determined by a complex interaction of factors. These factors include person factors such as perceived need, environmental factors such as the physical design of the environment and demands of a task, sociocultural factors such as social attributes related to devices, and the design of the device in terms of ease of use, aesthetics, quality, and durability. The next section will discuss the role of human factors engineering in ensuring that technology is useable by older people.

THE HUMAN FACTORS OPPORTUNITIES IN PROMOTING TECHNOLOGY FOR OLDER ADULTS

Human factors engineering can make a number of important contributions toward ensuring that older people are able to use technology to safely, effectively, and independently perform home tasks. One critical role for human factors engineers is to gather information about the needs of older people and the types of problems they encounter at home. While data are available regarding the types of tasks, such as meal preparation, difficult for the elderly, such data are not sufficient in terms of identifying design solutions. To appropriately identify intervention strategies, data are needed on the specific aspects or demands of tasks that are problematic for older people. Human factors task analytic techniques would be extremely useful in providing this type of data. Further we need information on the types of technologies or devices older people desire and need. As indicated, technology is much more likely to be used if it is perceived as useful.

A second role of human factors engineering is to provide data to product designers on the characteristics of older adult populations. Designers need specific information on the abilities and limitations of older people and the implications for the design process. Clearly human factors engineers should play a major role in the design of technology in terms of specifying design parameters that allow the technology to be used effectively by older people.

Additionally, human factors engineers need to be involved in the evaluation of technology. We need data regarding the overall appropriateness of technological products for older users and the extent to which these technologies meet the needs and preferences of this population. To gather this type of data, disabled and healthy elderly must be involved in product design and testing. In too many instances, designers make assumptions about user needs and preferences that are untested in the design process. As discussed a survey of designers of remote control units indicated that none of them had considered older adults in the design process. Finally, human factors engineering should be involved in the design of training programs to ensure that older people are able to acquire the skills to successfully interact with "high-tech" products and devices.

CONCLUSIONS

Technology holds the promise of improving the quality of life and enhancing the independence of older adults. If properly designed, technology could allow older people to perform routine tasks with greater ease and independence and also provide them with enhanced opportunities for learning and social interaction. This is especially true for older people who are frail or homebound. A number of technologies are available that could be very beneficial to older people, and future technologies offer even greater potential benefit. Older people are receptive to using technology; however, it must be useful, useable, affordable, and available.

To maximize the benefits of technology for older people, we need to carefully evaluate the role of and need for technology in the lives of the elderly. We also need to ensure that products are designed so that they are usable by this population. This is not to suggest that older people require specially designed products; accommodating the needs of the elderly in the design process typically accommodates the needs of all users, both young and old. Failure to design for a diverse population limits the use of technology and prevents it from achieving the goal of improving the quality of life for people of all ages. Designers need to perceive of older people as active users of technology and recognize that there are many ways in which technology can be applied to improve the lives of this population.

Enormous opportunities and challenges for human factors engineers lie in the area of technology and aging. Although progress has been made, research in this area is rather limited. As discussed in this and other chapters in this handbook, a number of unanswered questions remain. For example, how do we best train older people to use new technology, or are synthetic speech systems usable by this population and, if so, how should they be designed? What type of input device is optimal for older people, and how well do older people navigate within a windows environment? What types of technologies are most useful for this population? Answers to these and other questions are needed before we can successfully integrate technology into the lives of older adults. Given that older people represent an increasingly large segment of the population designers and researchers must expand their focus and include the needs and concerns of the elderly within the scope of their activities.

References

Bouma, H. (1993). Gerontechnology: A framework on technology and aging. In H. Bouma & J. A. M. Graafmans (Eds.), *Gerontechnology* (pp. 1–6). Amsterdam: ISO Press.

Brickfield, C. F. (1984). Attitudes and perceptions of older people toward technology. In P. K. Robinson & J. E. Birren (Eds.), *Aging and technological advances* (pp. 31–38). New York: Plenum Press.

Chute, D. L., & Bliss, M. E. (1994). Prosthesis ware: Concepts and caveats for microcomputer-based aids to everyday living. *Experimental Aging Research, 20,* 229–238.

Collins, S. C., Bhatti, J. Z., Dexter, S. L., & Rabbit, P. M. A. (1993). Elderly people in a new world: Attitudes to advanced communications technologies. In H. Bouma & J. A. M. Graafmans (Eds.), *Gerontechnology* (pp. 227–282). Amsterdam: ISO Press.

Czaja, S. J., Guerrier, J., Nair, S., & Landauer, T. (1993). Computer communication as an aid to independence for older adults. *Behavior and Information Technology, 12,* 197–207.

Czaja, S. J., Hammond, K., Blascovich, J., & Swede, H. (1989). Age-related differences in learning to use a text-editing system. *Behavior and Information Technology, 8,* 309–319.

Czaja, S. J., Weber, R. A., Nair, S., & Clark, C. (1993). A human factors analysis of ADL activities: A capability-demand approach. *Journals of Gerontology, 48,* 44–50.

Danowski, J. A., & Sacks, W. (1980). Computer communication and the elderly. *Experimental Aging Research, 6,* 125–135.

Dawson, D., Hendershot, G., & Fulton, J. (1987). Aging in the eighties: Functional limitations of individuals aged 65 years and older. *National Center for Health Statistics Advance Data 1987, 133,* 1–11.

Dyck, J. L., & Smither, J. A. (1994). Age difference in computer anxiety: The role of computer experience, gender and education. *Journal of Educational Computing Research, 10,* 239–247.

Edwards, R., & Engelhardt, K. G. (1989). Microprocessor-based innovations and older individuals: AARP survey results and their implications for service robotics. *International Journal of Technology and Aging, 2,* 45–55.

Eilers, M. L. (1989). Older adults and computer education: "Not to have the world a closed door." *International Journal of Technology and Aging, 2,* 56–76.

Engelhardt, K. G. (1989). Health and human service robotics: Multidimensional perspectives. *International Journal of Technology and Aging, 2,* 6–41.

Faletti, M. V. (1984). Human factors research and functional environments for the aged. In A. Altman, M. P. Lawton, & J. F. Wohlwill (Eds.), *Elderly people and the environment* (pp. 191–237). New York: Plenum.

Furlong, M. S. (1989). An electronic community for older adults: The SeniorNet network. *Journal of Communication, 39,* 145–153.

Gallienne, R. L., Moore, S. M., & Brennan, P. F. (1993, December). Alzheimer's caregivers: Psychosocial support via computer networks. *Journal of Gerontological Nursing,* pp. 15–22.

Garbe, D., Stockler, F., & Wald, R. (1993). The state of the art: Telecommunication and the elderly. In H. Bouma & J. A. M. Graffmans (Eds.), *Gerontechnology* (pp. 283–292). Amsterdam: ISO Press.

Gitlin, L. N. (1995). Why older people accept or reject assistive technology. *Generations, 19,* 41–46.

Hahm, W., & Bickson, T. (1989). Retirees using e-mail and networked computers. *International Journal of Technology and Aging, 2,* 113–124.

Harkins, J. E., Levitt, H., & Peltz-Strauss, K. (1994). Technology and telephone relay service. *Technology and Disability, 3,* 173–194.

Harper, D. (1995). Ease and independence without stigma: Three products that work. *Generations, 19,* 58–60.

Holmes, D., Teresi, J., & Holmes, M. (1990). Computer applications in health care planning and practice. *International Journal of Technology and Aging, 3,* 69–78.

Jay, G. M., & Willis, S. L. (1992). Influence of direct computer experience on older adults attitudes toward computers. *Journal of Gerontology: Psychological Sciences, 47,* 250–257.

Kane, R. L., Ouslander, J. G., & Abrass, I. B. (1994). *Essentials of clinical geriatrics* (3rd ed.). New York: McGraw-Hill.

Kart, C. S. (1990). *The realities of aging: An introduction to gerontology* (3rd ed.). Boston: Allyn & Bacon.

Krauss, I. K., & Hoyer, W. J. (1984). Technology and the older person: Age, sex, and experience as moderators of attitudes toward computers. In P. K. Robinson, J. Livingston, & J. E. Birren (Eds.), *Aging and technological advances* (pp. 349–350). New York: Plenum Press.

LaPlante, M., Hendershot, G., & Moss, A. (1992). *Assistive technology devices and home accessibility features: Prevalence, payment, needs, and trends* (DHHS Publication No. PHS-92-1250). Hyattsville, MD: National Center for Health Statistics.

Lawton, P. (1990). Aging and the performance of home tasks. *Human Factors, 32,* 527–536.

Leirer, V. O., Morrow, D. G., Tanke, E. D., & Pariante, G. M. (1991). Elders nonadherence: Its assessment and medication reminding by voice mail. *Gerontologist, 31,* 514–520.

Mann, W. C. (1994a). Environmental problems in homes of elders with disabilities. *Occupational Therapy Journal of Research, 14,* 191–211.
Mann, W. C. (1994b). Technology. In B. R. Bonder & M. B. Wagner (Eds.), *Functional performance in older adults* (pp. 323–338). Philadelphia: Davis.
Mann, W. C. (1995). Rehabilitation engineering: The national institute on disability and rehabilitation research focuses on assistive technology for elders. *Generation, 19,* 49–53.
Moss, M., & Lawton, M. P. (1982). The time budgets of older people: A window on four lifestyles. *Journal of Gerontology, 37,* 115–123.
Nair, S. (1989). *A capability-demand analysis of grocery shopping problems encountered by older adults.* A thesis submitted to the Department of Industrial Engineering, State University of New York at Buffalo in partial fulfillment for the requirements for Master of Science.
Neugarten, B. L. (1977). Personality and aging. In J. E. Birren & K. W. Schaie (Eds.), *Handbook of the psychology of aging* (pp. 626–649). New York: Van Nostrand-Reinhold.
Norburn, J. E., Bernard, S. L., Konrad, T. R., Woomert, A., DeFriese, G. H., Kalsbeek, W. D., Koch, G. G., & Ory, M. G. (1995). Self-care assistance from others in coping with functional status limitations among a national sample of older adults. *Journal of Gerontology: Social Sciences, 50B,* S101–S109.
Office of Technology Assessment. (1985, June). *Technology and aging in America* (OTA-BA-264). Washington, DC: U.S. Congress, Office of Technology Assessment.
Parsons, H. M., Terner, J., & Kearsley, G. (1994). Design of remote control units for seniors. *Experimental Aging Research, 20,* 211–218.
Robinson, S. (1993). Support for elderly people using videotelephony: The Frankfurt pilot. In H. Bouma & J. A. M. Graafmans (Eds.), *Gerontechnology* (pp. 305–316). Amsterdam: ISO Press.
Smither, J. A. (1993). Short term memory demands in processing synthetic speech by old and young adults. *Behavior and Information Technology, 12,* 330–335.
Sterns, H. L., Barrett, G. V., & Alexander, R. A. (1985). Accidents and the aging individual. In J. E. Birren & K. W. Schaie (Eds.), *Handbook of the psychology of aging* (2nd ed., pp. 703–724). New York: Van Nostrand-Reinhold.
Stewart, L. M., & Kaufman, S. B. (1993). High-tech home care: Electronic devices with implications for the design of living environments. In *Life-span design of residential environments for an aging population* (pp. 57–65). Washington, DC: American Association for Retired Persons.
Struyk, R., & Soldo, B. (1980). *Improving the elderly's housing.* Cambridge, MA: Ballinger.
Swartz, J. (1988). The computer market. *American Demographics, 10,* 38–41.
Tanke, E. D., & Leirer, V. O. (1993). Use of automated telephone reminders to increase elderly patients' adherence to tuberculosis medication appointments. In *Proceedings of the Human Factors and Ergonomics Society 37th annual meeting* (pp. 193–196). Santa Monica, CA: Human Factors and Ergonomics Society.
Tobias, J. (1994). Shared resource assistive systems. *Technology and Disability, 3,* 213–217.
U.S. Senate Subcommittee on Aging, American Association of Retired Persons, Federal Council on Aging, and the U.S. Administration on Aging. (1991). *Aging America: Trends and projections* (DHHS Publication No. (FCoA)91-28001). Washington, DC: U.S. Department of Health and Human Services.
Willis, S. (1985). Towards an educational psychology of the older adults learner: Intellectual and cognitive bases. In J. E. Birren & K. W. Schaie (Eds.), *Handbook of the psychology of aging* (2nd ed, pp. 703–724). New York: Van Nostrand-Reinhold.
Wylde, M. A. (1995). How to size up the current and future markets: Technology and the older adult. *Generations, 19,* 15–19.

Chapter 14

Designing Written Instructions for Older Adults: Learning to Use Computers

Roger W. Morrell
Katharina V. Echt

INTRODUCTION

Electronic technology is prevalent in almost every aspect of our daily lives. Preschool children and teenagers entertain themselves with computer games. Many facets of business are routinely conducted on-line by young and middle-aged adults. Millions of people surf the Internet intermittently throughout the day. It would appear, however, that the information highway has bypassed the elderly. Results from several surveys conducted over the last 10 years indicate that adults over the age of 65 report using electronic devices less often and have less experience with personal computers than younger adults (Brickfield, 1984; Kerschner & Hart, 1984; Rogers, Walker, Gilbert, Fraser, & Fisk, 1994; Schwartz, 1988). Furthermore, the older adults who use computers and electronic devices to any degree represent a select segment of the elderly: those older individuals who have higher incomes and

Handbook of Human Factors and the Older Adult

higher educational achievements (Kerschner & Hart, 1984). The implication of this skewed distribution of older users is that a large portion of the older age group is most likely not able to access important sources of information, communication, and service opportunities.

Therefore, the purpose of this chapter is to explore how to increase the use of electronic technology by the elderly. We argue that one of the primary reasons for low utilization by older adults is that few instructional materials are available that can effectively teach older adults to use electronic devices. We begin our discussion by focusing on how computers may be used in the everyday lives of older adults. Second, we investigate how age-related changes in vision may necessitate a number of considerations for the design of printed instructional material for the elderly. We follow this discussion with a set of guidelines derived from research in the area that may be applied when designing printed instructional materials for older adults in general, as well as when constructing computer manuals. Finally, the past research on computer training with older adults and studies on general instructional design for the elderly are examined. In this section we explore how age-related deficits in the cognitive processes of working memory and spatial ability may specifically affect the design of printed instructional materials for teaching computer skills to older adults.

We focus on directions in print because printed manuals are the most common form of instruction currently provided with computer hardware and software. Printed material can also be readily produced by most individuals without extensive expertise because of recent advances in desktop publishing, innovations in laser printers, and the proliferation of "copy shops" that offer services that include layout design and production and printing at an affordable price. Overall, we suggest that findings from studies in cognition and aging, education, as well as concepts from human factors may be integrated to establish a set of recommendations to follow for the design of printed instructions specifically for older adults for learning how to use computers. Such design considerations might, in turn, motivate the elderly to increase their use of technology.

Finally, it is important to note that we focus on the development of instructional materials for computer use as a practical example of how our recommendations may be utilized. There is a definite need to develop instructional materials for computer use that are "elderly friendly." The present guidelines for designing written instructions may well transfer to other domains and may also be employed whenever relevant over a wide range of everyday situations. Although we focus on older adults specifically, it is also likely that the guidelines will extend over computer users of other ages in many instances.

THE POTENTIAL OF COMPUTER INTERACTION WITH THE ELDERLY

It is surprising that the use of computers is low among the elderly, because little systematic evidence is available to support the contention that older individuals are more resistant to learning how to use computer technology than young adults or that they experience insuperable problems when using electronic technology in general (Ansley & Erber, 1988; Garfein, Schaie, & Willis, 1988; A. A. Hartley, Hartley, & Johnson, 1984; Krauss & Hoyer, 1984; McNeely, 1991). Furthermore, it has been shown that computers may be easily integrated in the everyday lives of older adults (Hahm & Bikson, 1989). Results from several studies have demonstrated that computers have been introduced successfully into a variety of environments, such as institutional settings with frail elderly (Weisman, 1983), adult day care centers (Fisher, 1986; Zemke, 1986), senior residential and community facilities, as well as into the homes of healthy community-dwelling older adults (Czaja, Guerrier, Nair, & Landauer, 1993; Furlong & Kearsley, 1986). Advanced age also does not appear to interfere with usage as Hollander and Plummer (1986) have reported that the most consistent users of computers in their research were individuals over the age of 76. Ryan and Heaven (1986) suggest that they key to acceptance of new technologies by the elderly is to present these as useful tools and allow the older users to acquire computer skills through actual experience.

Additionally, results have indicated many uses of computers in the everyday lives of older adults, and such utilization can be beneficial for the elderly (Ramm & Gianturco, 1973). For example, electronic communication (bulletin board) systems may offer a valuable means of social interaction and mental stimulation for the elderly by providing links to other users of the systems, as well as to information and services outside the home (Czaja et al., 1993; Kerschner & Hart, 1984). These types of electronic networks have been shown to minimize isolation and loneliness for older individuals with restricted mobility (Furlong, 1989). McConatha, McConatha, and Dermigny (1994) further report that general interaction with computers may improve the performance of activities of daily living, increase cognitive functioning, and decrease levels of depression among older residents of long-term care facilities.

Computer training classes in community senior centers have been shown to increase activity among those older individuals who participated in the learning sessions on several domains. These include increased interaction among the older adults who use the centers, greater community involvement, and more intergenerational social interaction (Chin, 1985; Eilers, 1989). Eilers (1989) suggest that participating in classes for learning how to use computers offered in senior centers might also ease the transition of using these types of facilities by the 50- and 60-year-old groups who traditionally avoid using them. Furthermore, a number of researchers have observed that computer use by the elderly results in increased feelings of accomplishment, self-confidence, autonomy, competency, self-esteem, and sense of mastery among the older participants in their studies (Eilers, 1989; Fuchs, 1988; Kautzmann, 1990; McConatha et al., 1994).

Finally, tremendous innovations in health care provision for the elderly have taken place because of direct application of electronic technology. Examples range from providing effective interfaces between older patients and clinicians (Holmes, Teresi, & Holmes, 1990) to reducing medication noncompliance problems through computerized voice mail (Leirer, Morrow, Pariante, & Sheikh, 1988; Leirer, Morrow, Tanke, & Pariante, 1991; Leirer, Tanke, & Morrow, 1993; Leirer, Tanke, & Morrow, in press; Tanke & Leirer, 1993). Other interventions include those designed to compensate for age-related decline in functional aspects, such as using computers to circumvent the loss or impairment of speech (Chappell, 1993). The use of computer technology has been especially instrumental in rehabilitation processes with older adults (Frydenberg, 1988). Personal application of electronic technology for assistance in health-related matters also seem to concern older adults, as Kerschner and Hart (1984) have reported overwhelming interest expressed by the elderly respondents to a survey for products or services that would contact authorities in case of a medical emergency in the home. Therefore, the potential application of electronic technology to assist older adults in health-related matters appears to be ever-increasing.

From this discussion, it is clear that older adults are capable and motivated to use computers and other types of electronic technology, as many individuals over the age of 65 are presently using these products for a variety of reasons. Furthermore, many benefits are to be gained by older adults by using this technology. Why is it, then, that older adults do not use computers or electronic technology as much as younger adults?

There are several reasons for the discrepancy in the use of computers by younger and older individuals. The first reason is that the cohort of individuals over the age of 65 matured during a time when opportunities for them to learn how to use electronic technology were usually unavailable. Historically, instructional materials have been geared toward the younger learner. A second reason older adults may make less use of electronic technology than younger adults is that computer hardware and software manufacturers have traditionally focused the majority of their marketing attention on the recreational or educational pursuits of younger populations or on business applications because these groups of consumers were assumed to be the only viable target markets for such products (Hoot & Hayslip, 1983). Another possible reason for the difference in usage between age groups is that few attempts have been made in the public domain to adjust instructional materials for learning how to use computers (or the operation of any device for that matter) that take into consideration age-related changes in vision. Similarly, little systematic applied research has been conducted on how to design instructional materials for the elderly that accounts for age-related changes in cognition that might affect the acquisition of the skills needed for older adults to operate these types of devices. Furthermore, the range of topics that have been investigated and the types of computer tasks employed are relatively small in the research that has been completed in this area.

Hence, there is a paucity of evidence to guide the development of training materials for electronic devices for the older population. Consequently, older adults who have been interested in learning about how to operate electronic technology have, to a large degree, had to search for training opportunities or master the material on their own using instructions designed for much younger people.

In the next two sections of this chapter we will review two age-related aspects that are important when considering instructional design for the elderly. First, we will look at age-related changes in vision and provide general suggestions on how to design instructions that may mediate changes in sight that surface as we age. Second, we examine the computer training studies that have been conducted with older adults as well as findings on general instructional design. We explore this second body of research because no research is available that specifically investigates designing instructional material for teaching computer skills to older adults. In this segment we suggest that age-related changes in cognition must be considered when designing instructional materials for older computer users.

THE EFFECTS OF AGE-RELATED CHANGES IN VISION ON INSTRUCTIONAL DESIGN

Computer manuals or written instructional material of any type are a visual media and directions that cannot be seen easily are basically useless. For the researcher, it is also difficult to evaluate the effectiveness of a particular instructional strategy with older adults if the to-be-learned information is not being perceived accurately by sensory and perceptual modalities. This is especially important when designing instructions for older adults because one implication of visual loss in the elderly is an increased reliance on memory to compensate for the decreased quantity and quality of the information entering the visual system (Hiatt, 1987). A large body of evidence is available, however, that reliably documents age-related declines in memory (see Craik & Salthouse, 1992, for extensive discussions of these findings). Consequently, older adults may be particularly disadvantaged in learning how to perform some types of tasks when the design of instructional material does not account for age-related decrements in vision. To effectively design instructions for use by the elderly, it is crucial to gain a basic understanding of how aging affects vision. Next, we review some of the visual changes that become pronounced with increased age.

Structural Changes in Vision with Age

Changes in the visual system may commence as early as middle age. The greatest losses, however, occur in later life, as it has been estimated that only 15% of persons between the ages of 75 and 79 have 20/20 vision (Verillo & Verillo, 1985). Age-related decline in visual acuity is also noted to exist even with correction (Charness & Bosman, 1992). Kline and Schieber (1985) have compiled findings from a number of researchers and suggest seven structures of the eye are responsible in part for some of the age-related changes in vision that have been documented. These structures are the cornea, anterior chamber, iris and pupil, lens, vitreous body, and the retina. We have briefly summarized points from their discussion that are relevant to this chapter in the following list (for elaboration on this topic, see Kline & Scialfa, this volume; Fozard, 1990; Kline & Schieber, 1985):

1. The cornea is the clear, front surface of the eyeball, whose purpose is to bend light and focus it on the retina. Age-related structural changes of the corneal surface may degrade the quality of light entering the eye to and thus affect its refractive power.
2. The anterior chamber lies behind the cornea and in front of the lens and holds a clear fluid, the aqueous humor, which supplies nutrients to the lens and removes wastes. Changes in the aqueous humor's efficiency to transport nutrients and wastes have been associated with the development of glaucoma.
3. The iris and pupil work together to regulate the amount of light entering the eye. The iris is a muscle that contracts and expands affecting the size of the pupil. Because the iris's dilator muscles may become atrophied with increased age, the pupillary diameter may be reduced. Hence, the amount of light that can enter the eye and reach the retina may be lessened. This condition is referred to as *senile meiosis*.
4. The lens is responsible for the fine adjustments that allow focused and

clear vision at different distances, or accommodation. As the lens grows older it becomes less flexible, larger, more opaque, and generally more yellow. These changes result in decreased amounts of light entering the eye, loss of accommodative ability, and possibly difficulty in color discrimination.

5. The vitreous body lies behind the lens and in front of the retina, and it is responsible for the shape of the eyeball. It is composed of liquid, gel, and microfibrils. Age-related changes in the proportion of the components that form the vitreous may reduce the transparency of the vitreous, which results in increased scattering of light on its way to the retina.

6. The retina is the structure toward the back of the eye that holds the photoreceptors. These photoreceptors, or cones and rods, can be classified in terms of function. The cones are responsible for color vision and function best in high levels of illumination. There is also a concentration of these cones toward the center of an area of the retina called the macula. This area is responsible for the discrimination of fine spatial detail. Rods are responsible for low-illumination vision. Because there is a general loss in the number of photoreceptors with increased age, such losses may influence visual acuity and perceptual abilities.

The various structural changes that occur with increased age are characterized by a gradual onset (Verillo & Verillo, 1985). There is usually no sudden change in vision as one ages. The changes just discussed generally are not solely responsible for an overwhelming loss of visual functioning, but they often precede diseases that are more devastating to the visual system. These diseases include cataracts, glaucoma, and senile macular degeneration.

Implications for Instructional Design

Although severe disease-related visual impairment is often irreversible, it is possible that we may be able to compensate for normative losses in vision associated with age-related structural changes in the eye. This can be accomplished by the manner in which bodies of text in instructional materials are designed. Charness and Bosman (1992) suggest that the visual decrements that are most salient to the design of instructions for use by the elderly are those related to light sensitivity, contrast sensitivity, acuity (or spatial resolution), and color vision. We noted that changes in the cornea, pupil and iris, lens, and vitreous body may substantially decrease the amount of light that effectively reaches the retina. To mediate this problem, it has been recommended that a compromise of increased illumination and reduction of glare should be achieved in the environments of elderly adults (Charness & Bosman, 1992). The loss of contrast sensitivity with age is another concern when designing instructional materials in print for older adults. Consequently, it may be necessary to increase the degree of contrast between the focal object and its background for greater detectability by older readers. Hiatt (1987) suggests that this can be accomplished not only by increasing the difference of the two on a gray scale by at least 2–3 values but also by careful use of color, texture, and size variations (see Charness & Bosman, 1992, for a more in-depth discussion on illumination, glare, and contrast sensitivity).

The primary source of decreased visual performance in older adults is related to the loss of acuity. Therefore, the size and arrangement of relevant graphic details are important considerations in the design of printed instructional materials for use by the elderly whether the directions be used for computer instruction or for other types of procedural tasks. Unfortunately, many typographical and graphic design decisions are made by "designers who believe that any type style they choose is correct and attractive" (Bell, 1993, p. 12). It has been shown, however that various characteristics of type may affect the reader's ability to glean information and to effectively interpret ideas from printed material, particularly for textual materials intended to provide instruction. The findings from a number of studies that have examined the effects of type variables on the comprehension of textual materials by visually impaired individuals and persons of different ages without sight abnormalities also suggest that these layout attributes may have an extreme impact on the readability of text. Therefore, interventions in the form of text design changes may compensate, at least in part, for some losses in visual acuity in older adults. In the next section we will explore how text design attributes may be used to make instructions easier to read for the elderly.

Designing Text for the Elderly

Typeface

A typeface is the distinctive design of an alphabet of letters and related characters (Conover, 1985). Three general typefaces are found in printed materials (Bell, 1993): serif, sans serif, and novelty types, as shown in Figure 1. Serif typefaces are characterized by strokes at the end of some letters of the alphabet. Sans serifs typefaces do not exhibit these strokes and generally have a monotone appearance (Prust, 1989). Novelty typefaces are characterized by stylistic and sometimes unusual variations; they are used primarily for distinctive headings.

In general, typefaces have not received an enormous amount of empirical attention in the aging literature. J. Hartley (1994) recommends that novelty typefaces should be totally avoided in the design of instructional text for

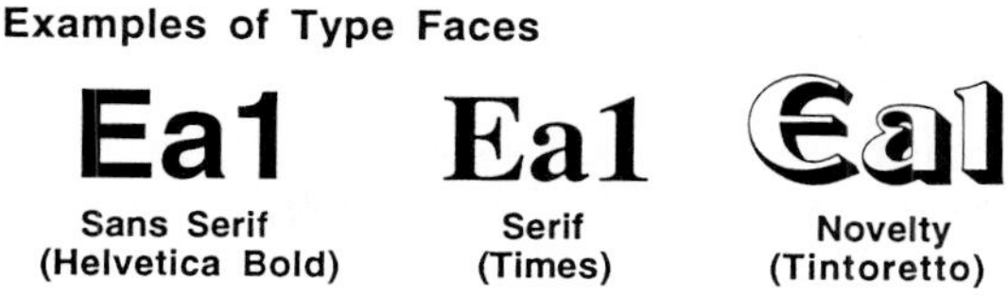

Examples of Type Faces

Ea1 Ea1 Eal

Sans Serif (Helvetica Bold) | Serif (Times) | Novelty (Tintoretto)

FIGURE 1 Examples of type faces.

older adults. Most other authors simply conclude that a typeface should be "easily readable" without disclosing the distinguishing attributes that might make one typeface more preferable for use than another. Shaw (1969), however, has reported reading improvements in the performance of visually handicapped readers with materials that used a sans serif typeface. This finding was particularly pronounced for the older participants in this study. In addition, Sorg (1985) has also examined typeface preferences among older adults. Findings from her research suggest that Helvetica (a sans serif typeface) was the easiest to read by her elderly participants compared to Century Schoolbook (a serif typeface). Finally, although Century Schoolbook was found easier to read by older adults in the study by Vanderplas and Vanderplas (1980), the participants were able to read lines of text set in Helvetica faster than other sans serif typefaces and faster than several other serif typefaces. So, taken together, there is some evidence to suggest that a sans serif typeface and specifically Helvetica might facilitate reading for older adults relative to other type designs.

Type Size

In general, findings have shown that type size should be increased to maximize text legibility (Conover, 1985; J. Hartley, 1994; Shaw, 1969). But the question remains: how much should the type be enlarged for easier reading by older adults and under what conditions should this be done?

Headings in print are generally greater than 14 points in size and are usually large enough to be visible by adults with mild to moderate visual impairment (see Figure 2 for examples of type sizes). Headings are also composed of few words, which adds to their ability to be seen. Therefore, when considering what type size promotes greater legibility, we are primarily concerned with the size of type that makes up the text of a printed piece or the body copy, such as the paragraph you are now reading (Adams, Faux, & Rieber, 1988). Several researchers have examined how the size of body copy can affect how efficiently it is read by individuals of different ages. Tinker (1963) examined small, medium, and large types sizes for reading efficiency in the general population. The findings indicated that medium size printed materials (11 point) yielded better performance than either smaller

Examples of Type Sizes

10 Point	This is the size of the type.
11 Point	This is the size of the type.
12 Point	This is the size of the type.
14 Point	This is the size of the type.

FIGURE 2 Examples of type sizes.

or larger type sizes in young participants. Vanderplas and Vanderplas (1980) compared several typefaces on reading efficiency in adults aged 60–83. Their results indicated that more text per unit was read as type size increased and performance was found to be superior for 12–14 point type, particularly for the older readers. Sorg (1985) interviewed 52 residents of long-term care facilities to determine how type size affected legibility. Her findings suggested that the older adults preferred 14 point type and also found this size of type to be the easiest to read compared to 12 point typefaces. Finally, J. Hartley (1994), in his review of 18 studies that had examined various aspects of type design with older adults, concludes that 12–14 point type size is preferable for use by the elderly and the visually impaired.

It has, however been shown that bigger type is not necessarily better (more readable) for body copy. Extreme increases in type size may counter any benefits derived from such increases and may actually affect the integrity of the text and hinder legibility of the to-be-learned text. Although it is usually recommended that text should be set in 10–12 point for ease of prolonged reading by the general population, it would appear from these findings that body copy set in 12–14 point type would be most easily read by older adults.

Type Weight

The weight of a letter in type refers to its image area. The three most common type weights are light, medium, and bold as shown in Figure 3. Although type weight should be an important consideration when presenting instructional text to older readers because of poorer contrast sensitivity, no research is available that specifically investigates this topic with the elderly. Medium or boldface type on white backgrounds, however, are most commonly presented for use by visually impaired individuals, in order to maximize contrast, and light typefaces are generally discouraged for use by individuals with impairments in sight (J. Hartley, 1994).

In addition, the use of directive cues, or elements that call special atten-

Examples of Type Weights

abcdefghijklmnopqrstuvwxyz
ABCDEFGHIJKLMNOPQRSTUVWXYZ
Helvetica Light

abcdefghijklmnopqrstuvwxyz
ABCDEFGHIJKLMNOPQRSTUVWXYZ
Helvetica Medium

abcdefghijklmnopqrstuvwxyz
ABCDEFGHIJKLMNOPQRSTUV WXYZ
Helvetica Bold

FIGURE 3 Examples of type weights.

tion to key words, phrases, or sections of text may facilitate the performance of elderly individuals (Grabinger, 1993). Directive cues include boldface type, and may also take the form of underlining, upper case letters, and italics. Balan (1989) has noted that directive cues, when applied properly, can improve the instructional value of text. For example, Taub (1984) examined recall performance of older readers with selected portions of underlined text. Findings indicated that use of underlining facilitated text recall performance in elderly adults. Much like the use of type size, there are also upper limits to the extent that the use of directive cues are beneficial as an excessive combination of boldface type, italics, and underlining may nullify their effectiveness (Balan, 1989).

Capital and Lowercase Letters

Although little systematic evidence is available on the effects of capital and lowercase letters on the readability of text in older adults, some data are available on what kind of type older adults prefer to read. Sorg (1985) reported that the older participants in her study preferred bodies of text presented in all capital letters relative to other formats. It is generally believed, however, that body copy set entirely in capital letters suffers a loss of legibility (J. Hartley, 1994). The preference observed by Sorg may be the result of participants viewing only a small amount of text (primarily extended headings). The use of all capital letters has usually been found to severely retard reading more than any other legibility factor, because the use of all capitals does not provide readers with the necessary visual cues that make words recognizable. Text set in upper- and lowercase letters, however forms words that are distinct, based upon their irregular word shape and internal pattern (Carter, Day, & Meggs, 1993). The use of lowercase letters also increases reading speed and has been found to be more pleasing to the reader (Conover, 1985). Therefore, the use of all capital letters in body copy should be avoided when designing for textual materials for individuals of all ages. Capital letters, however may be used for typographic coding, such as to distinguish two parts of a page. Capitals may also be beneficial when presented in headlines or for indicating when new paragraphs begin (Van Nes, 1986).

Physical Spacing

The physical spacing of text is directly related to the legibility of printed materials. In general, the physical spacing of text refers to the spacing between lines, the spacing between letters on a line, and the manner in which these lines are laid out. Spacing between sections of text has been shown to aid in documenting the underlying structure and organization of the to-be-learned material (J. Hartley, 1994).

Leading, or line spacing, determines the distance separating each line of type and is usually in the form of a single or double space (Hooper & Hannafin, 1986). It has been noted that lines that are closely presented, as in single spaced text, may increase the occurrence of lateral masking or a distraction that occurs as a function of the proximity of other letters (Kruk & Muter, 1984; Tinker, 1963). Peripheral vision is important in reading printed materials, as it serves to guide eye movement over the text characters and allows for integration of information from one fixation point in text to the next (Raynor, 1978). The peripheral vision of elderly individuals is especially susceptible to lateral masking. Masking effects, however, can be readily reduced by increasing the physical spacing between lines (Hooper & Hannafin, 1986). J. Hartley (1994) recommends that the design of instructional text reflect spacing between lines that equals the type size plus the spacing between words for visually impaired individuals. Hooper and Hannafin (1986) also suggest that decreasing the number of characters per line will decrease the likelihood of masking effects and improve text legibility.

Justification and Line Width

Justification refers to how lines of type are positioned between side margins on a printed page. Full or forced justification refers to the spacing of text lines so that the margins on either side of a line of type are equal. Center justification (or centering) is the balancing of text around a central axis. Nonjustification or left justification allows for an even left margin and an uneven right margin. Each of these types of justification is illustrated in Figure 4. It is generally recommended that nonjustified (or left justified) text

Examples of Type Justification

Full or Forced Justification

Full or forced justification refers to the spacing of text lines so that the margins on either side of a line of type are equal. Center justification (or centering) is the balancing of text around a central axis. Non justification or left justification allows for an even left margin and an uneven right margin.

Center Justification

Full or forced justification refers to the spacing of text lines so that the margins on either side of a line of type are equal. Center justification (or centering) is the balancing of text around a central axis. Non justification or left justification allows for an even left margin

Non justification or Left Justification

Full or forced justification refers to the spacing of text lines so that the margins on either side of a line of type are equal. Center justification (or centering) is the balancing of text around a central axis. Non justification or left justification allows for an even left margin

FIGURE 4 Examples of type justification.

is optimal for the layout of printed materials because the original spacing and configuration of the typeface used is preserved and is, thus, more readable (Balan, 1989; J. Hartley, 1994). Text that is full or forced justified often results in lines that are characterized by words and spaces that are stretched or condensed as needed to maintain even left and right margins. The distortion that results from full or forced justification may disadvantage visually impaired individuals. Similarly, centered justification increases line length variability and may also present particular problems for people with sight limitations.

Line width, is the distance between the right and left sides of a line or body of type. When the eye has completed its movement over a line of text it will perform a return sweep to the beginning of the next line. If the beginning of the next line is not immediately distinct (directly and evenly positioned below) from that of the previous line the eye is required to compensate and correct to align the new information into foveal vision, which allows for vision of distinct and fine detail (Keenan, 1984). *Saccade* is the term used to define this eye movement or correction required to bring distinct text into foveal vision (Van Nes, 1986). Consequently, as the number of saccades required to perceive text increases, so does the time required to read a particular passage. Therefore, line length should remain relatively constant to reduce visual confusion.

Huey (1968) found that shorter lines of type, defined as being 9–10 cm in length, are less likely to yield inaccuracy on the return sweep. Similarly, Gregory and Poulton (1970) maintain that participants ranging in age from 20 to 80 with poor reading ability performed better when line length was approximately seven words. It has also been reported that short lines were preferred by undergraduate college students when studying (Grabinger, 1986). On the other hand, Tinker (1963) suggests that the optimal line length is dependent on the size of the type and how it is set. Finally, Conover (1985) suggests that the optimal width of a line can be achieved by measuring the lowercase alphabet (all letters lined up from *a* to *z*) and adding one-half to this. In summary, there appears to be little consensus on what constitutes the optimal line length of type that might facilitate legibility in elderly adults or individuals of any age. J. Hartley (1994), however, notes that 50 to 65 characters per line is optimal for visually impaired individuals. Hence, this rule, which was derived from a Royal National Institute for the Blind data-based report, might serve as a guideline for designing text for older adults as well until systematic research can be conducted in this area with older adults.

Color

In general, findings from studies focused on the use of color in instructional materials are mixed, because there is concern that color may be a source of distraction. Some researchers maintain that color adds to the number of physical elements presented simultaneously in a message or visual complexity and, therefore, may require greater mental effort to process. In contrast, results from some of the studies support the notion that the use of color in pictures may actually speed visual processing as color photos may heighten the realism of an image. Gilbert and Schleuder (1990) conducted a study comparing color and black and white photo advertisement clippings. They concluded that images in color were more readily remembered than those without. In addition, their findings suggest that images with color were processed with greater speed.

A major concern when using color in printed material for the elderly is the difficulty older adults have with color discrimination. Results indicate that the ability to discriminate between colors decreases with age and is particularly pronounced for the blue–green wavelengths (Fozard, 1990; Kline & Schieber, 1985). Decline in color sensitivity also appears to become particularly marked by 70 years of age (Verillo & Verillo, 1985). Therefore, the general strategy used to decrease errors in performance as a result of this decrement is to avoid instructional designs that require discrimination of colors in the blue–green range and/or discrimination of colors in the same hue (Charness & Bosman, 1992; Hiatt, 1987). Hiatt (1987) also suggests the use of texture and patterns in conjunction with color may make color discriminations more readily apparent for older adults.

Summary

In the preceding paragraphs on typographical and graphic design of instructional materials, we provided several recommendations for the general design of printed instructional material for older adults. These suggestions may be applied to the design of printed instructional material for teaching older adults to use computers, as well as the performance of other procedural tasks. We feel it is safe to assume that body copy presented in 12–14 points, in a sans serif typeface (probably Helvetica), in capital and lowercase letters, and in a medium to boldface may be more readable for older adults compared to other type design alternatives. Adequate spacing between bodies and lines of text, justification that results in similar line lengths, and the judicious application of color may also facilitate readability for the elderly.

It is important to realize, however, that many of these recommendations stem from studies concerned with facilitation of reading in individuals with severe visual impairments or low verbal ability. Most elderly individuals are not severely visually impaired nor do they have low verbal ability. It is important to note, however, that elderly users are likely to have some degree of age-related visual impairment and, therefore, may be hindered by design decisions that are inappropriate for this age group. Therefore, it is clear that more research is needed on the effects of typography and graphic design techniques on the comprehension of printed materials in the normal elderly with mild to moderate visual impairment.

An area of caution also lies when applying the information we know about printed materials to computer displayed text. Such a generalization cannot be easily made for a number of reasons (see Gould, Alfaro, Barnes, & Haupt, 1987, and Rieber, 1994, for more in-depth discussions). Primarily, information is perceived differently on the computer screen than on the printed page as a result of reflected light versus emitted light. As a whole, however, some researchers such as Kerr (1986) maintain that some of the same rules for page design can be applied to screen design, especially when certain aspects of the design resemble similar features on paper (Gould, Alfaro, Finn, & Haupt, 1987).

DESIGNING INSTRUCTIONS FOR COMPUTER USE IN OLDER ADULTS

Computer Training and the Elderly

Most of the results from the few studies that have focused on computer training methods with the elderly suggest that older adults are slower than younger adults in acquiring computer skills and that older adults usually make more mistakes and require more assistance than younger adults when learning how to perform computer tasks (Charness & Bosman, 1992; Charness, Schumann, & Boritz, 1992; Elias, Elias, Robbins, & Gage, 1987; Zandri & Charness, 1989). Some researchers, however, have shown minimal age differences in the performance of computer tasks or none at all (e.g., A. A. Hartley et al., 1984, with young and older adults and Garfein et al., 1988, with middle-aged and older adults). It also appears that trainees of all ages learn how to perform computer tasks better when paired with a partner or when they are taught in small groups relative to individual instruction (Danowski & Sacks, 1980; Zandri & Charness, 1989).

The standard methodology in computer training studies with the elderly consists of the manipulation of various training contingencies to isolate a technique that might facilitate skill acquisition in this population. Results from studies conducted with young and older individuals suggest that both age groups show similar benefits from improved training conditions as no age by training condition interaction has surfaced in any of the findings that have been reported. For example, in one study two different methods of training (video modeling versus a computer-based technique) were compared for teaching young and older adults how to use a spreadsheet program (Gist, Rosen, & Schwoerer, 1988). The modeling condition was found to increase performance relative to the tutorial condition for both age groups. Similarly, Czaja, Hammond, Blascovich, and Swede (1986) investigated using a standard manual, computer-based instruction, and instructor-based training for teaching older adults to perform a series of text editing tasks. Although, findings revealed that the on-line instruction was inferior to the other instructional conditions and the other conditions did not differ from each other in their effects on performance, none of the methods was found truly effective in teaching people word processing. In related research, Charness and his group of researchers (1992, Experiment 2) controlled the nature of the training session by manipulating whether the learner was actively (self-paced condition) or passively (fixed-paced condition) involved in a training tutorial on acquiring word processing skills. Better performance was achieved in the self-paced condition relative to the fixed-paced condition for both age groups. In another study, Kelley, Charness, Mottram, and Bosman (1994) compared a keystrokes-only condition, where computer commands were accessed by pressing combinations of keys and a menus condition for teaching young and older adults to perform word processing tasks. Young and old subjects performed better when using the menus interface than when using only keystrokes to operate the computer.

It is interesting to note that findings from two of these studies suggest that, when a training method is specifically designed to significantly lower cognitive demands, it will be successful in facilitating performance in both young and old adults relative to other training techniques. For example, the modeling sequence employed by Gist and colleagues (1988) demonstrated the steps of the procedure. The model's demonstration integrated the procedures by showing how the step-by-step instructions were actually performed, which ultimately reduced demands on working memory and, thus, enhanced performance above the level achieved by the computer-based instruction. In the study by Kelley et al. (1994) the menus condition was found to be superior to the keystrokes-only condition. In this instance the authors likened the superior format to a cued recall paradigm, which is considered by researchers in cognition to reduced memory demands relative to a recall condition (or the condition that required learners to remember keystrokes to perform computer procedures).

Therefore, it would seem that instructions or training methods that extensively reduce cognitive demands are likely to enhance performance of computer tasks for the elderly. It is often found that, if a technique improves the performance of a special population, then the general population will also benefit. Therefore, it is probable that instructions or training materials that extensively reduce cognitive demands will also improve performance for individuals of all ages. Furthermore, some evidence indicates that instructions for older adults should be designed to reduce demands on certain underlying cognitive mechanisms that have been shown to evidence age-related decrements.

Age-Related Changes in Cognition

A majority of researchers in aging and cognition agree that most component processes of cognition decline with advanced age. We have chosen to briefly emphasize two of the underlying cognitive processes (among others) that undergo age-related changes likely to be influential in the acquisition of computer skills in older adults: working memory and spatial ability. These and other cognitive aspects are more fully discussed in other chapters included in this volume. We will also propose suggestions that may be incorporated into instructional design that may be used to mediated age-related declines in these cognitive processes in the next sections of the chapter.

Working Memory

Working memory has been described as a cognitive system that consists of a "central executive" (or processor) capable of attention, selection, and manipulation (Baddeley, 1986). The "central executive" is assumed to have a limited amount of processing capacity, some portion of which may be devoted to the short-term storage of information. Other storage demands may be divided into two subsidiary slave systems: the "articulatory loop," which is able to maintain verbal information by subvocal rehearsal (verbal working memory), and the "visuospatial scratch pad," which performs a similar function through the visualization of spatial material (spatial working memory) (see Baddeley, 1986, for more discussion of this topic). There is general agreement among cognitive aging researchers that working memory evidences substantial declines with age (Baddeley, 1986; Craik & Jennings, 1992; Hultsch & Dixon, 1990), the cause of which may be due to decreased storage capacity (Foos, 1989; Light, Zelinski, & Moore, 1982), processing capacity (Cohen, 1981; Craik, Morris, & Gick, 1990; Wright, 1981), or both (Babcock & Salthouse, 1990; Foos & Sabol, 1981). Although there is debate about the source of the decline, most evidence indicates that older adults are inordinately affected by increases in task complexity as older adults have exhibited greater impairments of performance than have younger adults when the complexity of both verbal and spatial working memory tasks has increased (Light & Anderson, 1985; Salthouse, Mitchell, Skovronek, & Babcock, 1989; Wright, 1981).

Spatial Ability

Results from a number of studies suggest that spatial abilities increase during adolescence, reach their peak during the second or third decade of life, and decrease steadily thereafter (Salthouse, 1982). Furthermore, increased age has been found to be associated with lower levels of performance on tests of spatial visualization ability, tasks requiring the integration of spatial information, and performance tests that require a high degree of working memory operations or ongoing information processing (Salthouse, 1991). Older adults are able to use certain visual–spatial characteristics because memory performance for such attributes has been shown to be well above chance in work by Smith and Park (1990). Higher accuracy, however has been reported for young adults than for older adults on measures of memory for spatial location (e.g., Park, Cherry, Smith, & Lafronza, 1990), and older adults in general do not remember visual–spatial characteristics of presented items as well as younger adults (see Salthouse, 1991, for a discussion). Therefore, some declines must exist.

Charness has noted that a computer mouse operates in a plane that is different from the plane of the computer screen (Charness, Bosman, & Elliott, 1995). Because older adults may have trouble with spatial relations due to age-related declines in spatial ability, it is likely that they will experience greater difficulties when using a mouse than younger adults. The recent rapid development of mouse-driven software (such as windows programs) may also exacerbate the spatial requirements that are needed to perform computer procedures because the user must place the cursor on numerous predetermined locations on the computer screen (and then click or double click) or drag icons to specific sites to successfully execute many types of computer procedures. Thus, using a computer may become more and more difficult for older adults because of age-related cognitive declines, especially as the computer tasks become increasingly complex.

Implications on Instructional Design

At a basic level, using a computer is analogous to understanding how to perform a series of simple procedural tasks. We must also remember how to perform these simple actions because effective usage demands that we combine several simple operations in a strict procedural manner to accomplish more complex computer tasks. Because most instructions for using computers are presented in written form, the comprehension process requires the learner to translate written instructions (in working memory) into representation(s) of one or more physical actions (keyboard or mouse actions) and then to actually perform the physical action(s).

How can we design instructional materials for teaching older adults to use computers that take into consideration age-related declines in working memory and spatial ability? No studies are available that specifically take into account age-related deficits in these two cognitive factors when designing instructions for teaching older adults how to use computers. However, some research has considered how the working memory demands of instructional text may be lessened to increase comprehension in the elderly, which may aid in this discussion. Findings from research in educational psychology, primarily concerned with younger adults, may also assist in forming the basis for possible solutions. More specifically, some results suggest that working memory demands of bodies of text may be lessened by the manner in which the text is composed and structured. Furthermore, the addition of illustrations to text might also facilitate the comprehension of printed instructions by reducing both working memory and spatial requirements. These issues are discussed in the next section of the chapter.

Reducing the Working Memory Demands of Text

A few researchers have provided guidelines on how to make simple text more understandable for older adults. Morrow, Leirer, and Sheikh (1988) recommend that simple instructions (such as those found on the prescription signatures of medicine bottles) be clearly printed. The information should be presented in an explicit and familiar manner to increase comprehension of the material by older adults. Also suggested, other ways to facilitate understanding of written information in older adults is by (1) organizing the material in a standard format (usually in relatively small discrete segments), (2) writing the text in simple language, (3) avoiding negatives and inferences, and (4) phrasing the text in the active rather than the passive voice (Morrow et al., 1988; Park, 1992). Furthermore, presenting procedural instructions for taking medications in a list format has been shown to not only improve comprehension in older adults but to also be preferred by the elderly compared to medical information that has been traditionally formatted in paragraph form (Morrow, Leirer, & Altieri, 1995). Morrow and his colleagues (1995) suggest that providing procedural instructions in a list allows each step of a task to appear on a separate line, which ultimately emphasizes the procedural arrangement of the task.

In related research, Morrell, Park, and Poon (1989) compared medication-taking instructions as they were originally presented on a prescription signature from an actual pharmacy to revised versions of the same material in which the instructions were simply, clearly, and explicitly stated. Each procedural aspect of the instructions (when the medication was to be taken, number of pills to be taken each time, and any special instructions that were to be followed when taking the medication) was also presented on a separate line of the prescription signature in the revised versions. Their findings demonstrated that the young adults remembered and understood more of the information than the older adults on immediate testing. Both age groups, however, understood and retained more of the information when it was clearly structured and organized than when it was viewed in its original form. Similarly, James, Lewis, and Allison (1987) redesigned tax forms by clarifying the introductory letter, by asking questions in a more consistent manner, and by revising the layout of the material. Older respondents reported that they had less difficulty in completing the revised forms and further found the new material more helpful than the original versions.

Overall, these results and recommendations suggest that simple text may be revised easily to make it more understandable for older adults. Theoretically speaking, precise written instructions presented in a standard manner require less organization and integration of the concepts on the part of the reader, which may subsequently reduce the working memory demands of the text and thus, enhance comprehension.

The Addition of Illustrations to Text

In opening the discussion of how illustrations may enhance comprehension of text, it is important to note that illustrations not directly congruent with the presented information may serve as a source of distraction and, therefore, may interfere with learning (Rieber, 1994). Distraction of this type may present a particular disadvantage for older adults. For example, Lippman and Caplan (1992) have reported findings that suggest that diagrams may facilitate comprehension for young adults but worsened the performance of the older adults when used to remember a particular journey or route during a taped slide presentation. Similarly, results from a study conducted by Morrell, Park, and Poon (1990) revealed that older participants remembered less information about a medical regimen when the information was presented in text and graphics than when it was presented in text alone. The younger participants in this research remembered more when the medical information was presented with graphics and text than when it was presented in text alone.

However, considerable evidence is available that indicates that it is more likely material will be elaborately encoded and consequently retrieved when both a verbal code and a visual code are provided compared to a purely verbal code (Paivio, 1971). Researchers in education also strongly advocate the use of illustrations, especially for learners who are novices, as images have been shown to integrate and clarify new concepts in meaningful ways (Kerr, 1986). Furthermore, the use of illustrations may motivate, interest, and in general, obtain and maintain the attention of the learner (Rieber, 1994). Finally, it has also been shown that memory for pictures (in the form of simple and complex line illustrations of objects and scenes) is better than for words by individuals of all ages in a series of studies by Park and her colleagues (i.e., Park, Puglisi, & Smith, 1986; Park, Puglisi, & Sovacool, 1983; Smith & Park, 1990). Therefore, another way to reduce the working memory demands of procedural text and also lessen the spatial requirements of using a mouse is to add realistic text-relevant illustrations to the text. Such illustrations may be able to demonstrate spatial relationships embedded within steps of a procedure (such as how to attach component parts when assembling a bicycle or where to place the cursor on the computer screen) impossible to portray in words. Illustrations may also translate or organize and integrate the information included in the written instructions, thus reducing working memory and spatial demands, which, in turn, may enhance comprehension.

A review of the results from studies over a variety of types of procedural tasks reveals that in all instances the addition of illustrations to written instructions have been shown to facilitate performance relative to text alone formats with children and young adults (i.e., Booher, 1975; Frank, Wacker, Berg, & McMahon, 1985; Hayes & Henk, 1986; Kieras & Bovair, 1984; Stone & Glock, 1981; Wacker & Berg, 1983). Only one study of this type, however, has included a group of older adults. Morrell and Park (1993) supplied young and old individuals with instructional sets composed of text only, illustrations only, or the combination of text and illustrations for constructing a series of three-dimensional objects out of Lego blocks. The results indicated that participants of both age groups who received the instructions composed of both text and illustrations made fewer errors in performance than those individuals assigned to the other instructional format conditions. The authors suggested that the addition of illustrations to text reduced the working memory demands of the task, thus enhancing the performance of the participants relative to the text only or illustrations only conditions. Measures of spatial working memory and verbal working memory were also shown to be primary predictors of performance.

Taken together, the results from this research suggest that the addition of realistic text-relevant illustrations to written procedural instructions for computer usage may facilitate procedural task performance in the elderly because the illustrations may reduce the processing demands inherent in textual instructions. What is particularly interesting about the study by Morrell and Park is that the authors considered age-related differences in vision and cognitive factors when designing their instructional sets. All of the text was presented in either 18 or 24 point bold Helvetica type to reduce visual demands. In addition, the colors used in the illustrations (which mapped onto the actual building materials) were easily distinguishable from one another. Furthermore, the procedural steps consisted of individual clusters of short sentences that were clearly and simply written to reduce cognitive demands. The steps were also presented in a list format.

CONCLUSIONS

In this chapter, we have chosen the design of instructional materials for computer use by the elderly as an example of how to design written instructions to alleviate a practical problem in the everyday lives of older adults. As stated earlier, the guidelines may well be applied to the design of other types of instructional materials. We argue that one of the primary reasons that older adults use computers less often than younger adults is that few instructional materials have been designed that take into consideration age-related changes in vision and cognition. We suggest to designers of instructional materials for older adults that type variables such as size, face, and weight and factors associated with paragraph formatting such as justification and line length may be altered to compensate for some of the loss of visual acuity in the elderly. Additionally, it is possible that age-related declines in working memory and spatial ability may be mediated by the manner in which text is structured and organized and that the addition of realistic text-relevant illustrations may increase the comprehensibility of procedural text for older adults. Above all, we have tried to stress the need for more research on this topic, as few findings are available from which to base more definitive guidelines for designing instructional materials for older adults. We have attempted to demonstrate that making instructions easier to understand for older adults is not an insurmountable undertaking. Finally, it is likely that the guidelines we propose may also extend over other user populations.

Acknowledgments

This chapter was supported by Grant P50 AG11715 from the National Institute on Aging of the National Institutes of Health to Roger W. Morrell as director of a research project conducted through the Center for Applied Cognitive Research on Aging, University of Michigan, one of the Edward R. Roybal Centers for Research in Applied Gerontology. We thank Denise C. Park for her contributions to our current work in this area and Lisa A. Howard for her assistance in acquiring the reference materials that were used in preparation of this chapter.

References

Adams, J. M., Faux, D. D., & Rieber, L. J. (1988). *Printing technology.* Albany, NY: Delmar Publishers, Inc.

Ansley, J., & Erber, J. T. (1988). Computer interaction: Effect on attitudes and performance in older adults. *Educational Gerontology, 14,* 107–119.

Babcock, R. L., & Salthouse, T. A. (1990). Effects of increased processing demands on age differences in working memory. *Psychology and Aging, 5,* 421–428.

Baddeley, A. D. (1986). *Working memory.* Oxford: Clarendon.

Balan, P. (1989, August). Improving instructional print materials through text design. *Performance & Instruction,* pp. 13–18.

Bell, T. P. (1993, May, June). Beyond visual communication technology. *Technology Teacher,* pp. 9–12.

Booher, H. R. (1975). Relative comprehensibility of pictorial information and printed words in proceduralized instructions. *Human Factors, 17,* 266–277.

Brickfield, C. F. (1984). Attitudes and perceptions of older people toward technology. In P. K. Robinson, J. Livingston, & J. E. Birren (Eds.), *Aging and technological advances* (pp. 31–38). New York: Plenum.

Carter, R., Day, B., & Meggs, P. (1993). *Typographic design: Form and communication.* Van Nostrand: New York.

Chappell, N. (1993). Technology and aging. *Journal of Canadian Studies, 28,* 45–58.

Charness, N., & Bosman, E. A. (1992). Human factors and aging. In F. I. M. Craik & T. A. Salthouse (Eds.), *The handbook of aging and cognition* (pp. 495–545). Hillsdale, NJ: Erlbaum.

Charness, N., Bosman, E. A., & Elliott, R. G. (1995, August). *Senior-friendly input devices: Is the pen mightier than the mouse?* Paper presented at the 103rd annual convention of the American Psychological Association, New York.

Charness, N., Schulmann, C. E., & Boritz, G. M. (1992). Training older adults in word processing: Effects of Age, Training Technique, and Computer Anxiety. *International Journal of Technology and Aging, 5,* 79–106.

Chin, K. (1985). The elderly learn to compute. *Aging, 348,* 4–7.

Cohen, G. (1981). Inferential reasoning in old age. *Cognition, 9,* 59–72.

Conover, T. E. (1985). *Graphic communications today.* St. Paul, MN: West Publ. Co.

Craik, F. I. M., & Jennings, J. M. (1992). Human memory. In F. I. M. Craik & T. A. Salthouse (Eds.), *The handbook of aging and cognition* (pp. 51–110). Hillsdale, NJ: Erlbaum.

Craik, F. I. M., Morris, R. G., & Gick, M. L. (1990). Adult age differences in working memory. In G. Vallar & ST. Shallice (Eds.), *Neuropsychological impairments of short-term memory* (pp. 247–267). Cambridge, UK: Cambridge University Press.

Craik, F. I. M., & Salthouse, T. A. (Eds.). (1992). *The handbook of aging and cognition.* Hillsdale, NJ: Erlbaum.

Czaja, S. J., Guerrier, J. H., Nair, S. N., & Landauer, T. K. (1993). Computer communication as an aid to independence for older adults. *Behaviour and Information Technology, 12,* 197–207.

Czaja, S. J., Hammond, K., Blascovich, J. J., & Swede, H. (1986). Learning to use a word-processing system as a function of training strategy. *Behaviour and Information Technology, 5,* 203–216.

Danowski, J. A., & Sacks, W. (1980). Computer communication and the elderly. *Experimental Aging Research, 6,* 125–135.

Eilers, M. L. (1989). Older adults and computer education: "Not to have the world a closed door." *International Journal of Technology and Aging, 2,* 56–76.

Elias, P. K., Elias, M. F., Robbins, M. A., & Gage, P. (1987). Acquisition of word-processing skills by younger, middle-age, and older adults. *Psychology and Aging, 2,* 340–348.

Fisher, S. (1986). Increasing participation with a computer in an adult day care setting. *Activities, Adaptation, & Aging, 6,* 31–36.

Foos, P. W. (1989). Adult age differences in working memory. *Psychology and Aging, 4,* 269–275.

Foos, P. W., & Sabol, M. A. (1981). The role of memory in the construction of linear orderings. *Memory & Cognition, 9,* 371–377.

Fozard, J. L. (1990). Vision and hearing in aging. In J. E. Birren & K. W. Schaie (Eds.), *Handbook of the psychology of aging* (3rd ed., pp. 150–170). San Diego, CA: Academic Press.

Frank, A. R., Wacker, D. P., Berg, W. K., & McMahon, C. M. (1985). Teaching selected microprocessor skills to retarded students via picture prompts. *Journal of Applied Behavior Analysis, 18,* 179–185.

Frydenberg, H. (1988). Computers. *American Behavioral Scientist, 31,* 595–600.

Fuchs, B. (1988, Winter). Teaching elders to be computer-friendly. *Generations,* p. 57.

Furlong, M. (1989). An electronic community for older adults: The SeniorNet network. *Journal of Communication, 39,* 145–153.

Furlong, M., & Kearsley, G. (1986, Fall). Computer instruction for older adults. *Generations,* pp. 32–34.

Garfein, A. J., Schaie, K. W., & Willis, S. L. (1988). Microcomputer proficiency in later-middle-aged and older adults: Teaching old dogs new tricks. *Social Behaviour, 3,* 131–148.

Gilbert, K., & Schleuder, J. (1990). Effects of color and complexity in still photographs on mental effort and memory. *Journalism Quarterly, 67,* 749–756.

Gist, M., Rosen, B., & Schwoerer, C. (1988). The influence of training method and trainee age on the acquisition of computer skills. *Personnel Psychology, 41,* 255–265.

Gould, J. D., Alfaro, L., Barnes, V., & Haupt, B. (1987). Reading is slower from CRT displays than from paper: Attempts to isolate a single-variable explanation. *Human Factors, 29,* 269–299.

Gould, J. D., Alfaro, L., Finn, R., & Haupt, B. (1987). Reading from CRT displays can be as fast as reading from paper. *Human Factors, 29,* 497–517.

Grabinger, R. S. (1986). *Relationship among test format variables in computer-generated text.* Paper presented at the annual convention of the Association for Educational Communications and Technology, Las Vegas, NV.

Grabinger, R. S. (1993). Computer screen designs: Viewer judgments. *ETR&D, 41,* 35–73.

Gregory, M., & Poulton, E. C. (1970). Even versus uneven right-hand margins and the rate of comprehension reading. *Ergonomics, 13,* 427–434.

Hahm, W., & Bikson, T. (1989). Retirees using EMail and networked computers. *International Journal of Technology and Aging, 2,* 113–123.

Hartley, A. A., Hartley, J. T., & Johnson, S. A. (1984). The older adult as computer user. In P. K. Robinson, J. Livingston, & J. E. Birren (Eds.), *Aging and technological advances* (pp. 347–348). New York: Plenum.

Hartley, J. (1994). *Designing instructional text.* London: Kogan Page Limited.

Hayes, D. A., & Henk, W. A. (1986). Understanding and remembering complex prose augmented by analogic and pictorial illustrations. *Journal of Reading Behavior, 18,* 63–78.

Hiatt, L. G. (1987). Designing for the vision and hearing impairments of the elderly. In Regnier & Pynoos (Eds.), *Housing the aged* (pp. 341–371). New York: Elsevier.

Hollander, E. K., & Plummer, H. R. (1986). An innovative therapy and enrichment program for senior adults utilizing the personal computer. *Activities, Adaptation, & Aging, 6,* 59–68.

Holmes, D., Teresi, J., & Holmes, M. (1990). Computer applications in health care planning and practice. *International Journal of Technology and Aging, 3,* 69–78.

Hooper, S., & Hannafin, M. J. (1986). Variables affecting the legibility of computer generated text. *Journal of Instructional Development, 9,* 22–28.

Hoot, J. L., & Hayslip, B. (1983). Microcomputers and the elderly: New directions for self-sufficiency and life-long learning. *Educational Gerontology, 9,* 493–499.

Huey, E. B. (1968). *The psychology and pedagogy of reading.* Cambridge, MA: MIT Press.

Hultsch, D. F., & Dixon, R. A. (1990). Learning and memory in aging. In J. E. Birren & K. W. Schaie (Eds.), *Handbook of the psychology of aging* (pp. 259–274). San Diego, CA: Academic Press.

James, S., Lewis, A., & Allison, F. (1987). *The comprehensibility of taxation: A study of taxation and communications.* London: Avebury Aldershot.

Kautzmann, L. (1990). Introducing computers to the elderly. *Physical and Occupational Therapy in Geriatrics, 9,* 27–36.

Keenan, S. A. (1984). Effects of chunking and line length on reading efficiency. *Visible Language, 18,* 61–80.

Kelley, C. L., Charness, N., Mottram, M., & Bosman, E. (1994). *The effects of cognitive aging and prior computer experience on learning to use a word processor.* Paper presented at the Cognitive Aging Conference, Atlanta, GA.

Kerr, S. T. (1986). Instructional text: The transition from page to screen. *Visible Language, 20,* 368–392.

Kerschner, P. A., & Hart, K. C. (1984). The aged user and technology. In R. E. Dunkle, M. R. Haug, & M. Rosenberg (Eds.), *Communications technology and the elderly: Issues and forecasts* (pp. 135–144). New York: Springer.

Kieras, D. E., & Bovair, S. (1984). The role of a mental model in learning to operate a device. *Cognitive Science, 8,* 255–273.

Kline, D. W., & Schieber, F. (1985). Vision and aging. In J. E. Birren & K. W. Schaie (Eds.) *Handbook of the psychology of aging* (2nd ed., pp. 296–233). New York: Van Nostrand-Reinhold.

Krauss, I. K., & Hoyer, W. J. (1984). Technology and the older person: Age, sex and experience as moderators of attitudes towards computers. In P. K. Robinson, J. Livingston, & J. E. Birren (Eds.), *Aging and technological advances* (pp. 349–350). New York: Plenum.

Kruk, R. S., & Muter, P. (1984). Reading of continuous text on video screens. *Human Factors, 26,* 339–345.

Leirer, V. O., Morrow, D. G., Pariante, G. M., & Sheikh, J. I. (1988). Elders' nonadherence, its assessment, and computer assisted instruction for medication recall training. *Journal of the American Geriatrics Society, 36,* 877–884.

Leirer, V. O., Morrow, D. G., Tanke, E. D., & Pariante, G. M. (1991). Elder's nonadherence: Its assessment and medication reminding by voice mail. *Gerontologist, 31,* 514–520.

Leirer, V. O., Tanke, B. D., & Morrow, D. G. (1993). Commercial cognitive/memory systems: A case study. *Applied Cognitive Psychology, 7,* 675–689.

Leirer, V. O., Tanke, B. D., & Morrow, D. G. (in press). Designing automated voice message reminders for improving health care adherence. In D. Herrmann, M. Johnson, C. McEnvoy, C. Hertzog, & P. Hertel (Eds.), *Basic and applied memory: Research on practical aspects of memory.* Hillsdale, NJ: Erlbaum.

Light, L. L., & Anderson, P. A. (1985). Working memory capacity, age, and memory for discourse, *Journal of Gerontology, 40,* 737–747.

Light, L. L., Zelinski, E. M., & Moore, M. (1982). Adult age differences in reasoning from new information. *Journal of Experimental Psychology: Learning, Memory, and Cognition, 10,* 46–60.

Lippman, P. D., & Caplan, L. J. (1992). Adult age differences in memory for routes: Effects of instruction and spatial diagram. *Psychology and Aging, 7,* 435–442.

McConatha, D., McConatha, J. T., & Dermigny, R. (1994). The use of interactive computer services to enhance the quality of life for long-term care residents. *Gerontologist, 34,* 553–556.

McNeely, E. (1991). Computer-assisted instruction and the older-adult learner. *Educational Gerontology, 17,* 229–237.

Morrell, R. W., & Park, D. C. (1993). The effects of age, illustrations, and task variables on the performance of procedural assembly tasks. *Psychology and Aging, 8,* 389–399.

Morrell, R. W., Park, D. C., & Poon, L. W. (1989). Quality of instructions on prescription drug labels: Effects on memory and comprehension in young and old adults. *Gerontologist, 29,* 345–354.

Morrell, R. W., Park, D. C., & Poon, L. W. (1990). Effects of labeling techniques on memory and comprehension of prescription information in young and old adults. *Journal of Gerontology, 45,* 166–172.

Morrow, D. G., Leirer, V. O., & Altieri, P. (1995). List formats improve medication instructions for older adults. *Educational Gerontology, 21,* 163–178.

Morrow, D. G., Leirer, V. O., & Sheikh, J. (1988). Adherence and medication instructions: Review and recommendations. *Journal of the American Geriatrics Society, 36,* 1147–1160.

Paivio, A. (1971). *Imagery and Verbal Processes,* Holt, R Rinehart, and Winston: New York.

Park, D. C. (1992). Applied cognitive aging research. In F. I. M. Craik & T. A. Salthouse (Eds.), *The handbook of aging and cognition* (pp. 449–494). Hillsdale, NJ: Erlbaum.

Park, D. C., Cherry, K. E., Smith, A. D., & Lafronza, V. (1990). Effects of distinctive context on memory for objects and their locations in young and older adults. *Psychology and Aging, 5,* 250–255.

Park, D. C., Puglisi, J. T., & Smith, A. D. (1986). Memory for pictures: Does an age-related decline exist? *Journal of Psychology and Aging, 1,* 11–17.

Park, D. C., Puglisi, J. T., & Sovacool, M. (1983). Memory for pictures, words, and spatial location in older adults: Evidence for pictorial superiority. *Journal of Gerontology, 38,* 582–588.

Prust, Z. A. (1989). *Graphic communications: The printed image.* South Holland, IL: The Goodheart-Willcox Company.

Ramm, D., & Gianturco, D. (1973). Computers and technology: Aiding tomorrow's aged. *Gerontologist, 13,* 322–325.

Raynor, K. (1978). Eye Movements in Reading and Information Processing. *Psychological Bulletin, 85,* 618–660.

Reibel, L. P. (1994). *Computers, Graphics, & Learning,* Wm. C. Brown Communications: Dubuque, IA.

Rogers, W. A., Walker, N., Gilbert, D. K., Fraser, E., & Fisk, A. D. (1994, August). *A questionnaire study of automatic teller machine usage by adults of all ages.* Paper presented at the annual meeting of the American Psychological Association, Los Angeles.

Royal National Institute for the Blind. (1993). *See it right: Clear print guidelines* (Fact Sheet 2). London: Public Policy Office, RNIB.

Ryan, E. B., & Heaven, R. K. B. (1986). Promoting vitality among older adults with computers. *Activities, Adaptation, & Aging, 6,* 15–29.

Salthouse, T. A. (1982). *Adult cognition: An experimental psychology of human aging.* New York: Springer-Verlag

Salthouse, T. A. (1991). *Theoretical perspectives on cognitive aging.* Hillsdale, NJ: Erlbaum.

Salthouse, T. A., Mitchell, D. R., Skovronek, E., & Babcock, R. L. (1989). Effects of adult age and working memory on reasoning and spatial abilities. *Developmental Psychology, 26,* 845–854.

Schwartz, J. (1988). The computer market. *American Demographics, 10,* 38–41.

Shaw, A. (1969). *Print for partial sight library.* London: Library Association.

Smith, A. D., & Park, D. C. (1990). Adult age differences in memory for pictures and images. In E. A. Lovelace (Ed.), *Aging and cognition: Mental processes, self-awareness, and interventions, 69-96.* Amsterdam: North-Holland.

Sorg, J. A. (1985). *An exploratory study of type face, type size, and color paper preferences among older adults.* Unpublished masters thesis, Pennsylvania State University, University Park.

Stone, D. E., & Glock, M. D. (1981). How do young adults read directions with and without pictures? *Journal of Educational Psychology, 73,* 419–426.

Tanke, E. D., & Leirer, V. O. (1993). Use of automated telephone reminders to increase elderly patients' adherence to tuberculosis medication appointments. In *Proceedings of the Human Factors and Ergonomics Society 37th annual meeting.* Santa Monica, CA: Human Factors and Ergonomics Society.

Taub, H. A. (1984). Underlining of prose material for elderly adults. *Educational Gerontology, 10,* 401–405.

Tinker, M. A. (1963). *Legibility of print.* Ames: Iowa State University Press.

Vanderplas, J. M., & Vanderplas, J. H. (1980). Some factors affecting the legibility of printed materials for older adults. *Perceptual and Motor Skills, 50,* 923–932.

van Nes, F. L. (1986). Space, colour and typography on visual display terminals. *Behaviour and Information Technology, 5,* 99–118.

Verillo, R. T., & Verillo, V. (1985). Sensory and perceptual performance. In N. Charness (Ed.), *Aging and human performance* (pp. 1–33). New York: Wiley.

Wacker, D. P., & Berg, W. K. (1983). Effects of picture prompts on the acquisition of complex vocational tasks by mentally retarded adolescents. *Journal of Applied Behavior Analysis, 16,* 417–433.

Weisman, D. (1983). Computer games for the elderly. *Gerontologist, 23,* 361–363.

Wright, R. W. (1981). Aging, divided attention, and processing capacity. *Journal of Gerontology, 36,* 605–614.

Zandri, E., & Charness, N. (1989). Training older and younger adults to use software. *Educational Gerontology, 15,* 615–631.

Zemke, R. (1986). Taking a byte of the apple: Computer activities in a senior day care center. *Physical and Occupational Therapy in Geriatrics, 4,* 39–48.

Chapter 15

The Older Worker

Paul E. Panek

INTRODUCTION

The United States and other industrialized nations are currently experiencing what is called the *graying* of the work force (Hayslip & Panek, 1993). For a variety of reasons, such as economic and personal factors, increased longevity, and federal legislation, more individuals are remaining longer in the work force. Between 1985 and the year 2000, the number of workers between the ages of 45 and 65 years is expected to grow by 41%, while the number of workers in the 16–35 years age group will decline slightly (Johnston, 1987). This trend is expected to continue into the next century (Rosen & Jerdee, 1988) and by the end of this century the median age of the labor force will be age 40. Also, extended and multiple careers will become the norm, and the prevailing retirement age will move toward 70 as a large number of older workers choose, either because of necessity or for fulfillment, to remain in the labor force (Kirkland, 1994). In addition to the work force getting older, it is increasingly female and diverse (Rix, 1990; Staats, Colbert, & Partlo, 1995).

Further, the enactment of the Age Discrimination and Employment Acts (ADEA) of 1967 (amended 1978, 1986) and the virtual elimination of mandatory retirement by Congress in 1986 has resulted in employers becoming more sensitive to using the worker's chronological age as a basis for

Handbook of Human Factors and the Older Adult

employment decision making (Avery & Foley, 1988; Waldman & Avolio, 1993). The ADEA defines *older workers* as individuals age 40 years old and older (Sterns & Alexander, 1987; Waldman & Avolio, 1993). Additional implications of these demographic trends can be found in chapter 1 of this handbook by Howell.

A result of these facts and trends has been an increase in interest in "industrial gerontology," which is the study of aging and work, focusing on a variety of employment, working environment, retirement, and related issues pertinent to middle-aged and older workers, such as training and retraining, job performance, and the like (Hayslip & Panek, 1993; Sterns & Alexander, 1986; 1987).

The issues associated with aging and work fall naturally into the domain of human factors, since the human factors approach focuses on adapting the work environment to the work force, in such areas as training, workplace design, job design and equipment design (Sterns, Barrett, Czaja, & Barr, 1994). For this reason, the human factors approach is particularly relevant to issues regarding the older workers, and its principles can be applied to enhance and facilitate employment opportunities for older adults as well as the organizations that employ them. In this chapter we plan to highlight and discuss factors and issues pertinent to older workers or the "aging" worker in a multidimensional perspective.

Dimensions Affecting the Older Worker

To adequately discuss the older worker, we need to view her or him during all phases of the adult life span within the context of a number of dimensions; that is, a multidimensional perspective. These dimensions are (1) sensory–perceptual, (2) biological–physiological, (3) cognitive, (4) personal–interpersonal, and (5) cultural–environmental. Examples of dimensions and factors affecting older workers are presented in Table 1. The factors presented should be considered illustrative and not exhaustive and are those particularly relevant to the older worker functioning in the work environment.

During the course of the life span normal changes occur in each of these dimensions that may have an effect on one or more of the other dimensions. For example, declines with age in the sensory–perceptual dimension (e.g., decreased hearing ability) can lead to changes in the cognitive dimension (e.g, incorrect interpretation of verbal instructions regarding the task), which can effect the cultural–environmental dimension (e.g., ineffective job performance), which subsequently affects the personal–interpersonal dimension (e.g., criticism from coworkers as a result of workers poor job performance, which reflects on the entire department). Therefore, to understand the older worker, we must recognize that he or she is affected by many

TABLE 1
Dimensions Affecting the Older Worker

Dimensions	Examples of affecting factors
Sensory–perceptual	Vision
	Hearing
	Taste and smell
	Somesthesis
	Selective attention
	Vigilance
	Perceptual style
	Perceptual–motor reaction time
Biophysiological	Musculoskeletal system
	Cardiovascular system
	Respiratory system
	Central nervous system
	Health and physical condition
Cognitive	Cognitive–intellectual processes
	Problem solving
	Learning and memory
Personal–interpersonal	Personality (traits and processes)
	Motivation
	Self-concept
	Stress and coping
	Interpersonal relationships
Cultural–environmental	Ethnicity and culture
	Occupation or job
	Work environment
	Organizational demands and climate

Source: Adapted from Hayslip and Panek (1993).

interacting factors of a sensory–perceptual, biophysiological, cognitive, personal–interpersonal, and cultural–environmental nature. Each factor affects and is affected by each other factor during the course of the life span (see Hayslip & Panek, 1993).

Person–Environment Interaction

A framework that will illustrate the significance and implications for each of these dimensions with regard to both the aging process and the older worker (and workers of any age) is the concept of "person–environment interaction" and the "transactional model" of Lawton and Nahemow (1973). The concept of person–environment interaction suggests that all aspects of behavior and performance are the result of the interaction or transactions between the individual and the environment (Pervin, 1968), such as the workplace. A match, or "best fit," in terms of abilities, skills, and performance levels of the individual to the environment expresses itself as high performance, job satisfaction, and little stress for the worker, while a mismatch leads to poor performance and stress for the worker (Hayslip & Panek, 1993; Jahoda, 1961).

To perform successfully on the job and adapt, individuals must match their ability levels to the demands of their work environment. This can be illustrated by the transactional model of Lawton and Nahemow (1973). The components of the transactional model are presented in Table 2.

TABLE 2
Components of the Transactional Model

Component	Description and example
Degree of individual competence	The diverse collection of abilities and skills the worker possesses; e.g., sensory processes. Each of these abilities or skills levels is unique to the worker and varies over time between minimum and maximum limits that are specific to each worker
Environmental press	The demands from the environment impinging on and affecting the individual; e.g., demands or requirements of the task or job
Adaptive behavior	The outer manifestation of individual competence. In the work environment, adaptive behavior can be considered the observable (measurable) performance on the task or job
Affective responses	The inner, unobservable aspects of the individual–environmental transaction, including the worker's evaluation and emotional reaction to the environment. For example, persons who are critical of their performance or feel they have let their boss or co-workers down may respond by becoming angry or depressed
Adaptation level	The point or level where the worker is functioning at a comfortable level relative to the external demands. Beyond this comfort zone, positive affect decreases and becomes negative as the demands push the worker past his or her adaptation level. For example, if the worker's adaptation level is making 6 items per hour, 7 might be challenging, attempting or required to make 10 items per hour would cause the worker discomfort and result in errors

Source: Adapted from Hayslip and Panek (1993) and Lawton and Nahemow (1973).

Prevalent Beliefs Regarding Older Workers

Business and industry hold a number of common, and generally negative stereotypes regarding older workers (see Hayslip & Panek, 1993; Rix, 1990; Speas & Obenshain, 1995). These include the productivity of workers declines with age; job performance declines with age; "you can't teach an old dog new tricks," in other words, older workers do not do well in training and retraining; "older workers are not comfortable with new technologies"; "older workers are rigid, not flexible and have difficulty in adapting to change"; and "older workers lack the desire or motivation to get ahead." Throughout this chapter we will address the facts regarding each of these beliefs.

The many unfounded attitudes and beliefs about older workers generally stem from a lack of knowledge and understanding about the aging process (Lindley, 1989) and, in many instances, are not supported by research. Moreover, it is important to remember that attitudes toward older workers are multidimensional and can occur at a number of different levels, as well as, being moderated by a number of different factors.

SENSORY–PERCEPTUAL DIMENSION

In terms of the older worker and the effects of normal aging, the most pertinent sensory processes perhaps, are, vision, audition, olfaction, and somesthesis (touch, vibration, temperature, kinesthesis, and pain). Regarding perceptual processes, the most relevant perceptual processes are selective attention, perceptual style, and perceptual–motor reaction time. Depending upon the specific occupation, the changes associated with the normal aging process may have potential affects upon the older worker, his or her co-workers, and the work environment.

Vision

Declines in visual functioning can significantly affect the quality and quantity of the visual information available to the older worker, and subsequently their interaction with, and performance in, the work environment (see Kline & Scialfa, Chapter 3). Some examples include difficulty in reading instructions, requiring higher levels of illumination on the work site, reading dials on equipment and machinery, driving, etc.

Audition

Changes in the ability to hear are a function of both normal aging processes and external factors such as exposure to noise (see Kline & Scialfa, Chapter

3). Hearing ability decreases dramatically over the course of the adult life span to the point that, by late adulthood, many individuals have some form of hearing disorder (Olsho, Harkins, & Lenhardt, 1985).

In terms of implications for the older workers, decreases in hearing ability can lead to inaccurate hearing of instructions, difficulties in carrying on conversations, difficulty in hearing the telephone, and so forth. Therefore, many industries require workers, when working in environments with high noise levels, such as municipal street workers and airline baggage handlers, to wear protective ear plugs. Further, as the ambient noise level of the work environment increases, older workers would most likely experience greater difficulty in accurately hearing auditory information, which can be attributed to either stimulus overload or decreases in sensitivity.

Olfaction

Research (see Hayslip & Panek, 1993) suggests that decrements in our ability to smell (detect odors) is due primarily to environmental factors, such as substances or chemicals at the industrial site or airborne toxic agents, rather than age per se. The decrease in the ability for older workers to detect odors with increasing age would have the most pronounced effect in jobs or occupations where failure to detect low levels of substances can lead to health risks; for example, due to hazardous chemicals or gas.

Somesthesis

Our sensitivity to touch, vibration, temperature, kinesthesis, and pain are collectively known as *somesthesis* and result from normal and intensive stimulation's of the skin and viscera. Declines in sensitivity in each of these somesthetic senses can be attributed to a decreased number of sensory receptors for each sense. The primary result of decreased sensitivity is an inability to correctly detect stimulation from the working environment. Possible examples include exposure to potentially dangerous temperature levels, susceptibility to falls, and an inability to discriminate among different materials.

Selective Attention and Vigilance

Selective attention, vigilance and aging are discussed in detail in this handbook in the chapter by Kline and Scialfa (Chapter 3). These abilities are very important in jobs or occupations where the worker must maintain attention for extended periods of time. Research suggests that there is very little attenuation of age differences, with practice, in vigilance (Parasuraman & Giambra, 1991).

Depending upon the job or occupation, the declines in selective attention and vigilance ability may or may not have significant implications for the older worker. The effects of the decrease in selective attention ability and vigilance would be most pronounced in jobs or positions where the worker must focus attention for extended periods of time, such as radar operators, air traffic controllers, long distance truck drivers, and inspectors for errors or defects in items moving along an assembly line.

Perceptual Style

The construct of perceptual or cognitive style has been developed to explain individual differences in perception and is discussed in detail in this handbook in the chapter by Rogers (Chapter 7). One aspect of perceptual–cognitive style is field dependence or independence.

Extensive cross-sectional research suggests a shift toward field dependence during old age, which has numerous implications for interacting with the environment (see Rogers, Chapter 7). For example, perceptual style has been found to be related to accidents in a group of older commercial drivers (Barrett, Mihal, Panek, Sterns, & Alexander, 1977).

Perceptual–Motor Reaction Time

One of the most reliable changes with increasing age is a slow down in performance and behavior (see Hayslip & Panek, 1993; Vercruyssen, Chapter 4). Specifically, from age 40 onward, accuracy appears to be emphasized at the expense of speed in performing a psychomotor task. For example, Panek, Barrett, Alexander, and Sterns (1979) investigated age and self-selected performance pace on a visual monitoring inspection task. Results indicated no significant differences between older and younger individuals in performance accuracy but significant differences in terms of the pace at which they elect to perform the task; that is, older individuals preferred a slower pace.

The effects of the slowdown in performance and the older worker vary as a function of the occupation or job. See Chapter 4 in this handbook by Vercruyssen for a detailed discussion of movement control and speed of performance with age.

BIOPHYSIOLOGICAL DIMENSION

Beginning in early adulthood, a number of internal biological and physiological changes take place and, by middle and late adulthood, begin to affect us functionally. That is, these changes can potentially influence our behavior and adaptation to the work environment.

In terms of the older worker and the work environment, the most relevant biological and physiological changes occur in the musculoskeletal system, cardiovascular system, respiratory system, and the central nervous system. Other factors of note on this dimension include the older workers health and physical condition.

Musculoskeletal System

The muscular system begins to change during middle adulthood. For example, changes in overall muscle strength and muscle mass begin during the mid-30s; at age 45, muscle strength is approximately 90% of the level at age 25; and 75% at age 65. Further, muscle tone changes; and there is a redistribution of fat and subcutaneous tissue with aging.

All of the skeleton within the body has been ossified by age 18. Thereafter, due to increased loss of calcium, increased porosity, and erosion, the bones start to become brittle and the articulating surfaces begin to deteriorate. After reaching its peak, bone mass for both men and women then begins to drop by about 1% a year. Due to the settling of bones within the spinal column, changes in body curvature, and shrinkage of the intervertebral disks and vertebrae, individuals may shrink one to two inches in height over the life span, usually beginning during their 50s.

The age changes in this system has significant implications for individuals engaged in jobs or occupations with relatively high "physical activity or strength" demands.

Cardiovascular System

The cardiovascular system undergoes systematic changes with age. At approximately age 25, the heart rate is at its peak efficiency; by age 45, the heart rate is at 94% of peak efficiency; and by age 65, the heart rate is at 87% peak efficiency. Although the structures within the cardiovascular system show signs of change and degeneration with age, these disorders are highly dependent on both genetic and environmental factors such as smoking, stress, diet, and exercise.

Curing middle adulthood, the frequency of heart disease, cardiovascular failure, and hypertension begins to increase. These conditions can require older workers to modify their life styles both at home and at work, such as to avoid stress. Again, changes in this system would have the most pronounced effects on persons employed in stressful occupations and occupations with high physical demand components. For example, Szafran (1965, 1970) found that speed and accuracy of decision-making performance of older pilots appeared to be highly dependent upon the individual's cardio-vascular–pulmonary status rather than chronological age.

Respiratory System

The maximum breathing, or vital, capacity of the lungs decreases progressively between 20 and 60 years of age. The lungs lose, on average, 30–59% of their maximum breathing capacity between the ages of 30 and 80 years.

However, the primary harmful effects on the lungs are caused by environmental factors. These include smoking and the inhalation of noxious agents such as asbestos, which have been liked to disorders of the respiratory system such as lung cancer, asthma, emphysema, and pneumonia. As one would suspect, changes in this system would have the most pronounced effect on persons in occupations with high physical demand components or in work environments where constant clean air flow and circulation may be a problem.

Central Nervous System

Our ability to think, reason, and act in response to incoming information from the environment depends on the integrity of our central nervous system, specifically the brain and spinal cord. Changes in the structure and function of the central nervous system play a major role in a variety of behavioral and performance changes that occur with the normal aging process.

The principal changes in the central nervous system occur in the brain. The normal aging of the central nervous system occurs at different rates for different people, and different regions of the brain change differentially. Generally, the number of cells in the central nervous system decreases, and the overall size of the brain decreases with age.

It is important to realize that age changes in brain structure and function are highly subject to, and moderated by, disease. Though there are changes in brain structure and functioning with normal aging processes, most people can compensate for deficits in memory, fine motor coordination, or learning new information by relying on their experience, planning, and organizational skills to maintain effective functioning in the workplace.

Health and Physical Condition

Physical limitations increase sharply with age, as does the severity of the limitations. For example, workers aged 65–69 are three times as likely as workers 45–54 and six times as likely as those 35–44 to report severe functional limitations (Berkowitz, 1988; Rix, 1990). These limitations include impairments in vision, hearing, speaking, lifting or carrying, walking, using stairs, and getting around outside as well as inside and obviously can affect work performance.

Research reported by Rix (1990) suggests a steady increase in both the presence and severity of work disability with age. A *work disability* is defined as a health problem or disability that prevents someone in the household from working or that limits the type or amount of work in which the person can engage. Berkowitz (1988) suggests that, while health and functioning may not improve with age, people may improve in knowledge and wisdom, which might well offset some of the physiological changes that could potentially affect job performance.

COGNITIVE DIMENSION

The life span literature regarding various cognitive process such as intelligence, learning, memory, and problem solving is quite extensive (see Howard & Howard, Chapter 2; Rogers, Chapter 7). However, very little of this research has focused directly on the older worker or issues related to the older worker.

Cognitive–Intellectual Processes

A fairly large number of cross-sectional and longitudinal research studies have focused on differences in cognitive test performance during the adult phases of the life span (see Avolio & Waldman, 1990; Salthouse, 1988). A variety of topics regarding cognitive aging are discussed in detail and can be found in this handbook in chapters by Rogers (Chapter 7) and Morrow and Von Leirer (Chapter 9). However, although the typical job of the future will be more intellectually demanding, very little research in the area of cognitive aging has focused directly on the older worker or issues related to the older worker.

Avolio and Waldman (1990) examined job complexity and occupational type as potential moderators of the relationship between age and cognitive ability. These researchers used general, verbal, and numerical ability scores for 21,646 individuals in the General Aptitude Test Battery (GATB) data base. Results indicated differences in the relationship between age and cognitive ability test scores across occupational types but not for different levels of job complexity. Findings from Avolio and Waldman (1990) indicate that contextual factors such as job complexity and the type of occupation account for a much greater share of the variance in cognitive ability test performance than either age or experience.

Problem Solving

Research (see Porterfield & St. Pierre, 1992; Rybash, Hoyer, & Roodin, 1986) generally suggests that older individuals often approach and solve problems differently. Further, although there appears to be some decline in problem-solving ability with normal aging processes, when problem-solving abilities decline before the late 50s, it is not usually the result of normal aging processes. However, we need to distinguish between ability and performance. That is, although observable performance may decline, ability, which we infer from performance, in fact may remain unchanged.

Learning and Memory

Research in learning and memory during the adult phases of the life cycle is extensive and are discussed in detail in this handbook by Howard and Howard (Chapter 2), Park and Jones (Chapter 11) and Tun and Wingfield (Chapter 6). The focus of the research and program efforts pertaining to older workers in this area has been training and retraining. That is, "Can you teach an old dog new tricks?"

Training

Because we live in a highly technological, rapidly changing world, both on and off the job, training and retraining are important issues for workers of all ages (Sterns & Hayslip, 1990). Although we know that older adults are capable of learning and acquiring new skills, industry, for the most part, has held to the belief that older adults cannot learn or be retrained. Also, older workers often fail to recognize threats of obsolescence and are reluctant to pursue training or retraining (Fletcher, Hansson, & Bailey, 1992). Finally, some older workers fear they are not capable of learning new skills, while others see no advantage in learning new technologies (Rosen & Jerdee, 1989). However, available research suggests that training can enhance and improve the performance of older workers in some occupations, particularly where experience, judgment, and maturity are important.

The growing awareness that older adults can be trained and retrained in both the laboratory and industrial settings has led to the development of training principles and methods that recognize the unique attributes of the older adult worker (Sterns, 1986; Sterns & Alexander, 1987; Sterns & Sanders, 1980). Consequently, one major issue today is assuring equitable access to training opportunities for older adult workers, since current policies and practices regarding training may exclude older employees (Sterns & Alexander, 1987).

Training of older adult workers may require changes in traditional training methods to accommodate the special needs, different motivations, and limitations of some individuals. A number of training approaches such as the discovery method, activity learning, and programmed instruction (see Sterns, 1986, for an in-depth discussion of these and other methods) have been effective with older workers. Also, certain techniques, such as self-paced learning, experiential training, on-the-job coaching, or pragmatic training are more effective in teaching older workers. Rosen and Jerdee (1985) report that in-service training and retraining provide older adult workers with the opportunity to strengthen knowledge and skills.

Factors that should be considered in the development of training programs for older adults are presented in Table 3. Particularly important are a thorough task analysis and training-needs analysis when developing training methods. The use of a task-analysis approach has been found to be a strong predictor of the success of a training program.

Overall, research suggests that older workers are able to learn and to adapt to job change (Sterns, 1986). In some cases, industrial training can

TABLE 3
Factors to Be Considered in the Design of Training Programs for Older Workers

Factor	Description and Example
Motivation	Older workers need to be encouraged and motivated to participate in training programs. Older workers have often been out of school for many years and may have a fear of failure or an inability to compete against better or more recently educated younger workers
Structure	A careful task analysis should be carried out to develop the training material and content, as well as determine the sequence of training. The training sequence should be in terms of increasing complexity, that is, after mastery of the basic skill, more difficult or complex aspects are then introduced; this increases self-confidence and reduces fear of failure
Familiarity	The use of former and familiar elements and skills on a new task facilitates the acquisition of new learning. Therefore, whenever possible training programs should be constructed on the basis of past knowledge and abilities
Organization	Research indicates that many older workers have been found to have difficulty organizing information adequately. Therefore, training programs should be organized so that the knowledge can be built on at each step or phase in the program
Time	Older workers often take longer to learn a new task, but when given sufficient time, older workers usually perform as well as younger workers. Therefore, training programs for older workers should have a slower presentation rate and longer periods of study

Source: Adapted from Sterns (1986), Sterns and Alexander (1987), and Valasek and Sterns (1981).

moderate any adverse effects of age on job performance for middle-aged and older workers (Welford, 1985).

PERSONAL–INTERPERSONAL DIMENSION

A variety of factors in the personal–interpersonal dimension play a critical role in the selection of an occupation and, often, in the successful performance of that occupation. Some of these factors include personality, rigidity, cautiousness, motivation, self-concept, stress and coping, friendships, marital relations, and loss of a spouse.

Personality

Personality has a major impact on our health, survival, intellectual functioning, and a number of other factors during adulthood (Hayslip & Panek, 1993), including functioning in the workplace, and is discussed in greater detail in this handbook in the chapter by Rogers (Chapter 7). Several aspects or traits of personality such as rigidity, cautiousness, coping style, and reaction to stress affect workers of all ages.

Cautiousness

Cautiousness and conservatism in behavior and decision making have often been considered manifestations of psychological and biological aging. This increased cautiousness in behavior and decision making is often considered an overall behavioral or personality characteristic of the aging individual, which is thought to affect all areas of behavior and performance.

Although alternative explanations for behavior described as "cautiousness" are available, such as compensation for declining or reduced skills or abilities, increased cautiousness on the part of older workers can either be a strength or weakness, depending on the job or occupation. For example, in positions that require "fast" or "risky" responses, such as operating machinery or trading commodities, it is a possible deficit. However, in positions such as investment bankers and upper level management, cautiousness may be a strength.

Rigidity

As we get older, it is often assumed that we will find it difficult to shift from one activity or behavior to another. We may perseverate rather than act, or we may adhere rigidly to a routine and become more inflexible. These characteristics, plus others, are often thought to be typical of middle-aged and older adults and is called the *rigidity hypothesis;* this is also one of the most common generalizations regarding the older worker.

The concept of rigidity is pertinent to industrial gerontology because, to function effectively in our work environment, we must constantly change, adapt, and be flexible to new situations, events, and demands from the work environment and other people. However, support for the rigidity hypothesis in the literature is mixed, at best, since other explanations for behavior described as rigid are available, e.g., compensation for real or imagined deficits (see Hayslip & Panek, 1993).

Motivation

Although the findings are somewhat mixed, age has generally been found to be positively related to factors such as job involvement, internal work motivation, and organizational commitment. Also, older workers have a stronger belief in the "Protestant work ethic" than do younger workers (Aldag & Brief, 1977; Johnson & Johnson, 1982). Additionally, with increasing age, workers tend to have higher needs for security and affiliation and lower needs for self-actualization and growth on the job (Rhodes, 1983).

Concerning the motivational aspects of pay, older workers value the financial rewards of work more than younger workers (Johnson & Johnson, 1982). In addition, both male and female older workers are motivated more by monetary compensation. Older workers of both genders often report that they continue to work in order to (1) remain active and engaged, (2) enhance meaningful life experiences, and (3) socialize (Johnson & Johnson, 1982).

Self-Concept

Work, or our occupation, generally occupies a central position in our lives during adulthood, often serving as a basis for our self-concept, feelings of self-esteem, and our very identity (Hayslip & Panek, 1993). Consequently, any factors that would negatively affect a person's self-concept during any segment of the life span would most likely affect the person's job performance, and vice versa.

Perhaps the three most pertinent issues affecting the self-concept of older workers are midcareer job change, job loss (dislocation), and interpersonal relations, such as friendship patterns, marital relations, loss of spouse through divorce or death.

Midcareer Job Change Middle adulthood can either be a period of career satisfaction, a time of advancement and being fulfilled by the job, or a time of career dissatisfaction, leading one to change jobs. However, research does not single out middle adulthood as a time of career crisis, although some people do change careers in middle adulthood. These changes may be horizontal, from one career to another, or vertical, to a higher level of responsibility (Osipow, 1983). Both types of changes come about for a variety or reasons, such as family changes (divorce, death of spouse); a desire for more income, status, or security; philosophical differences with one's employer; and, dissatisfaction with how ones skills are being used, rather than age per se.

Job Loss (Dislocation) Current cohorts of older workers are concentrated in declining industries and often have firm-specific skills that do not readily transfer to other firms. This make them especially vulnerable to job loss through plant shutdowns or layoffs (Rix, 1990).

The personal impact of job loss or unemployment on individuals can be very debilitating, leading to declines in physical health, self-esteem, depression, and anxiety (DeFrank & Ivancevich, 1986) for workers of all ages. Moreover, job loss has potential psychological, economic, and social effects on all members of the family (McLloyd, 1989).

The unemployment rate for men 55–64 years of age is higher than for those aged 25–54 years, a trend that has been common for the past 20 years (see Hayslip & Panek, 1993). Moreover, once out of work, older workers are likely to remain unemployed much longer than younger workers (Quinn & Burkhauser, 1990). When re-employed, they often find jobs at lower pay, requiring less skill, and at lower occupational levels, or in new occupations (Love & Torrence, 1989; Ruhm, 1989).

Sheppard (1976) studied laid-off professional men, engineers and scientists, and found age to be the most significant variable related to employment status. Wachtel (1966) studied 2,000 hard-core unemployed individuals in Detroit and found age to be the major reason for their unemployment.

Since older adults experience more prolonged unemployment, they are also more likely to become discouraged and drop out of the work force altogether (Hansson, Briggs, & Rule, 1990). In a study of the impact of a plant closing and subsequent move, Love and Torrence (1989) found the median length of unemployment for those age 55 and over to be 27 weeks, compared to 13 weeks for workers under age 45. Discouraged unemployed older workers are different in many ways from unemployed older workers who are actively searching for a job. Discouraged unemployed older workers tend to have significantly lower job-search self-efficacy expectations, more disorderly work histories, longer periods of current unemployment, and higher reported levels of depression, social isolation, and psychological discouragement (Rife & Kilty, 1989–1990).

Older workers tend to be unemployed longer than younger workers, for a number of reasons: (1) due to seniority, they tend to remain in declining industries and occupations until the jobs finally disappear as a result of economic or technological change (Johnson & Johnson, 1982); (2) current cohorts of older workers tend to have lower levels of formal education and, therefore, are excluded from positions with high educational requirements; (3) older workers have less mobility, due to greater responsibilities and obligations, compared to younger workers, so subsequently, they cannot easily move and relocate should their plant close and move to another area of the country; (4) older workers have less well-developed and obsolete job seeking skills compared to younger workers, due to the fact that they may have not interviewed for a job in 10 or 15 years (Johnson & Johnson, 1982); (5) since 1982, changes in health insurance have made it all but impossible for an older worker (who may have an "ongoing" health condition, however mild) to retain health insurance at less than excessive prices ($300+ per month). And prospective employers see the older adult as an insurance drain, too.

Interpersonal Relations

Interpersonal relationships play a vital role in affecting the quality of our lives in adulthood. Our relationships with others are critical to our satisfaction with life, our self-concepts, and our physical health. In adulthood, important sources of emotional, social and psychological support are friends and our spouse (significant other). As you would expect, the quality of our relationships with others can effect our job performance, at all phases of adulthood. Therefore, divorce, providing care for a member of the family, and death of spouse can be potentially disruptive to job performance or result in a return to or entry into the work force (see Staats, Partlo, Armstrong-Stassen, & Plimpton, 1994, for discussion of older working widows).

Middle-aged workers are part of the "sandwich generation"; that is, they often have the responsibility for caring for their own children as well as their aging parents. Data reported by Harris (1995) indicates that more than half of the persons in the work force care for an aging parent or another elderly relative, and nearly two-thirds of these employees are women. Research indicates (see Hayslip & Panek, 1993) that most caregiving activities are performed by the wife or adult female members of the family. Caregiver problems and requirements are often translated into workplace problems such as tardiness, absenteeism, changed work schedules, impaired work performance, and job turnover. Harris (1995) reports that 90% employed caregivers indicate that their responsibilities adversely affect their work, and 55% report increased financial strain. Further, they are nearly three times as likely as their coworkers to experience depression. In fact, as suggested by Staats et al. (1994) organizations have generally focused attention on needs pertinent to younger women workers, such as child-care services, as opposed to the needs of middle-aged or older women, such as elder-care services.

Absenteeism and Job Turnover For men, avoidable absenteeism tends to decrease slightly with increasing age. Avoidable absences are those where an employee is absent without prior approval. For women, there is little evidence for a consistent relationship between avoidable absences and age. Unavoidable absence (due to illness or accidents) tends to show a much more variable pattern of relationship with age and is likely to be a function of the job performed (Sterns & Alexander, 1987). Generally, for men, a higher rate of unavoidable absences occur for younger and older workers. The fewest unavoidable absences occur for middle-aged workers. The sex differences in the age–avoidable-absence relationship is most likely the result of working women serving as the primary caretaker of the family. Therefore, when another member of the family is ill or needs to go to see the physician, it is most likely the woman who misses work to take care of the child, spouse, or aged parent (Hayslip & Panek, 1993; Staats et al., 1994). Overall, older workers have lower absenteeism (Rhodes, 1983). Also, there is a negative relationship between age and job turnover.

Re-entry Typical re-entry workers are either women who left the labor force to raise families and then returned to work after varying periods of time (Jacobson, 1980) or are returning to work as a result of divorce or death of a spouse. These women, having lost their primary source of support, need to secure employment (Rix, 1990).

Re-entry women are clearly at a different stage of work life than men of the same age (Shaw, 1988). Their lack of work experience results in limited opportunities and lower earnings. A majority of employed midlife and older women work in retail sales, administrative support, and services, occupations for which the average wages are often below those of the total work force (Rix, 1990).

Widows also qualify as displaced homemakers, but for them, employment does not appear to be a "highly desirable alternative" (Morgan, 1984). Census data reported by Staats et al. (1994) indicate that there are 13.7 million widowed workers in the United States and 11.3 of that number are women. These researchers also reported that the income of the working widow is lower than other older workers. Finally, younger widows and widows who experience declines in their standard of living are more likely than other widows to seek employment.

Displaced homemakers, because of age, lack of work experience, and updated skills, generally face multiple barriers upon labor force re-entry.

Such women need training, advice on how to find jobs, other supportive services, and income (Rix, 1990).

Stress and Coping

Day-to-day stress and coping with major life changes in our lives is a normal part of life. Stress can be found on the job, at home, and in our personal lives. There are vast individual differences in the perception and significance of stressors as well as individual reactions to stress (Krause, 1994).

With regard to stress on the job and aging, Osipow, Doty, and Spokane (1985) studied pressures at work of over 300 employed men and women in five age ranges: below age 25; 25–34; 35–44; 45–54; and 55+. These researchers feel that the pressures of work and one's response to these pressures vary across the life span, and such pressures can affect work performance. Osipow et al. (1985) found that, while gender did not influence occupational stress, strain, or coping, workers under age 25 experienced the most psychological and interpersonal strain. For workers over age 25, stress in general declined consistently with age. It was suggested that older workers are either better at coping or have left jobs that they perceived as stressful. Staats et al. (1995) found the "quality of life" of older working widows, operationally defined in terms of work uplifts and work hassles, is lower than that of other older workers when the effects of age are controlled.

With regard to the distinct causes of stress at work, younger workers reported such causes as having unchallenging work, experiencing a conflict between the values or objectives of different people at work, or being in an aversive physical environment. Older workers reported that work overload and being responsible for others at work were the main causes of stress at work.

Finally, with increased age, people tended to change their coping styles to such activities as recreation, better self-care, and more effective use of time. Also, with increased age, people made better use of social support to cope with job stress.

Greenglass (1988) found that women experienced greater job related stress that men in similar managerial positions. Specifically, some women experience what is termed *multiple-role strain* due to the stress associated with the demands of various roles (Repetti, Matthews, & Waldron, 1989). That is, stress arises when the demands of one role (e.g., worker) interfere with the fulfillment of another role (e.g., mother). Multiple-role strain is greatest for mothers of young children, those employed full-time, married women whose husbands contribute relatively little to household labor and child care, and single parent women.

CULTURAL–ENVIRONMENTAL DIMENSION

Numerous factors in the cultural-environmental dimension significantly affect older workers and subsequently their job performance. These factors, such as ethnicity–culture, occupation, and factors related to the work environment (e.g., accidents, job satisfaction) and the organizational demands or climate, generally interact with the factors in the other five dimensions.

Ethnicity–Culture

In 1982, 74.9% of Japanese men between the ages of 60 and 64 were working, in contrast to 67.5% in Great Britain, 56.4% in the United States, and 39.7% in France (American Association of Retired Persons, 1988). For the age group 65–69 years, Japan's labor force includes 38.9% of these individuals, compared to the 17.1% rate in the United States and single-digit percentages in Great Britain, Germany, and France. These percentages are even more striking because more than 95% of Japanese firms have a mandatory retirement age of 60 or under.

Despite the prevailing mandatory retirement age in Japan, three out of four Japanese firms rehire retired workers or continue their employment beyond the official retirement age. As a rule, these rehired or retained workers step down from managerial or supervisory positions to posts of lesser responsibility. Japanese employers, with government encouragement, also actively help recent retirees search for new jobs if necessary.

Japanese employers are generally willing to make work adjustments to maintain the older worker's productivity and interest in the job. Approximately 55% of firms have a formal policy to help older workers remain healthy and productive through job transfers, reduced working hours, or changes in work operation and physical environment.

Often, in Japan, changes from physically demanding jobs such as assembly line work to less physically stressful positions often occur as early as the late 40s for Japanese workers. Toyota Motor, Nissan Motor, and Matsushita Electric (Panasonic) are among the many corporations engaged in job redesigning for an aging labor force. In doing so employers are responding to current and anticipated labor shortages, government pressure to increase older workers' labor force participation, and the perceived need to heighten morale among workers.

Business and industry is beginning to address the demands of the changing and aging work force. For example, the Volvo plant in Uaddevalla, Sweden, is being ergonomically designed, such as designing tools that are less physically demanding, to accommodate a work force in which 25% will be over age 45 and 40% are women.

In the United States, during the past 20 years, due to a variety of factors such as demographic changes, economic reasons, and legal decisions, more organizations have begun the practice of rehiring and utilizing retirees. Although a majority of organizations hire retirees for stable, ongoing assignments, there is considerable diversity in the occupational placement of these retirees (Hirshorn & Hoyer, 1994).

Occupations

As previously reported, the same chronological age can take on different meaning relative to the age distribution of the job or occupation in which it is embedded and jobs and occupations have "age norms" (Avolio, Panek, & Harcar, 1992; Waldman & Avolio, 1993). The age grading that goes on in organizations as well as by individuals themselves can lead to the blocking of advancements, restriction of training and development activities, not being offered more challenging job assignments, and higher incidences of obsolescence (Waldman & Avolio, 1993).

Age norms may shape both the expectations of the individual and the group (Rosen & Jerdee, 1988). Age norms involve the classification or categorization of individuals into groups based on age, which result in shared beliefs regarding the "appropriate" age an individual either should or should not occupy a particular role or position, including occupational roles and positions (Avolio et al., 1992; Cleveland & Hollmann, 1990; Lawrence, 1988). Researchers have reported that the determination of an individual's career success or progress is based partly on the age norm characterizing various career tracks. For example, Kanter (1977) reported specific age norms for occupations that designated whether individuals were considered "fast trackers" or "reached a plateau" in their careers. Neugarten and Datan (1973) have shown that chronological age plays an important role in determining whether one is perceived as being "on time" with respect to career progression or advancement.

By way of illustration, Gordon and Arvey (1986) found that many occupations, such as security guard, jeweler, and mayor, were classified as "old age jobs," while other occupations, such as file clerk, hospital attendant, and dental hygienist, were classified as "young age jobs." Further, Gordon and Arvey reported a positive correlation between the actual age distribution in an occupation and the classification of the occupation based on chronological age.

Data indicates that the proportion of older men employed in executive and managerial occupations tends to be reasonably high, reflecting, undoubtedly, age-related gains in experience that make these men attractive as managers and executives. The proportion of workers employed in what might be considered more physically arduous occupations, such as operatives and laborers, shows a drop with age, although almost as many middle-aged men can be found in this occupational category as among executives and managers. The oldest male workers are usually in farm occupations. Age differences in occupational distribution are somewhat less pronounced among women, who, regardless of age, show a clear tendency toward concentration in a very few occupations, most notably those classified as service or administrative, which includes clerical work (Rix, 1990).

Job Performance and Experience

The relationship between age and performance has been studied for more than a century (Schulz, Musa, Staszewski, & Siegler, 1994). In fact, one of the key issues in industrial gerontology focuses on intraindividual changes (changes within an individual over time). Specifically, does ability or job performance change as a function of age or the aging process (Avolio, Waldman, & McDaniel, 1990; McEvoy & Cascio, 1989)? However, the available literature on aging and work performance is limited, especially for technology-based jobs (Sterns et al., 1994), and could be described as ambiguous or mixed, at best (Cascio, 1986; Rhodes, 1983; Stanger, 1985). Further, most of the literature on aging and work performance has focused on whether a relationship between age and performance exists, without consideration of various dispositions and situational factors that may affect the relationship between aging and work performance that individuals accrue as they develop in their careers or jobs (Waldman & Avolio, 1993). To date, many questions still remain in the literature regarding the various dispositional and situational factors that may affect the relationship between aging and work performance (Waldman & Avolio, 1993).

Therefore, these and other contextual factors, such as the nature of one's job, characteristics of coworkers, and quality of supervision, can all directly or indirectly affect performance over time and, therefore, they should be taken into account when examining the relationship between chronological age and work performance. Similarly, Sparrow and Davies (1988) report that numerous factors, such as length of service (tenure), training, level, and job complexity, can mediate age differences in job performance. Katz (1980) postulated that sources or determinants of work performance change with the actual length of time a person has occupied a given job. Other sources include the availability of challenging assignments, working for an exceptional or mentoring supervisor, being provided opportunities to upgrade job knowledge and skills (Waldman & Avolio, 1993).

The most generally investigated or considered contextual factors are experience, job complexity, and the method of performance assessment or evaluation (e.g., supervisory ratings vs. productivity measures).

Waldman and Avolio (1986) conducted a meta-analysis of the literature on the relationship between age and work performance to examine the mixed results reported in previous reviews (e.g., Rhodes, 1983; Stanger, 1985). Briefly, Waldman and Avolio's meta-analyses indicated a tendency for age-related increases in performance, particularly for jobs in which performance was measured using nonjudgmental, productivity measures. However, for studies that used supervisory ratings as the measure of performance, there was a tendency toward slight declines in performance with increasing age. Further, Waldman and Avolio's findings indicated that the type of work performed may act as a moderator of the age and work performance relationship; that is, a more negative relationship was found between age and supervisory ratings of performance for nonprofessional jobs as compared to professional jobs.

McEvoy and Cascio (1989) extended the work of Waldman and Avolio (1986) by including all previous studies found in the literature that reported an age–performance correlation, whether the study focused on that relationship or not. Similarities and differences with previous research were found. First, as found by Waldman and Avolio (1986), McEvoy and Cascio's meta-analysis indicated relatively low relationships between age and work performance. However, no support was found regarding the variations in the relationship between age and work performance for different performance criteria, nor was there support for the finding that job type moderated the relationship.

Avolio et al. (1990) reported differences in the age and work performance relationship for five occupational groupings derived from the General Aptitude Test Battery data base. The relationship between age and work performance was found to be nonlinear. Finally, job experience was found to be a better predictor of work performance than age.

Longitudinal studies (see Waldman & Avolio, 1993) that examined the age and performance relationship generally report that performance may initially increase with age, plateau in mid life, and then remain constant, or in some cases decrease for older workers.

However, it is important to note that the definition and conceptualization of experience is difficult; that is, time in current job, seniority, time in organization, and so forth. But, generally, as in the case of age, experience has been shown to be nonlinearly related to performance across a wide range of occupations (Avolio et al., 1990; McDaniel, Schmidt, & Hunter, 1988). Basically, the contribution of experience to the prediction of performance tends to plateau or even drop at higher levels of experience, and additional experience on a job beyond a certain necessary minimum level may eventually result in diminishing returns for the individual and the organization (Waldman & Avolio, 1993).

Therefore, although the effects of experience at a job may counteract the effects of age (e.g., Sparrow & Davies, 1988), the existing research is too equivocal to draw conclusions on whether age differences in performance can be reduced or eliminated with task experience. Therefore, additional data are also needed to clarify the role of practice and experience in the relationship between aging and work performance (Sterns et al., 1994).

In conclusion, the assumption that age is generally related to work performance has not received wide support in the literature (Waldman & Avolio, 1993). Yet, a common belief remains that job performance declines with increasing age in the absence of definitive research support. Further, there are individual differences among older workers as well as intraindividual differences in ability or performance levels within older workers (as well as younger workers) at any point in time. We strongly encourage those interested in the age–performance relationship to read Waldman and Avolio (1993), who present a model of aging and work performance that suggests how both work and nonwork contextual experiences can accrue over time in their influence on work performance.

Work Environment

Accident Involvement

An accident can be considered the result of the dynamic and interactive relationship between the individual and the constantly changing demands of the environment. The literature indicates a specific, yet complex, relationship between age and frequency of accidents in the workplace (Sterns, Barrett, & Alexander, 1985). Older workers (age 45+ years) are injured less frequently than younger workers (less than 25 years of age) and about as often as adult workers (age 25–44 years). However, this is a generalization, and there are known differences in terms of the type of job, industry, and numerous other factors.

The most extensive study in the area of life-span trends in industrial accidents was conducted by Root (1981), which was based on data from over a million worker compensation records in 30 states. This represented approximately 40% of the American wage and salary work force.

Root found that occupational injuries occurred at a lower rate for older workers than for younger workers. Generally, the highest work injury rates for almost all types of industries were for workers 20–24 years of age, and the lowest were for workers 65 years and older. One factor that was observed in the data reported by Root was experience. Specifically, a significant number of injuries occur during the first year of the individual's employment on the position, regardless of age. It appears, with added experience in the job, that the worker gains experience in how to avoid accidents and how to perform the job more efficiently.

Overall, research indicates that older workers appear to be less likely to be injured on the job and accident rates for most occupations tend to decrease for older employees (Rhodes, 1983). However, when illness or injury do occur, they are more likely to be associated with longer-term absence or are more likely to be fatal or lead to permanent disability (Sterns et al., 1985).

Job Satisfaction

The research regarding the relationship between age and job satisfaction yields mixed results. Rhodes (1983) suggests a positive and linear relationship between age and overall satisfaction until at least age 60. That is, as age increases, the individual's overall satisfaction with the job increases. This relationship holds for both blue-collar and white-collar jobs, and both men and women. However, we know very little about sources of job satisfaction for older, nontraditional workers (Staats et al., 1995). Though there are mixed findings, research has generally reported that job satisfaction increases in a linear function for women and a curvilinear function for men (Kacmar & Ferris, 1989). However, although the exact relationship between age and job satisfaction is complex, the research generally is supportive of positive relationship between age and job satisfaction.

There is extensive research documenting that attitudes toward work, organizational commitment, and job satisfaction are progressively more positive with increasing age (Rhodes, 1983; Sterns & Alexander, 1987). Further, older workers have been shown to be a stable and productive element in the work force (Doering, Rhodes, & Schuster, 1983). Older workers appear to experience greater involvement, control, and satisfaction on their jobs relative to younger persons (Remondt & Hansson, 1991; Warr, 1992).

Regarding the job itself, younger workers often respond very unfavorably to jobs they see lacking in significance or meaning; older workers do not. Further, older workers do not like jobs with a high degree of complexity (Welford, 1985).

Updating and Obsolescence

Two serious problems for older workers are (1) reaching a plateau in their position and (2) obsolescence (Rix, 1990). Workers who have essentially stopped advancing on the job, that is, their career progression has leveled off, are considered to have reached a plateau. Career obsolescence pertains to workers who have fallen behind in the ability to use new techniques or master new skills in present jobs (Rix, 1990). On the other hand, professional competence is the ability to function effectively in the tasks considered essential within a given profession (Willis & Dubin, 1990). The negative consequences associated with workers who have reached a plateau and obsolescence include clogged channels of promotion, lower morale among other workers, and lower overall productivity of the department or unit.

Sterns and Hayslip (1990) state that a major issue for the 1990s is the question of how long a worker's skills will remain current. With the rapid technological changes occurring today, workers may find it necessary to continually update their knowledge, skills, and abilities or they may become obsolete. Obsolescence occurs when the demands of a job become incongruent with a worker's knowledge, skills, and abilities. According to Sterns et al. (1994) many factors have been empirically and theoretically related to obsolescence, such as aspects of the person (age) as well as the job setting (organizational climate).

There are various perspectives on how workers will engage in updating and retraining opportunities during the life span. Fossum, Arvey, Paradise, and Robbins (1986) suggested that individuals can be expected to pursue updating and retraining opportunities when they believe that training will lead to the development of relevant knowledge, skills, and abilities that will lead to valued outcomes. Fossum et al. (1986) suggest that obsolescence may increase with age. The importance of outcomes changes with increasing age, and there is decreased expectancy of obtaining valued outcomes through updating the person's knowledge, skills, and abilities. Therefore, with age, individuals should be less willing to invest in training, and this will be true not only for chronological age but also for job and occupational tenure.

Willis and Dubin (1990) take a developmental approach, which views maintaining professional competence through updating as a continual process, starting as soon as an individual enters the work force—continually putting an effort into staying up-to-date in one's job throughout his or her career. The remedial approach views updating as a process done to compensate for obsolescence that has already occurred.

Regardless of which perceptive is correct, as suggested by McLaughlin (1989), major challenges for organizations, now and in the future, will be to retain employees with potential for important work contributions, to retrain employees whose skills have become obsolete, and to create career paths and incentives to help senior employees avoid and break out of career plateaus.

Organizational Demands and Climate

Selection

Given the prohibition against age discrimination in employment, the possibility of age-related bias in employee selection is quite important. Many current personnel selection, ability or aptitude tests, and interview procedures may be unfairly discriminating against older job applicants (Sterns & Alexander, 1987). For example, selection tests may not have norms for older workers or may measure abilities that decline with age but have nothing to do with actual job performance (Stanger, 1985).

Changing Jobs for the Older Worker

On the basis of the factors affecting older workers in each of the six dimensions, jobs or job requirements may need to be changed to meet the needs of an "aging work force." These job changes or modifications can include equipment design and redesign, as well as job redesign. For example, equipment design efforts might include redesign of displays and controls or equipment. Job redesign changes might include alternative work–rest schedules or changing pacing requirements. Equipment redesign might include changing the lighting or the layout of the workplace.

Moreover, what appears to be an age-related performance decline may actually be the result of a mismatch between the job and the worker, which suggests that better matching of workers and jobs could result in a more productive workforce (Rix, 1990).

Discrimination

Even in light of federal legislation the problem of age discrimination continues to be a problem. By way of illustration, Sterns and Alexander (1987) cited that a national work force survey reported that more than 80% of American workers believe that employers discriminate against older employees.

The Age Discrimination in Employment Act (ADEA) of 1967 specified protection of workers from age discrimination between the ages of 40 and 65 and promotion of employment opportunities for older workers capable of meeting job requirements. In 1974, the act was amended to include coverage of government employees at the local, state, and federal levels. In 1978 it was amended to change coverage to age 70 and to abolish mandatory retirement altogether for federal employees. In 1986, the act was further amended to remove the maximum age limitation, with certain exceptions. Since January 1987, older persons, with few exceptions, have been legally entitled to remain at work for as long as they wish, assuming their performance is adequate (Rix, 1990). Further, it is a violation for employers to fail or refuse to hire, to discharge, or in other ways to discriminate against any individual with respect to compensation or other terms or conditions of employment because of age. Finally, workers cannot be limited, segregated, or classified in a way that might adversely affect their status as an employee because of age. (Sterns & Alexander, 1987).

Discrimination against older workers did not evaporate with the passage of the ADEA (Rix, 1990). In fact, the age of a worker can affect how an organization processes selection, promotion, and termination decisions and still stay within the letter of the law; that is, age is a bona fide occupational qualification (B.F.O.Q.) (Waldman & Avolio, 1993).

Because age discrimination can be subtle, there are no reliable statistics on how many middle-aged and older workers experience age discrimination and under what circumstances (Rix, 1990). However, information from the Equal Employment Opportunity Commission indicates that perceived "unlawful discharge" was mentioned in over 50% of the cases filed by older workers, the next two most frequent claims were "hiring and/or terms and conditions of employment," and "layoffs" (Rix, 1990). Finally, the number of discrimination lawsuits filed under the ADEA has risen dramatically in recent years (McEvoy & Casio, 1989). Personal reports of alleged discrimination against midlife workers by companies and the effects of downsizing can be found in Lewis (1994).

CONCLUSIONS: CAPABILITIES OF OLDER WORKERS

The core perspective of this chapter was that to adequately understand the older worker we must recognize that he or she is affected by many interacting factors of a sensory–perceptual, biophysiological, cognitive, personal–interpersonal, and cultural–environmental nature. Each factor affecting and being effected by each other factor during the course of the life span. In this chapter we have highlighted and discussed some of the factors and issues pertinent to older workers from a multidimensional perspective.

On the basis of the literature reviewed in this chapter, a number of general conclusions regarding older workers are possible. First, the work force in the United States and other industrialized nations is getting older, and by the year 2000 the median age of a worker in the work force will be 40 years, the age at which a person is considered an "older worker." Hence, business and industry needs to give careful consideration to the needs and abilities of older workers (Johnson & Johnson, 1982; Meier & Kerr, 1976; Rhodes, 1983; Sterns & Alexander, 1987).

Second, organizations and other workers often still hold negative views toward older workers, such as "they cannot learn new skills," in spite of "common knowledge" regarding the merits of older workers (Hirshorn & Hoyer, 1994). However, despite a lack of evidence, organizations continue to give credence to many of these negative views, resulting in policies and procedures that may indirectly or directly discriminate against older workers. But, given the fact that current cohorts of older workers are in better health, are better educated, and are more politically active than previous cohorts of older workers (Staats et al., 1994), many of these myths and generalizations may soon dissipate.

Third, older workers can benefit from training and retraining programs. Additionally, they possess a number of traits and attitudes valued by business and industry. For example, older workers are loyal and dedicated to the company, they have good attendance and punctuality records, and they are less likely to leave the organization.

Fourth, the assumption that age is generally related to work performance has not received wide support in the literature. Additionally, many contextual factors such as the nature of one's job, characteristics of coworkers, quality of supervision, experience, job complexity, the method of performance assessment or evaluation, and the like can all directly or indirectly affect the age–performance relationship. Finally, additional data are needed to clarify the role of practice and experience in the relationship between aging and work performance.

Fifth, the issues associated with aging and work naturally fall into the domain of human factors, since the human factors approach focuses on adapting the work environment to the work force. Consequently, the human factors approach is particularly relevant to issues regarding the older worker and its principles can be applied to enhance and facilitate employment opportunities. As noted in this chapter, business and industry are beginning to address the demands of the aging work force.

Finally, there is still a need for additional research pertaining to the older worker on many of the topics and issues discussed in this chapter. For example, it is not clear how the influx of technology, as well as new technology and information, into workplace settings affects the older as well as the younger worker. Also, are there alternatives to chronological age for assessing occupational performance for both older and younger workers (Avolio, Barrett, & Sterns, 1984)?

Acknowledgments

The author thanks Dr. Pat Raymark, Dr. John Skowronski, and Dr. Sara Staats, The Ohio State University at Newark, and Christine Franklin-Panek, coordinator, Back-on-Track (Displaced Homemaker Program), Licking County Joint Vocational School for their comments on an earlier draft of this manuscript.

References

Aldag, R. J., & Brief, A. P. (1977). Age, work, values, and employee relations. *Industrial Gerontology, 4,* 192–197.

American Association of Retired Persons. (1988, March/April). Japanese love of work a lifelong affair. *Working Age, 3*(5), 6–7.

Avery, R. D., & Foley, R. H. (1988). *Fairness in selecting employees,* New York: Addison-Wesley.

Avolio, B. J., Barrett, G. V., & Sterns, H. L. (1984). Alternatives to age for assessing occupational performance capacity. *Experimental Aging Research, 10,* 101–105.

Avolio, B. J., Panek, P. E., & Harcar, V. (1992). Occupational risk in retirement ages recommended for sixty occupations. *Psychological Reports, 71,* 1315–1330.

Avolio, B. J., & Waldman, D. A. (1990). An examination of age and cognitive test performance across job complexity and occupational types. *Journal of Applied Psychology, 75,* 43–50.

Avolio, B. J., Waldman, D. A., & McDaniel, M. A. (1990). Age and work performance in nonmanagerial jobs: The effects of experience and occupational type. *Academy of Management Journal, 33,* 407–422.

Barrett, G. V., Mihal, W. L., Panek, P. E., Sterns, H. L., & Alexander, R. A. (1977). Information processing skills predictive of accident involvement for younger and older commercial drivers. *Industrial Gerontology, 4,* 173–181.

Berkowitz, M. (1988). Functioning ability and job performance as workers age. In M. E. Borus, H. S. Parnes, S. H. Sandell, & B. Seidman (Eds.), *The older worker.* Madison, WI: Industrial Relations Research Association.

Cascio, W. F. (1986). *Managing human resources.* New York: McGraw-Hill.

Cleveland, J. N., & Hollmann, G. (1990). The effects of age-type of tasks and incumbent age composition on job perceptions. *Journal of Vocational Behavior, 36,* 181–194.

DeFrank, R. S., & Ivancevich, J. M. (1986). Job loss: An individual-level review and model. *Journal of Vocational Behavior, 28,* 1–20.

Doering, M., Rhodes, S. R., & Schuster, M. (1983). *The aging worker: Research and recommendations.* Beverly Hills, CA: Sage.

Fletcher, W. L., Hansson, R. O., & Bailey, L. (1992). Assessing occupational self-efficacy among middle-aged and older adults. *Journal of Applied Gerontology, 11,* 489–501.

Fossum, J. A., Arvey, R. D., Paradise, C. A., & Robbins, N. E. (1986). Modeling the skills obsolescence process: A psychological/economic integration. *Academy of Management Review, 11*(2), 363–374.

Gordon, R. A., & Arvey, R. D. (1986). Perceived and actual ages of workers. *Journal of Vocational Behavior, 28,* 21–28.

Greenglass, E. R. (1988). Type A behavior and coping strategies in female and male supervisors. *Applied Psychology: An Internal Review, 37,* 271–288.

Hansson, R. O., Briggs, S. R., & Rule, B. L. (1990). Old age and unemployment: Predictors of control, depression, and loneliness. *Journal of Applied Gerontology, 9,* 230–240.

Harris, D. (1995, June). Parental guidance. *Working Woman,* p. 37.

Hayslip, B. J., Jr., & Panek, P. E. (1993). *Adult development and aging* (2nd ed.). New York: HarperCollins.

Hirshorn, B. A., & Hoyer, D. T. (1994). Private sector hiring and use of retirees: The firm's perspective. *Gerontologist, 34,* 50–58.

Jacobson, B. (1980). *Young programs for old workers: case studies in progressive personnel policies.* New York: Van Nostrand-Reinhold.

Jahoda, M. (1961). A social-psychological approach to the study of culture. *Human Relations, 14,* 23–30.

Johnson, D. R., & Johnson, J. T. (1982). Managing the older worker. *Journal of Applied Gerontology, 1,* 58–66.

Johnston, W. B. (1987). *Workforce 2000: Work and workers for the 21st century.* Indianapolis, IN: Hudson Institute.

Kacmar, K. M., & Ferris, G. R. (1989). Theoretical and methodological considerations in the age-job satisfaction relationship. *Journal of Applied Gerontology, 74,* 201–207.

Kanter, R. M. (1977). *Men and women of the corporation.* New York: Basic Books.

Katz, R. (1980). Time and work: Toward an integrative perspective. In B. M. Staw & L. L. Cummings (Eds.), *Research in organizational behavior* (Vol. 2, pp. 37–91). Greenwich, CT: JAI Press.

Kirkland, R. I., Jr. (1994, February). Why we will live longer . . . and what it will mean. *Fortune,* pp. 66–68, 70, 74–76, 78.

Krause, N. (1994). Stressors in salient social roles and well-being in later life. *Journal of Gerontology: Psychological Sciences, 49,* P137–P148.

Lawrence, B. S. (1988). New wrinkles in the theory of age: Demography, norms, and performance ratings. *Academy of Management Journal, 31,* 309–337.

Lawton, M. P., & Nahemow, L. (1973). Ecology and the aging process. In C. Eisdorfer & M. P. Lawton (Eds.), *The psychology of adult development and aging* (pp. 619–674). Washington, DC: American Psychological Association.

Lewis, R. (1994, November). Downsizing taking a higher toll. *AARP Bulletin, 35* (10), 1, 14–15.

Lindley, C. J. (1989). Assessment of older persons in the workplace. In T. Hunt & C. J. Lindley (Eds.), *Testing older adults: A reference guide for geropsychological assessments* (pp. 232–257). Austin, TX: Pro-Ed.

Love, D. O., & Torrence, W. D. (1989). The impact of worker age on unemployment and earnings after plant closings. *Journal of Gerontology: Social Sciences, 44,* S190–S195.

McDaniel, M. A., Schmidt, F. L., & Hunter, J. E. (1988). Job experience correlates of job performance. *Journal of Applied Psychology, 73,* 327–330.

McEvoy, G. M., & Cascio, W. F. (1989). Cumulative evidence of the relationship between age and job performance. *Journal of Applied Psychology, 74,* 11–17.

McLaughlin, A. (1989). *Older worker task force; Key policy issues for the future.* Washington, DC: U.S. Department of Labor.

McLloyd, V. C. (1989). Socialization and development in a changing economy: The effects of paternal job and income loss on children. *American Psychologist, 44,* 293–302.

Meier, E. L., & Kerr, E. A. (1976). Capabilities of middle-aged and older workers: A survey of the literature. *Industrial Gerontology, 3,* 147–156.

Morgan, L. A. (1984). Continuity and change in the labor force activity of recently widowed women. *Gerontologist, 24,* 530–535.

Neugarten, B. L., & Datan, N. (1973). Sociological perspectives on the life cycle. In P. W. Baltes & K. W. Schaie (Eds.), *Life-span developmental psychology: Personality and socialization* (pp. 53–69). New York: Academic Press.

Olsho, L. W., Harkins, S. W., & Lendardt, M. L. (1985). Aging and the auditory system. In J. E. Birren & K. W. Schaie (Eds.), *Handbook of the psychology of aging* (2nd ed)., pp. 332–377). New York: Van Nostrand-Reinhold.

Osipow, S. H. (1983). *Theories of career development.* Englewood Cliffs, NJ: Prentice-Hall.

Osipow, S. H., Doty, R. E., & Spokane, A. R. (1985). Occupational stress, strain, and coping across the life-span. *Journal of Vocational Behavior, 27,* 98–108.

Panek, P. E., Barrett, G. V., Alexander, R. A., & Sterns, H. L. (1979). Age and self-selected performance pace on a visual monitoring inspection task. *Aging and Work: A Journal on Age, Work and Retirement, 2,* 183–191.

Parasuraman, R., & Giambra, L. (1991). Skill development in vigilance: Effects of event rate and age. *Psychology and Aging, 6,* 155–169.

Pervin, L. A. (1968). Performance and satisfaction as a function of individual-environment fit. *Psychological Bulletin, 69,* 56–68.

Porterfield, J. D., & St. Pierre, R. (1992). *Healthful aging: Wellness,* Guilford, CT: Dushkin.

Quinn, J. F., & Burkhauser, R. B. (1990). Work and retirement. In R. Binstock & L. George (Eds.), *Handbook of aging and the social sciences* (3rd ed., pp. 304–327). San Diego, CA: Academic Press.

Remondt, J. H., & Hansson, R. O. (1991). Job-related threats to control among older employees. *Journal of Social Issues, 47,* 129–141.

Repetti, R. L., Matthews, K. A., & Waldron, I. (1989). Employment and women's health: Effects of paid employment on women's mental and physical health. *American Psychologist, 44,* 1394–1401.

Rhodes, S. R. (1983). Age-related differences in work attitudes and behavior: A review and conceptual analysis. *Psychological Bulletin, 93,* 328–367.

Rife, J., & Kilty, K. (1989–1990). Job-search discouragement and the older worker: Implications for social work practice. *Journal of Applied Social Sciences, 14,* 71–94.

Rix, S. E. (1990). *Older workers.* Santa Barbara, CA: ABC-CLIO.

Root, W. (1981). Injuries at work are fewer among older employees. *Monthly Labor Review, 104,* 30–34.

Rosen, B., & Jerdee, T. H. (1985). *Older employees: New roles for valued resources.* Homewood, IL: Dow-Jones-Irwin.

Rosen, B., & Jerdee, T. H. (1988). Managing older workers' careers. In G. R. Ferris & K. M. Rowland (Eds.), *Research in personnel and human resources management* (Vol. 6, pp. 37–74). Greenwich, CT: JAI Press.

Rosen, B., & Jerdee, T. H. (1989). Investing in the older worker. *Personnel Administrator, 34,* 70–74.

Ruhm, C. J. (1989). Why older Americans stop working. *Gerontologist, 29,* 294–300.

Rybash, J. M., Hoyer, W. J., & Roodin, P. A. (1986). *Adult cognition and aging.* Elmsford, NY: Pergamon.

Salthouse, T. (1988). Initiating the formalization of theories of cognitive aging. *Psychology and Aging, 3,* 3–16.

Schulz, R., Musa, D., Staszewski, J., & Siegler, R. S. (1994). The relationship between age and major league baseball performance: Implications for development. *Psychology and Aging, 9,* 274–286.

Sheppard, H. L. (1976). Work and retirement. In R. Binstock & E. Shanas (Eds.), *Handbook of aging and the social sciences.* (pp. 286–309). New York: Van Nostrand-Reinhold.

Shaw, L. B. (1988). Special problems of older women workers. In M. E. Borus, H. S. Parnes, S. H. Sandell, & B. Seidman (Eds.), *The older worker.* Madison, WI: Industrial Relations Research Board.

Sparrow, P. R., & Davies, D. R. (1988). Effects of age, tenure, training, and job complexity on technical performance. *Psychology and Aging, 3,* 307–314.

Speas, K., & Obenshain, B. (1995). *AARP images of aging in America* (Final report). Chapel Hill, NC: EGI Integrated Marketing.

Staats, S., Colbert, B., & Partlo, C. (1995). Uplifts, hassles, and quality of life in older workers. In M. J. Sirgy & A. C. Samli (Eds.), *New dimensions in marketing/quality-of-life research* (pp. 117–135). Westport, CT: Quorum Books.

Staats, S., Partlo, C., Armstrong-Stassen, M., & Plimpton, L. (1994). Older working widows: Present and expected expectancies of stress and quality of life in comparison to married workers. In G. Puryear Keita & J. J. Hurrell, Jr. (Eds.), *Job stress in a changing workforce:*

Investigating gender, diversity, and family issues (pp. 181–195). Washington, DC: American Psychological Association.

Stanger, R. (1985). Aging in industry. In J. E. Birren & K. W. Schaie (Eds.), *Handbook of the psychology of aging* (pp. 789–817). New York: Van Nostrand-Reinhold.

Sterns, H. L. (1986). Training and retraining adult and older adult workers. In J. E. Birren, P. K. Robinson, & J. E. Livingston (Eds.), *Age, health and employment* (pp. 93–113). Englewood Cliffs, NJ: Prentice-Hall.

Sterns, H. L., & Alexander, R. A. (1986). Industrial gerontology. In G. L. Maddox (Ed.), *Encyclopedia of aging* (pp. 349–351). New York: Springer.

Sterns, H. L., & Alexander, R. A. (1987). Industrial gerontology: The aging individual and work. *Annual Review of Gerontology and Geriatrics,* 243–264.

Sterns, H. L., Barrett, G. V., & Alexander, R. A. (1985). Accidents and the aging individual. In J. E. Birren & K. W. Schaie (Eds.), *Handbook of the psychology of aging* (pp. 703–724). New York: Van Nostrand-Reinhold.

Sterns, H. L., Barrett, G. V., Czaja, S. J., & Barr, J. K. (1994). Issues in work and aging. *Journal of Applied Gerontology, 13,* 1–19.

Sterns, H. L., & Hayslip, B. J. (1990, June). *Retirement and reentry: What should psychologists be doing?* Paper presented at the annual meeting of the American Psychological Society, Dallas, TX.

Sterns, H. L., & Sanders, R. A. (1980). Training and education in the elderly. In R. R. Turner & H. W. Reese (Eds.), *Life-span developmental psychology: Intervention* (pp. 307–330). New York: Academic Press.

Szafran, J. (1965). Age differences in sequential decisions and cardiovascular status among pilots. *Aerospace Medicine, 36,* 303–310.

Szafran, J. (1970). The effects of aging on professional pilots. In J. H. Price (Ed.), *Modern trends in psychological medicine* (pp. 37–71). New York: Appleton-Century-Crofts.

Valasek, D. L., & Sterns, H. L. (1981, November). *Task analysis and training: Applications from lab to the field.* Paper presented at the 34th annual scientific meeting of the Gerontological Society of America, Toronto.

Wachtel, H. (1966). Hard-core unemployment in Detroit: Causes and remedies. In *Proceedings of the Industrial Relations Research Association* (pp. 233–241). Madison, WI. Industrial Relations Research Association.

Waldman, D. A., & Avolio, B. J. (1986). A meta-analysis of age difference in job performance. *Journal of Applied Gerontology, 71,* 33–38.

Waldman, D. A., & Avolio, B. J. (1993). Aging and work performance in perspective: Contextual and developmental considerations. *Research in Personnel and Human Resources Management, 11,* 133–162.

Warr, P. (1992). Age and occupational well-being. *Psychology and Aging, 7,* 37–45.

Welford, A. T. (1985). Changes of performance with age: An overview. In N. Charness (Ed.), *Aging and human performance* (pp. 333–369). Chichester, UK: Wiley.

Willis, S. L., & Dubin, S. S. (Eds.), (1990). *Maintaining professional competencies,* San Francisco: Jossey-Bass.

Chapter 16

Robotic Technologies and the Older Adult

K. G. Engelhardt
Donald H. Goughler

NEW IDEAS FOR HELPING TO SOLVE OLD PROBLEMS

This chapter will discuss applications of robotic and advanced microprocessor technologies to assist older adults in maintaining their independence. The concept on which this chapter focuses, service robotics, can be defined as "robotic systems that can sense, think and act to benefit or enable humans" (Engelhardt and Edwards, 1986).

Service robotics are hybrid systems incorporating the repeatable and programmable flexibility of robotic and sensor technologies with the adaptability, judgment, and decision making of humans derived from the emerging capabilities of artificial intelligence. The vigor achieved by such integration exceeds the capabilities of any single component of the human–robot system.

Robotics began as products in the mid-1960s and became one of the paths from which service robotics emerged in the mid-1980s. Robots are made of integrated electromechanical components that are computer and

Handbook of Human Factors and the Older Adult

learning based. Their morphology has traditionally been that of an "arm" dedicated to repetitious tasks. Historically, the most prevalent use of robots has been in industry, including material handling, such as parts assembly in manufacturing; spray painting, usually in the automotive industries, and welding. Service robots are being designed for very different applications. They must work with and for humans to serve specific needs in human environments.

The potential for intervening with advanced technology to augment human independence has only begun to be explored. Sometimes, human oriented applications are not even considered a primary focus of technological development. Too often, the lag time between the development of an innovation and its adoption and acceptance is very long, particularly in terms of immediate human needs. To prevent such an outcome, we must ask appropriate questions about both the needs and the abilities of aging humans and the capabilities and potentials of the technologies that can be utilized to serve these identified needs (Engelhardt, 1989).

As a precursor to applying robotics to human benefit, it is important to demystify robotic technologies and conceptualize them as tools, similar to the context in which automobiles and wheelchairs are tools for assisting human mobility. The development of robotic applications to assist older adults can provide new "smart tools" that enable gerontologists, allied health care professionals, and family caregivers to provide better care. Smarter tools will also allow older adults to actively participate in their own care.

THE UNIQUE TECHNOLOGICAL NEEDS OF OLDER PERSONS

Smart Technology and Aging with Independence

As Americans live longer, the need for innovative interventions to care for older citizens is becoming increasingly evident. The Census Bureau in the United States predicts that the elderly population will more than double by the year 2050 (U.S. Department of Commerce, 1995). As the proportion of older adults in the population has increased, extensive services have been developed to prevent them from becoming unnecessarily or prematurely institutionalized. Past government policy, as well as current policy recommendations from advocates and professionals, has promoted informal or family caregiving as a preferred resource for assisting older persons to maintain independence (Pillemer, Moen, Krout, & Robinson, 1995; White House Conference on Aging, 1995). Families who provide care are regarded as a major factor in delaying or inhibiting the premature institutionalization of at-risk older adults (Chappell, 1983; Hooyman & Kiyak, 1988; LeVande, Bowden and Mollema, 1987). These informal systems, when available, are successful in meeting the basic physical and instrumental self-maintenance needs of the elderly (Feller, 1983; Shanas, 1979). Informal supports are also the base of elder care, since unpaid family members, about 75% of whom are women, provide 80% of the care received by older persons in the community (Coile, 1990).

The expanding proportion of older adults in the American population will challenge both professional and personal caregiving during the next four decades (Barrow, 1989; Kemper & Murtaugh, 1991; Torrey, 1994; U.S. Senate Special Committee on Aging, 1985). Demands on aging spouses and families, who sometimes have severe disabilities themselves, will increase (Brody, 1985; Cantor, 1992). The mobility of modern society, increased employment of women, and the stresses of family, finances, and housing are making family caregiving more difficult (Barrow, 1989). The cost to families of providing long-term care is the single largest cause of personal bankruptcy, affecting more than 1 million people each year (Halamandaris, 1994). As traditional modes of caregiving are threatened by these challenges, a complementary strategy that augments the remaining self-help capacity of older adults and permits them to extend the duration of their own self-help capacity is needed (Kane & Kane, 1991).

Recent rapid advances in robotic-related technologies offer the potential for new strategies that can help individuals extend or enhance their self-help capabilities and, therefore, their independence. The advanced assistive devices in this category have become smarter, more flexible, and robust systems that are becoming increasingly modular and adaptable to human needs. It is now possible to address problems of human need that would have been impossible until very recently because the technologies to fill these needs did not exist (Engelhardt, 1984, 1994). Unfortunately, most older persons who could benefit from technological interventions know little or nothing about its potential; and few policy makers, as well as formal and informal caregivers, have explored the service viability of advanced technologies (Clark & Gaide, 1986; Engelhardt, 1984). For development of the service potential of these technologies to be successful, roboticists, designers, and gerontologists need to collaborate with older persons in evaluating this resource.

First, we need to overcome the misconception that older adults are technophobic. On the contrary, today's older population has experienced a history of profound technological changes, including space exploration, and has constantly adopted new technologies during the decades of their lives. Recently, Engelhardt surveyed 58 households in rural Pennsylvania in which an older adult, with a disabling condition, was receiving personal care and identified the existing technologies these older adults use in their homes. Among these households, all had at least one TV and 71% had two or more, 22% had a VCR, 57% had at least one remote controller, all had telephones and 62% had two or more, 53% had a microwave oven, 69% had an electric coffee maker, 69% had an electric blender, and 93% had one or more vacuum cleaners (Engelhardt, 1988).

Even though the study location was a rural area of moderate income households, technologies that have been available during the last 40 years and have been perceived by the general public to be useful are regularly used by these older adults. They use technology and have espoused technological innovations that did not exist when they began to operate their households. One of these appliances, the microwave oven, has features similar to a robotic system. Both "think" and "act" to serve human needs. The microwave oven can "probe" the temperature of our favorite dish, "sense" when it has reached the desired temperature, then alert the human that the dish is ready to be removed from the oven. Microwave ovens, a technology once unfamiliar to this population, were perceived to be friendly and easy to use by the older adults in this study. As robotic technologies evolve into almost limitless numbers and configurations, the forms and images of robotics that are part of our present knowledge base will reach new understandings and become as familiar to the future elderly as the microwave oven is today.

Robotic Kitchens and Nutrition

The kitchen can be viewed as the interface between independence and institutionalization and is a potentially fertile locale for developing smart assistive technologies. Eating and meal preparation include manipulative tasks that challenge many older persons (Clark & Gaide, 1986; Faletti, 1984). When debility prevents older adults from preparing their own meals, they lose a basic gesture of personal freedom and dignity as well as their nutritional stability. They become dependent on family or professional helpers and may be forced to leave their homes and enter institutions.

Extensive public and private support systems have been developed to help elderly people with meals. On the public side, the Older Americans Act provided funding for more than 102 million home-delivered meals for 800,000 persons in fiscal year 1993 (U.S. Department of Health and Human Services, 1994). Numerous volunteers and family members also assist older adults with meal preparation. Nutrition support was one of the earliest and one of the longest standing objectives of the organized aging network. Its programmatic maintenance is also a challenge to students of gerontology who will be policy makers and program leaders. Because nutrition service delivery has become costly it has been a cost-cutting target of Congress.

Robotic-related technologies provide a special opportunity to address meal preparation. To gain fruitful guidance for technological development, Czaja (1990) has recommended that human factors task analysis techniques be applied to meal preparation behavior.

During 1992–1993 the authors conducted a project, funded by both the Pennsylvania Department of Aging and the Retirement Research Foundation, that explored the feasibility of utilizing microprocessor-based technology to relieve caregiver burden and augment care receiver independence in personal meal preparation.

Initially, our research assessed the daily living skills of 142 homebound older adults and investigated issues related to their family caregivers. Instruments used in this research included the Katz Index of Activities of Daily Living (ADL), Instrumental Activities of Daily Living Index (IADL), Pfeiffer's Short Portable Mental Status Questionnaire, Zarit's Caregiving Burden Interview, and Pennsylvania Care Management Assessment Form.

Results showed that, among this population of care receivers, *none* was able to score in the independent range of the IADL scale. While 11.2% were able to prepare meals if assisted by a helper, the other 88.8% were unable to contribute to meal preparation and required a caregiver to prepare meals for them. However, the IADL results did not provide the important insight into the reasons why these limitations are perceived. To identify functional deficits that limited the care receiver's meal preparation ability (and that could potentially be addressed by or were amenable to robotics technologies), we videotaped meal preparation processes of a subsample of seven caregiver–care receiver teams. These sessions were conducted in the participants' kitchens and focused on the functional analysis of meal preparation behavior and actions.

The caregiver–care receivers teams prepared a standard dinner meal that ensured a balanced diet. The preparation process replicated a wide range of preparation challenges that standard food packaging presents to older people. The meal consisted of lean steak wrapped in cellophane, whole potatoes packaged in a heavy paper with cord closure, a packaged frozen vegetable, fruit in a flip top can, juice in a half gallon container, rolls in a plastic bag that was knotted shut, and butter in a paper wrapper. Tapes were evaluated by an interdisciplinary team of nurses, geriatricians, roboticists, administrators, caregivers, and physical therapists. The videotaped trials

TABLE 1
Functions and Tasks

Functions		
Gathering	Preparing	Tending
Tasks	Tasks	Tasks
• Traversing room • Opening refrigerator, stove, microwave, drawer, cupboard • Walking while carrying • Bending, reaching for item, and removing from cupboard, etc.	• Cutting package or food • Tearing package with hands • Screwing or unscrewing container cup • Pouring liquid or seasoning • Placing food in container • Handling, manipulating, cleaning food	• Moving, manipulating food • Removing or placing lid on container • Adjusting appliance controls

were assessed at three increasingly specific levels of activity: functions, tasks, and movements. Functions referred to the most general descriptors of activity and included (1) gathering, (2) preparing, and (3) tending.

Tasks intrinsic to these functions were identified. Gathering, for instance, included tasks such as procuring food from the refrigerator or storage areas and assembling dishes and utensils. Preparing included tasks such as opening food packages, pouring, cleaning food, and placing food in cookware. Tending tasks included stirring, checking temperature, and turning meat. Table 1 shows some examples of the relationship between functions and tasks.

Finally, finite movements inherent in these tasks, such as grasping, lifting, rotation, and flexion of body parts were analyzed. Some examples of the relationship between tasks and movements are shown in Table 2.

A first concern was to determine how completely care receivers could

TABLE 2
Tasks and Movements

Task	Characteristic Movements
• Opening package	• Grasping • Finger flexion • Thumb to finger opposition movement
• Reaching	• Shoulder flexion • Bilateral range of motion

TABLE 3
Completion of Functions by Care Receivers

	Function Type		
Team	Gathering (CR completion)	Preparing (CR completion)	Tending (CR completion)
AG	9 (55.6%)	11 (63.6%)	3 (66.7%)
CD	9 (33.3%)	7 (28.6%)	2 (0%)
FR	7 (71.4%)	9 (88.9%)	4 (100%)
BB	7 (0%)	4 (100%)	5 (60%)
KK	6 (33.3%)	7 (71.4%)	5 (20%)
EE	8 (100%)	10 (80%)	2 (100%)
LL	6 (33.3%)	6 (66.7%)	9 (100%)
Totals	52 (51.9%)	54 (74.1%)	30 (70%)

perform meal preparation functions. The number of functions required to prepare the meal varied, from a low of 16 to a high of 23, mainly due to idiosyncratic customs of the participants such as the extent to which individuals washed food before cooking it.

Care receivers in the trial succeeded in completing a mean of 62.6% of all meal preparation functions while caregivers' assistance was needed to complete a mean of 37.4%. *Completion* of a function was defined as successfully performing all tasks inherent in that function.

Gathering (38.2%) and preparing (39.7%) were the most prevalent functions, while 22.1% of the functions were classified as tending. As shown in Table 3, care receivers were similarly successful in preparing (74.1%) and tending (70.0%) functions, but less successful (51.9%) in gathering functions. This difference appears attributable to the fact that most of the care receivers had mobility impairments.

Next, we assessed performance of 10 characteristic tasks, including (1) traversing the kitchen, (2) opening appliances, (3) transporting (walking while carrying), (4) cutting food or food package, (5) tearing packages, (6) manipulating container caps or closures (i.e., prying, twisting), (7) pouring liquids or solids, (8) bending or reaching, (9) handling or manipulating food (i.e., washing, sorting), and (10) manipulating appliance controls. The most frequent tasks were traversing (29.3%), bending or reaching (18.1%), and handling food (14%). The teams performed a mean of 65.3 tasks with a range from 59 to 71 tasks.

Care receivers successfully completed 64.8% of all tasks, ranging from an individual low of 35.2% completion to an individual high of 95.5%. The

TABLE 4
Cumulative Completion of Tasks by Care Receivers

Task	Frequency	Proportion of all tasks	CR performance	CR completion
Traversing room	126	29.3%	78	61.9%
Opening oven or refrigerator	40	9.3%	27	67.5%
Transporting materials	35	8.1%	23	65.7%
Cutting food or package	21	4.9%	18	85.7%
Tearing package	19	4.4%	15	78.9%
Manipulating container lid	16	3.7%	12	75.0%
Pouring liquid or solid	28	6.5%	23	82.1%
Bending or reaching	78	18.1%	41	52.6%
Handling, cleaning food	60	14.0%	43	71.7%
Manipulating controls	7	1.6%	5	71.4%
Total	430		305	64.8%

tasks performed most successfully by care receivers were generally those that could be completed while seated or in a stationary position. The three tasks that required ambulation or gross changes in body position—traversing, transporting, and bending or reaching—were less frequently performed successfully (60.6%) than the sedentary tasks (76.8%). Table 4 displays the cumulative completion of tasks by care receivers.

A review of the third criteria, movement capacity, consisted of clinical analysis of the movements performed by each care receiver during the trials. The following excerpts from the movement analysis of one care receiver, KK, illustrate this evaluation technique and provide a summary of findings.

KK's task completion score was 47.5%, including a score of 38.7% for traversing, transporting, and bending or reaching and 20% for twisting caps and pouring, compared to 57% for all other tasks. She had extreme difficulty with both ambulation and grip or lifting movements.

For example, regarding ambulation and reaching, KK displayed marked difficulty with sit-to-stand transfer, requiring maximal upper extremity assistance and trunk flexion to the right rather than normal use of leg muscles without trunk substitution.

Regarding her use of hands and arms, KK was unable to open a jar lid and displayed notable inability to pop the lid with fine motor grasps and was unable to grasp fully and roll the paper on the potato bag, which required wrist pronation and supination.

All seven care receivers displayed ambulation deficits; all but one displayed movement deficits related to bending and reaching; five were unable to open flip top lids, unscrew bottle caps, or tear open food packages.

In exploring potential solutions to performance shortcomings, robotics simulations of several representative movements were developed in a laboratory kitchen setting, using an off-the-shelf light industrial robot arm with a four pound payload to which a customized gripper was attached.

For instance, to demonstrate robotic augmentation of reaching, the robotic arm was programmed to reach upward and downward and to open and reach into overhead kitchen cabinets and secure items including plates, cups, and medicine containers. It also was programmed to reach downward and place these items on a table as well as to open a refrigerator, retrieve food items, place these items in a microwave, and operate dials and push buttons.

Although not tested in this particular project, the robot could address deficits in the pinch or grasp movement needed for opening packages or pulling tab containers. With the use of a secondary stabilizing device, the robot could open packages, pull-tab containers, and jars.

To augment ambulatory deficiencies, the subjects' most common barrier to full participation, the robot can be mounted on a commercially available track device or navigate autonomously, which would enable the robot to traverse the work area under software control and perhaps to lend a helping elbow to the older person.

This trial provided some insight into exciting possibilities for utilizing robotic technology to help older adults prepare meals. While further testing and resolution of factors such as cost are necessary, the potential for robotic technology in meal preparation is promising.

SERVICE ROLES FOR ROBOTICS

Robots as Important Tools for Caregivers

Robotic technology has the potential to relieve caregiver burden with other housekeeping tasks in addition to kitchen activities. Other examples are laundry, cleaning, and tending.

Robotic aids can perform manipulation tasks in an older person's home. For example, Engelhardt's research has shown that older people are successful in using a voice control (Engelhardt, Awad, Vander Loos, Boonzaier, & Leifer, 1984). This is particularly important for older adults whose hands are affected by arthritis or who, because of a stroke, have limited use of their hands and arms. For these individuals, a computer keyboard is a difficult challenge, which can be eliminated by voice control.

For older people, voice technology offers a natural approach to controlling objects and devices within their personal space. However, designers should be aware that they need a natural language interface that enables them to communicate with the system in everyday English as opposed to computerese or robotese.

Remote voice control of environmental objects such as televisions, appliances, stereos, doors, windows, and locks already exist. Security can be enhanced by voice-activated door locks and by using smoke detectors that have feedback designed for aged ears. Voice operation of entertainment items is important also.

Voice technology might play an important role in functions such as reminding older people to take their medicines. A buzzer or bell gives only one level of communication: sound without content. Voice messages act as more effective memory joggers by reminding people what they need to do.

We can apply principles already operating in natural-language data-base interfaces to this area. Several age-related considerations could be important in voice input and output and in a natural query language for older users. The jargon or slang of relevant decades could be stored and used to optimize a specific person's ability to communication by using familiar terms. For example, if you want to ask whether an older person wants to listen to a compact disc player, you might use words such as *record player* or *phonograph* to improve that person's understanding of the question.

Voice output could also be used interactively with human input to help maximize functional well-being. For instance, a smart system might ask its user "Can you hear this?" and, based on the response (or nonresponse), adjust volume levels of various output devices. The system could also decrease or increase its speech output rate to increase intelligibility. In this way, it could temporarily or permanently adapt to changing user or environmental characteristics. Redundancy and repetition may also play important roles in successful use. In one research situation with older persons with cognitive deficits, the rule was "everything in triplicate"—we repeated all instructions three times (Engelhardt & Edwards, 1986).

Another example of a robotic aid, a stationary system with some sensory capabilities such as force and tactile sensors, can help with some personal grooming and feeding tasks. A self-navigating robotic wheelchair can transport the care receiver, and an attached robotic arm can be used to perform manipulative tasks.

These applications of robotic technology have been introduced in concept and tested, to some extent, in limited resource applications. If adapted to the caregiving environment, these innovations could enhance an older adult's independence even after some of his or her functional capabilities are diminished, thereby simplifying caregivers' jobs.

Daily Living Expert Assistance Systems

Expert systems that offer cognitive assistance could help someone with physical or cognitive limitations to make the decisions required in everyday living. An expert system could aid in keeping people independent and in their own homes for a longer time. It could help remind older individuals to perform certain tasks. It could also alert a caregiver elsewhere should a change of status signal an emergency situation.

Development of a memory aid or "mind jogger" for specific activities can be a first step in creating an expert system for a wide spectrum of people with short-term memory deficiencies. Work on this problem has been explored at the University of Michigan (Levine, Kirsch, Fellon-Krueger, & Jaros, 1984) and at Carnegie Mellon University (Engelhardt, 1991). Development of an effective memory aid for those with declining cognitive abilities depends on the system's ability to communicate information to its user and on the user's ability to comprehend this information. The quality, form, and content of the information conveyed are important considerations.

What is the best way for a reminding aid to present information so that it is most likely to be understood? We know virtually nothing about how much and what kinds of information various user groups need. The range of choices varies, depending on the intended user. Whether we use visual or auditory reminders or both depends on the user's cognitive, perceptual, and motor demands (Pastalan, undated). Voorhees (1984) has demonstrated the importance of careful integration of multimodal information systems in designing airline cockpits. This analogy is applicable to in-home use since automated feedback, in both instances, serves a reminding function. In both cases, we must consider specific characteristics associated with visual and voice output. Our goal in working with older adults, as in Voorhees's cockpit design, is to deliver the "maximum amount of information transfer under conditions of minimum cognitive effort" (Voorhees, 1984). Determining requirements for devices that improve independence requires examining functional capabilities of older users. Their cognitive status, hearing loss, and visual abilities are three main factors in designing input control schemes and effective verbal or visual feedback (Czaja, 1990).

Lawton's concept of "centers of control" that older people create in their environments, analogous to "cockpit control," can be a starting point for considering technology's capability for increasing independence (Lawton, 1985). He observes that older people with decreased mobility generally have a favorite easy chair surrounded by those objects they consider essential:

tables, television, medicines, water and pitcher, and personal memorabilia. They usually face an entrance so they know who is entering and leaving. Since elderly individuals often spend greater amounts of time in their own homes, control over their home environments becomes increasingly important to their sense of independence (Lawton, 1985).

An airplane cockpit is the organized center for controlling an aircraft. Its design allows the pilot to maximize the interactive workspace. Work with older persons with decreased mobility, whose wheelchairs, in some cases, serve as their primary interactive lifespace, has brought a new meaning to this concept of "centers of control."

Robots as Personal Servants

Age-related deficits in mobility or strength, which affect an older individual's ability to function independently, are even more acute in chronically ill individuals in institutional settings. Robotic systems are now being created that can navigate autonomously in semistructured environments such as acute care hospitals and long-term care facilities. The potential uses for this class of service robotics are numerous, ranging from simple fetch and carry tasks to monitoring of the environment and the human to telepreserve for telemedicine. Robots are smart enough to identify problems and help seek solutions. For instance, if the robot is programmed to monitor the respiration or heart rate of the human it is assisting, any change in these indicators could be identified; then, if the situation demanded, the robot could use telephone lines to summon help for its human and could incorporate bidirectional, visual, and communication capabilities to allow for telemedicine activities.

Robots as Guardians and Protectors

Little research has been directed toward understanding technological interventions and how these interventions can be used to increase human safety, monitoring, and security. Advances in sensor technologies permit sensing capabilities that extend from smoke detection to monitoring of toxic gases, from automated temperature sensors for hot water to prevent burns to appliances that turn off automatically after an interval of time. The list of such small "roboticlike" technologies is long. These are not gadgets, these are safety devices that might be considered amoeba robots, small systems that sense, think, and act. In the smoke detector, a small sensor detects smoke and "knows" to sound an alarm that will alert humans to potential danger. These small systems can be further enhanced by adding light warnings for the hearing impaired. They can also be made more robotic by adding voice output that could convey meaningful alerting information. For instance, the system could direct humans to the safest exit, inform them where the fire was located, and of course, automatically alert the fire department and provide it with relevant information. If expanded, the system could monitor the whole house for numerous potential dangers and monitor the safety of the human occupants as well.

Another example of an integrated system for monitoring in an in-home setting or a long-term care facility might be an informed alerting system. Intelligent alerting systems can be created to monitor care receivers' safety and guard against nighttime wandering that may place the care receiver in danger (Engelhardt, 1989).

Many of the components of such a smart home that could create a forgiving environment exist today in product components, in laboratories, and in the knowledge bases of expert designers and developers. At this point, they have not been successfully brought together, along with mobile platforms and articulated manipulators, into integrated systems that would help support human independence and caregiver workloads. Such an environment can incorporate an "adapting life space" approach that could help compensate for declining human abilities.

Robots as Lifetime Career Assistants: Robotic Work Stations

Older adults, who begin to lose physical capabilities but who, otherwise, are able and desire to continue employment, are often forced to retire when they lose the ability to perform a small segment of their jobs. Now, the growth of microprocessor-based technologies, bolstered by the emphasis of the Americans with Disabilities Act of 1990 on creating innovative work accommodations, has facilitated a different scenario for aging Americans.

Robotic workstations have been under development for almost two decades. The ideas of using computers, manipulators, voice input, specially designed office components, and specific task analyses has been reported on extensively (Boonzaier, Engelhardt, & Awad-Edwards, 1985; Engelhardt, Awad, & Leifer, 1983; Engelhardt et al., 1984; Engelhardt, Edwards, Sample, & Sandrof, 1988; Fu, 1985). With communications technologies advancing at an exponential rate, integration of these different innovations provides even more power to the idea that robotic workstations can prove useful by allowing almost anyone to remain actively engaged in work; even if the person is homebound and even despite severe disabilities. Smart technologies can be designed to compensate for functional and cognitive impairments and will present new options for persons to continue to work longer despite declining physical capabilities.

One demonstration system, developed at Carnegie Mellon University by Engelhardt and associates, featured a modular design of the system environment that allowed five different configurations of three separate workstation modules. The primary station allowed voice control of office tasks during a portion of a 24-hour day. The station was reconfigurable to a second module, a stand-alone robot station that performed other tasks when it was not working with a person with disabilities. Conceivably, this could allow someone to use the robot for 8 hours then turn the robot station into an assembly station for another 16 hours and earn money with the robot when it is not being used for office or personal tasks. All three workstations are independently adjustable in height, which allows for accommodating the characteristics of a wide variety of user ergonomics and preferences. The height adjustment can be voice controlled. The third module, the office/computer station (without the robot) can be utilized also by someone who does not need robot assistance during that 16 hours. This versatile design tried to capture the flexible capabilities of the technologies and use them to augment or answer complex human needs. The modular, multipurpose design affords new ways to reduce barriers associated with the cost of purchasing the system. Designing robotic office systems in this flexible way allows them to be considered a capital equipment investment by an employer.

Before the fabrication of the robotic system, precise task taxonomies were developed to guide the design. Interactive evaluation research with potential end users was conducted. The research included instrumentation of the system and integration of specialized software to collect performance data for the robot. Evaluation data included the following: reliability (ratios such as up/down time and number of robots/day, safety (number of times the emergency stop buttons were activated), robot usage (amount of time and the time/day the robot was used and how it was used, such as real-time vs. preprogrammed subroutines), and telephone usage (amount of time/day and how it was used, such as autodialing vs. single digit dialing). Instrumentation also included the capacity to record a typical day for analysis of input rates and typical work output data sheets. Performance data for the human was collected. Videotaping selected user sessions as well as various instruments to collect user perceptions of their experiences and the robots performance allowed us to correlation and validation of the information derived from the instrumentation.

Robotics in Transportation

Automotive vehicles are rapidly becoming smarter. Their capabilities range from monitoring internal diagnostics to verbally warning passengers to buckle up. This is an important development for older drivers and may enable them to remain independently mobile longer.

In the future, proximity sensors will help with obstacle and accident avoidance. Vision systems could help with deciphering roadway signs (Czaja, 1990). Global position sensors are beginning to be utilized to help with navigation and destination tracking. Smart cars coupled with sensor embedded roadways could provide increased safety and extend the longevity of an older adults' driving ability by providing reserve "backup" sensory capabilities.

EVALUATING ROBOTIC TECHNOLOGIES INTERACTIVELY

The most important lesson to be drawn from the applications discussed in this chapter, and a guiding principle for designers of technologies for older adults, is that it is imperative to seek an appropriate match between the needs and the abilities of the older adult and the design and capabilities of the technologies. To integrate humans and robots into human environments, we need a strategy that considers numerous issues, such as feasibility, utility, and potential marketability, often in parallel. One methodology, which we call *interactive evaluation* (IE); Engelhardt, 1989) has been particularly useful in integrating robotic systems with the older adult. This model, shown in Figure 1, assumes that human factors are primarily and integrally related to technical and environmental factors. Interactive evaluation blends the research protocols of different fields to examine the human, robotic, and environmental factors relative to particular application domains. Research conducted within this framework allows us to benefit from the greater knowledge and experience base that can be derived from multiple perspectives.

The first step is to learn more about human needs, functional capabilities, attitudes, and perceptions as well as their physiological and psychological parameters. This needs research provides task identification that can be analyzed from various technical and clinical perspectives.

The next step is to design research questions and formulate simulations that can test the assumptions and discover answers. Utilizing perspectives from care receivers, family caregivers, formal caregivers, and robot researchers, desirable machine characteristic are determined by human performance with identified tasks in realistic environments. These interactions of humans and robotic technologies optimize the division of task actions between smart systems and intelligent humans. The design of robotic technol-

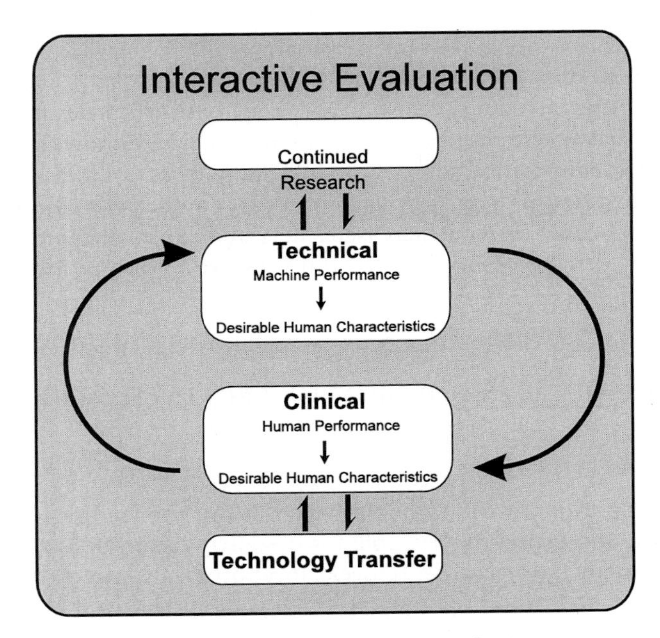

FIGURE 1 Model of interactive evaluation.

ogy for professional caregiving situations, as well as caregiving families, is defined by precise measurements of how adequately caregivers and care receivers, as a team and as individuals, perform tasks and where supplemental technology is needed.

FUTURE EXPECTATIONS

The accelerated development of technologies, coupled with changing demographics, presents new challenges to designers of service robotics. The challenging question is this: how do robotic scientists begin to research in a domain that is ill-defined and rapidly changing and for innovations that are not yet fully developed but rapidly evolving? This will require a process approach. Developers from various perspectives and disciplines must function integratively to identify needs by working directly with potential end-users and simultaneously examining whether existing or future planned technologies can address these needs. This is an approach to create a more effective human–environment–robot "fit."

As service sectors emerge as a dominant economic and social force in the coming decades, smart technologies in human services will become increasingly more important. With technologies that perform certain manipulative and mobile tasks in the home, institution, or workplace, older adults can remain independent longer. Smart technologies can offer new ways to facilitate autonomy and safety much like the telephone, television, airplane, and automobile afforded new opportunities for communication and transportation for previous generations. Systems designed in the next quarter century will require collaborative planning and evaluation to bring creative ideas to utilitarian fruition.

Beyond the mystique associated with high technology lies the potential for discovering useful tools to serve humans. For students or designers, exposure to smart assistive technologies and their potential use with the elderly humans provides a perspective of ability rather than disability. While textbooks on gerontology thoroughly describe the loss of control that older adults may experience as their physical disabilities decline, an understanding of robotic assistive technologies focuses on helping older adults remain in control by using technological tools to compensate for lost functional or cognitive abilities. With this perspective, the student may be able to understand the older adult as one who does not simply need to be cared for but as one who learns new techniques for caring for himself or herself. Such a perspective make the gerontologist a partner with the older adult as they use new tools to discover exciting new ways to expand the older adult's control of his or her environment.

References

Barrow, G. M. (1989). *Aging, the individual and society* (5th ed.). New York: West Publ. Co.

Boonzaier, D. A., Engelhardt, K. G., & Awad-Edwards, R. (1985). *Interactive evaluation of current voice in-put technologies for the physically disabled suggests new avenues for continued research. RESNA 8th annual Conference Proceedings,* Memphis, TN. pp. 323–325.

Brody, E. M. (1985). Parent care as a normative family stress. *Gerontologist, 25*(1), 19–29.

Cantor, M. H. (1992, Summer). Families and caregiving in an aging society. *Generations,* pp. 67–70.

Chappell, N. L. (1983). Informal support networks among the elderly. *Research on Aging, 5,* 77–79.

Clark, M. C., & Gaide, M. S. (1986, Fall). Choosing the right device. *Generations* pp. 67–70.

Coile, R. C., Jr. (1990). *The new medicine: reshaping medical practice and health care management.* Rockville, MD: Aspen Publications.

Czaja, J., Ed. (1990). *Human factors research needs for an aging population* (pp. 19–23). Washington, DC: National Academy Press.

Engelhardt, K. G. (1984, May 22). *High technology and its benefits for an aging population. Hearing before the Select Committee on Aging, House of Representatives* 98th Cong., 2d Sess. (1984) (Comm. Pub. No. 98–459).

Engelhardt, K. G. (1989). Computers, artificial intelligence, robotics, and aging humans. *International Journal of Technology and Aging, 2*(1), 4.

Engelhardt, K. G. (1991). *Development of a mind jogger.* Unpublished technical report, Carnegie-Mellon University, Pittsburgh, PA.

Engelhardt, K. G. (1988). *Rural Caregivers Technology Survey.* Southwestern Pennsylvania Family Caregivers' Support Program (unpublished report). Southwestern Pennsylvania Area Agency on Aging: Monessen, PA.

Engelhardt, K. G. (1994). *International issues and service robotics.* IEEE International Conference on Systems, Man and Cybernetics, Keynote Address, San Antonio, TX.

Engelhardt, K. G., Awad, R., & Leifer, L. (1983). *Progress in the development of an evaluation model suitable for application in the research and development environment.* Manuscript for the Proceedings of the Rehabilitation Engineering Society of North America, San Diego, CA.

Engelhardt, K. G., Awad, R. E., Vander Loos, H. F., Boonzaier, D. A., & Leifer, L. J. (1984, October). *Interactive evaluation of voice control for a robotic aid: Implications for training and applications. Proceedings of the Voice Input/Output Systems Application Conference,* Chicago.

Engelhardt, K. G., & Edwards, R. A. (1986, March). Increasing independence for the aging. *Byte, 1(3),* pp. 191–196.

Engelhardt, K. G., Edwards, R. A., Sample, W. S., & Sandrof, M. F. (1988). *The robotic vocational workstation. Annual research review* (pp. 67–79). Pittsburgh, PA: Carnegie-Mellon University, The Robotics Institute.

Falletti, M. V. (1984). Using technology. *Generations, 8*(4), 35–38.

Feller, B. A. (1983). Americans needing help to function at home. *Vital and health statistics of the National Center for Health Statistics.* Washington, DC: National Center for Health Statistics.

Fu, C. (1985). *A voice controlled workstation for handicapped individuals. Proceedings of the 2nd International Personal Robot Congress,* San Francisco.

Halamandaris, V. J. (1994). Long-term care as a bellwether. *Caring, 13*(3), 5–7.

Hooyman, N. R., & Kiyak, H. A. (1988). *Social gerontology: A multi-disciplinary perspective.* Boston: Allyn & Bacon.

Kane, R. L., & Kane, R. A. (1991). A nursing home in your future? *New England Journal of Medicine, 324,*(9), 627–629.

Kemper, P., & Murtaugh, C.M. (1991). Lifetime use of nursing home care. *New England Journal of Medicine, 324,* (9), 595–600.

Lawton, A. P. (1985, March). Keynote address on environment and the aging. Technology and Aging Conference, Palo Alto, CA.

Levande, D. I., Bowden, S. W., & Mollema, J. (1987). Home health services for dependent elders: The social work dimension. *Journal of Gerontological Social Work, 11*(3/4), 5–17.

Levine, S. P., Kirsch, N. L., Fellon-Krueger, M., & Jaros, L. A. (1984). The microcomputer as an orthotic device for cognitive disorders. In *Proceedings of the Second International Conference on Rehabilitation Engineering* (p. 130). Washington, DC: RESNA.

Pastalan, L. A. (undated). *The simulation of age related sensory losses: A new approach to the study of environmental barrier.* Unpublished research report, University of Southern California, Los Angeles.

Pillemer, K., Moen, P., Krout, J., & Robinson, J. (1995). Setting the White House conference on aging agenda: Recommendations from a expert panel. *Gerontologist, 35*(2), 258–261.

Shanas, E. (1979). The family as a social support system in old age. *Gerontologist, 19*(2), 169–174.

Torrey, B. B. (1994, March 17). *Demographic overview of America's elderly* (Congressional

Staff Briefing). Washington, DC: National Research Council, Commission on Behavioral and Social Sciences and Education.
U.S. Department of Commerce, Bureau of the Census. (1995). *Statistical brief: Sixty-five plus in the United States.* Washington, DC: Author.
U.S. Department of Health and Human Services, Administration on Aging, Office of State and Community Programs. (1994). *National summary of program activities as authorized under Titles III and VII of the Older American's Act: Fiscal Year 1993.* Washington, DC: Authors.
U.S. Senate Special Committee on Aging. (1985). *Developments in Aging: 1984; Vol. 2. Appendices.* Washington, DC: U.S. Government Printing Office.
Voorhees, J. W. (1984). The integration of voice and visual displays for aviation systems. *Journal of the American Voice Input/Output Society, 1,*(1), 48.
White House Conference on Aging. (1995). *Adopted resolutions* IRDS3 and IRDS14). Washington, DC: Author.

Index

O

P

R

S

T